Otolaryngology: An Evidence-Based Approach

Otolaryngology: An Evidence-Based Approach

Edited by Stephanie Madison

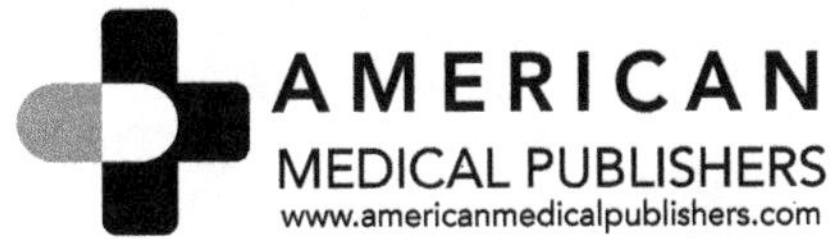

American Medical Publishers,
41 Flatbush Avenue,
1st Floor, New York,
NY 11217, USA

Visit us on the World Wide Web at:
www.americanmedicalpublishers.com

ISBN: 978-1-63927-412-3

Cataloging-in-Publication Data

Otolaryngology : an evidence-based approach / edited by Stephanie Madison.
p. cm.
Includes bibliographical references and index.
ISBN 978-1-63927-412-3
1. Otolaryngology. 2. Evidence-based medicine. 3. Otolaryngology--Practice.
4. Otolaryngology--Diagnosis. I. Madison, Stephanie.
RF46 .O86 2022
617.51--dc23

Table of Contents

Preface IX

Chapter 1 **Basal Cell Adenocarcinoma of the Parotid Gland in an Elderly Iranian Woman** 1
Zahra Sarafraz, Mohammad Hossein Azaraein, Mansour Moghimi and Seyyed Ali Musavi

Chapter 2 **Benign but Aggressive Tumors of Infancy Report of Two Cases** 6
Boutemeur S, Ramoul S, Azouani Y, Kabir A and Ferdjaoui A

Chapter 3 **Case Report of Huge Esthesioneuroblastoma** 9
Mouhannad Abdulber Fakoury

Chapter 4 **Cervical Schwannoma- A Case Report** 12
Jyotiranjan Das, Jayant Saha, Shantanu Dutta and Ajay Manickam

Chapter 5 **Combined Evaluation of FDG-PET/CT and CT Imaging Characteristics of Cervical Lymph Nodes to Increase the Interpretation Accuracy for Nodal Metastatic Involvement in Head and Neck Cancer** 15
Richard A Marshall, Peter M Som, Livnat Uliel, Eric Genden, Michael Buckstein, Vishal Gupta, Brett Miles, Neetha Gandikota, Idoia Corcuera-Solano, Krzysztof Misiukiewicz, Andrew G. Sikora and Lale Kostakoglu

Chapter 6 **Correlation Between Serum and Salivary House Dust Mite Specific Immunoglobulins in Allergic Rhinitis (AR) Patients and Non-Allergic Rhinitis Matched Controls** 23
Sethu T Subha, Loy Heng She, Wong Shew Fung, Davendralingam Sinniah and Valuyeetham Kamaru Ambu

Chapter 7 **Deciphering Tinnitus from the Shoulders of Giants: A Kuhnian Shift may be Required** 29
Sylvester Fernandes

Chapter 8 **Delayed Distant Metastasis of Tonsillar Squamous Cell Carcinoma Origin** 35
Hermann Simo, Louis De Las Casas, Vasuki Anandan, Michal Preis and Reginald Baugh

Chapter 9 **Documenting the Hypopharyngeal Environment of Patients Undergoing General Endotracheal Tube Anesthesia: A First Look at Intraoperative pH Characteristics** 38
Elliot Regenbogen, Slawomir P. Oleszak, Thomas Corrado, A. Laurie W. Shroyer, Elizabeth Vanner, Jordan Goldstein and Michael L. Pearl

Chapter 10 **Dynamics of Swallowing Tablets during the Recovery Period following Surgery for Tongue Cancer** 45
Yu Yoshizumi, Shinya Mikushi, Ayako Nakane, Haruka Tohara and Shunsuke Minakuchi

Chapter 11 **Endoscopic Repair of Carotid Artery Injury** 51
Irit Duek, Gill E Sviri, Moran Amit and Ziv Gil

Chapter 12 **Factors Affecting Recurrence of T1 and T2 Tongue Cancer Undergoing Intraoral Resection** 54
Takeshi Mohri, Yasuhiko Tomita, Takashi Fujii, Miki Tomoeda, Shota Kotani, Tomonori Terada, Nobuo Saeki, Nobuhiro Uwa, Kousuke Sagawa and Masafumi Sakagami

Chapter 13 **Functional Appliances in the Treatment of Sleep Apnea in Children** 59
Rosa Carrieri Rossi, Nelson Jose Rossi, Nelson Carrieri Rossi, Reginaldo Raimundo Fujiya and Shirley Nagata Pignatari

Chapter 14 **Giant Cystic Parathyroid Adenoma Masquerading as a Retropharyngeal Abscess** 66
Diom ES, Fagan JJ and Dhirendra Govender

Chapter 15 **Is Marriage a Risk Factor for Allergic Rhinitis?** 70
Sara Safar AlShehri and Kamal-Eldin Ahmed Abou-Elhamd

Chapter 16 **Juvenile Laryngeal Papillomatosis in Benin: Epidemiological, Diagnostic, Therapeutic and Evolutionary Aspects** 75
Lawson Afouda Sonia, Hounkpatin Spéro, Avakoudjo François, Brun Luc and Adjibabi Wassi

Chapter 17 **Mucosal Immune Responses Associated with NKT Cell Activation and Dendritic Cell Expansion by Nasal administration of α-galactosylceramide in the Nasopharynx** 78
Shingo Umemoto, Satoru Kodama, Takashi Hirano, Kenji Noda and Masashi Suzuki

Chapter 18 **Naopharyngeal Notochondroma- A Case Report and Literature Review** 85
Bibek Gyanwali, Hongquan Wu, Bunu Karmacharya, Meichan Zhu and Anzhou Tang

Chapter 19 **Nutritional Management for Patients with Head and Neck Cancer: The Second Step of an Italian Survey** 88
Marianna Trignani, Melissa Laus, Valentina Mastronardi, Olga Leone, Marilina De Rosa, Giulio Campitelli, Angelo Di Pilla, Giuseppe Santarelli, Albina Allajbej, Ambra Pamio, Domenico Genovesi and Adelchi Croce

Chapter 20 **Otosclerosis Surgery: Contribution of Imaging in Surgical Failures and Labyrinthine Complications Diagnosis** 92
Myriam Jrad, Asma Ben Mabrouk, Aymen Ben Othmen, Jihene Marrakchi, Anis Zaidi, Rym Zainine, Ghazi Besbes and Habiba Mizouni

Chapter 21 **Personal Music Devices: An Assessment of User Profile and Potential Hazards** 98
Virangna Taneja, Shelly Khanna Chadha, Achal Gulati and Ankush Sayal

Chapter 22 **Possibility for Allergy Immunotherapy with Long Synthetic Peptide of Bet V1** 102
Motoharu Uehara and Hiroyuki Hirai

Chapter 23 **Pregnancy and Dental Treatment** 106
ABI AAD Lamia and Dany Joseph Daou

Chapter 24 **Role of Elective Neck Management in Maxillary Sinus Squamous Cell Carcinoma** 112
Pauline Castelnau Marchand, Eleonor Rivin del Campo and Yungan Tao

Chapter 25 **Speech Perception and Subjective Preference with Fine Structure Coding Strategies** 116
Robert Mlynski, Michael Ziese, Thorsten Rahne and Joachim Müller-Deile

Chapter 26 **Sphenoid Aspergilloma: Diagnosed as a Malignancy** 123
Gray MR, Thrasher JD, Dennis Hooper, Dumanov MJ, Cravens R and Jones T

Chapter 27 **Sudden Sensorineural Hearing Loss after Total Thyroidectomy Surgery Under General Anesthesia** 131
Mitat Arıcıgil, Abitter Yucel, Mehmet Akif Alan, Fuat Aydemir and Suayp Kuria Aziz

Chapter 28 **Supraglottic Obstruction in an Adult with Inspiratory Arytenoid Cartilage Prolapse** 134
Amy L Rutt, James P Dworkin and Noah Stern

Chapter 29 **Evaluation of TSH And T4 Levels in Idiopathic Sudden Sensorineural Hearing Loss Patients** 138
Arıcıgil M

Chapter 30 **The Silent Sinus Syndrome: A Collaborative Approach between Rhinologists and Oculoplastics** 142
Yaser Najaf Abdulmohsen AlTerki and Adel Al-Buluoshi

Chapter 31 **The Effect of Novel Combination Therapy with Azelastine Hydrochloride and Fluticasone Propionate in Allergic Rhinitis** 145
Amtul Salam Sami, Nida Ahmed and Sabahat Ahmed

Chapter 32 **The Effects of N-Acetyl Cysteine on Nasal Mucociliary Clearance in Healthy Volunteers** 153
Morvarid Elahi and Homayoun Elahi

Chapter 33 **Tinnitus: An Evolutionary Symptom?** 156
Sylvester Fernandes

Chapter 34 **Utilizing Dehydrated Human Amnion/Chorion Membrane Allograft in Transcanal Tympanoplasty** 162
Griffith S Hsu

Chapter 35 **Variables that Effect Psychophysical Parameters and Duration to Stability in Cochlear Implant Mapping** 165
Maria CS and Maria PLS

Chapter 36 **Approach to the Patient with External Laryngeal Trauma: The Schaefer Classification** 169
Omakobia E and Micallef A

Chapter 37 **Advanced Bionics® Cochlear Implants in Patients with Prelingual Hearing Loss** 172
Henrique Furlan Pauna, Guilherme Machado de Carvalho, Alexandre Caixeta Guimarães, Luiz Henrique Schuch, Eder Barbosa Muranaka, Walter Adriano Bianchini, Agrício Nubiato Crespo, Edi Lucia Sartorato and Arthur Menino Castilho

Chapter 38 **Auditory Brainstem Response Characteristics of Children with Cerebral Palsy: Clinical Utility and Prognostic Significance** 176
Mohammad Shamim Ansari, Rangasayee Raghunathrao and Mohammad A Hafiz Ansari

Permissions

List of Contributors

Index

Preface

The purpose of the book is to provide a glimpse into the dynamics and to present opinions and studies of some of the scientists engaged in the development of new ideas in the field from very different standpoints. This book will prove useful to students and researchers owing to its high content quality.

The branch of medicine which deals with the surgical treatments of ear, nose and throat as well as related structures such as head and neck, is referred to as otolaryngology. Various sub-specialties of otolaryngology include pediatric otolaryngology, laryngology and voice disorders, facial plastic and reconstructive surgery. Pediatric otolaryngology deals with velopalatine insufficiency, cleft lip and palate, as well as vascular malformations. Laryngology and voice disorders include phono-surgery and swallowing disorders. Surgeries such as facial cosmetic surgery, maxillofacial surgery, traumatic reconstruction and craniofacial surgery fall under the category of facial plastic and reconstructive surgery. Another important field of otolaryngology is rhinology which deals with nasal obstruction, nasal septum deviation, sinusitis, environmental allergies, pituitary tumor and empty nose syndrome. This book attempts to understand the multiple branches that fall under the discipline of otolaryngology and how such concepts have practical applications. It includes contributions of experts which will provide innovative insights into this field. This book is a resource guide for experts as well as students.

At the end, I would like to appreciate all the efforts made by the authors in completing their chapters professionally. I express my deepest gratitude to all of them for contributing to this book by sharing their valuable works. A special thanks to my family and friends for their constant support in this journey.

Editor

1

Basal Cell Adenocarcinoma of the Parotid Gland in an Elderly Iranian Woman

Zahra Sarafraz*, **Mohammad Hossein Azaraein, Mansour Moghimi and Seyyed Ali Musavi**

Faculty of Medicine and Health Sciences, Unit of Otolaryngology Medicine, Department of Otolaryngology, Yazd University of Medical Sciences, Yazd, Iran

***Corresponding author:** Zahra Sarafarz, Faculty of Medicine and Health Sciences, Unit of Otolaryngology Medicine, Department of Otolaryngology, Yazd University of Medical Sciences, Yazd, Iran; E-mail: zahra.sarafraz@yahoo.com

Abstract

Basal Cell Adenocarcinoma (BCAC) is a rare subtype of carcinoma of salivary glands. It accounts for 1.6% of all salivary gland neoplasms and 2.9% of malignant salivary gland neoplasms. BCAC is especially rare in parotid glands. The biological behavior of BCAC is invasive and destructive, with perineural and vascular invasion. This paper presents a BCAC with multiple recurrences and wide local extension in a 71-year-old Iranian woman with a 30-year history of a large mass on the right side of her neck. The importance aspects of this case were its long duration, multiple recurrences, facial nerve involvement and the use of clinicopathological criteria for diagnosis.

Background

Basal Cell Adenocarcinoma (BCAC) is one of the rare subtypes of carcinoma of salivary glands. It is a salivary gland malignancy that was first recognized as a distinct neoplastic entity in World Health Organization's (WHO's) classification of salivary gland tumors in 1991. BCAC of the salivary gland is a rare neoplasm, especially in the parotid gland. It composes 1.6% of all salivary gland neoplasms and 2.9% of malignant salivary gland neoplasms. The most important differential diagnosis of BCAC is Basal Cell Adenoma (BCA), but the behavior of BCAC is invasive and destructive with perineural and vascular invasion [1,2]. The histopathology of BCAC shows two cell types, i.e., small basaloid epithelial cells at the periphery and larger epithelial cells in the center of the tumour clusters . Most cases of BCAC are de novo, but 25% of BCACs originate from pre-existing basal cell adenomas. In general, BCAC has a good prognosis. Metastasis is rare but may recur locally [3,4]. BCACs are categorized into four types on the basis of their growth patterns, i.e., solid, trabecular, tubular, and membranous; the solid type is the most common [2,5]. The BCAC in our 71-year-old patient had some interesting features that were different from those in previous case reports.

Case Presentation

A 71-year-old Iranian woman with a 30-year history of a large mass on the right side of her neck was referred to the Otolaryngology Department at Shahid Sadoughi Hospital in Yazd, Iran in 2012. She presented with a firm, fixed, non-tender mass on the right side of her neck that measured 10×15 cm with normal skin with no apparent invasion. The clinical examination provided no evidence of cervical lymphadenopathy. The patient complained about mild dysphagia, and the oropharyngeal exam revealed a bulging mass in the right side of the oral cavity. Facial movements were partially asymmetrical on the right side of the lower lip (other branches of facial nerve were intact). Also, a bulge was found on the anterior wall of the right external auditory canal. A superficial parotidectomy was performed 10 years ago; subsequently, the patient experienced five recurrences of masses on her neck, and the last recurrence occurred four years ago. Unfortunately, we don't have any documented pathology from her previous surgeries. An investigation of the patients' family history showed no occurrence of cancer.

Investigation

Imaging

Abdominal ultrasonography revealed no abnormality, and the chest X-ray indicated no signs of metastasis. The CT scan showed a large, irregular mass in the right parotid gland, bulging into the parapharyngeal space. It extended up to the base of the skull (Figure 1).

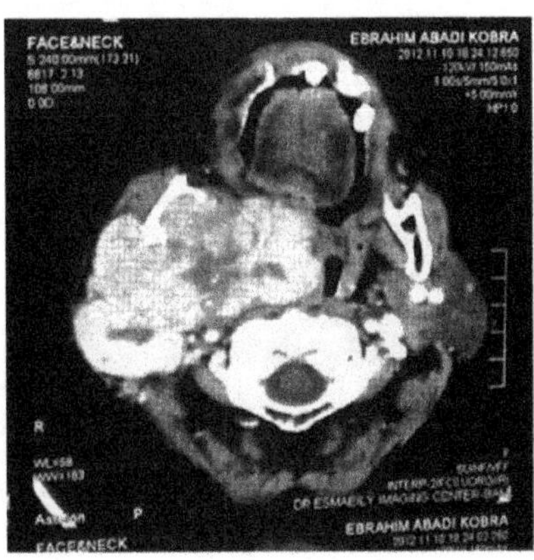

Figure 1: Mass extension in patient axial cut of neck CT scan

Antibodies	Clone	Class	Code	Antigen Unmasking Methods: Microwave Retrieval	Dilution
Monoclonal Mouse Anti-Human Muscle Actin (SMA)	1A4	IG2a, kappa	M0851	15 minutes heating-induced epitope retrieval (750 W) in 10 mmol/L citrate buffer, pH 6	1:75 in 0.02 M PBS, pH 7.2-7.6
Monoclonal Mouse Anti-Human Cytokeratin AE1/AE2	AE1 and AE3	AE1:IgG1, kappa; AE3: IgG1, kappa	M3515	15 minutes heating – induced epitope retrieval (750 W) in 10 mmol/L citrate buffer, pH 6	1:50 in 0.02 M PBS, pH 7.2-7.6
Polyclonal rabbit Anti-S 100	-	-	Z0311 Ig fraction	15 minutes heating – induced epitope retrieval (750 W) in 10 mmol/L citrate buffer, pH 6	1: 300 in 0.02 M PBS, pH 7.2-7.6
Polyclonal Rabbit Anti-Human Carcinoembryonic Antigen (CEA)	-	-	A0115 Ig fraction	15 minutes heating – induced epitope retrieval (750 W) in 10 mmol/L citrate buffer, pH 6	1:100 in 0.02 M PBS, pH 7.2-7.6
Monoclonal Mouse Anti-Human Vimentin (VIM)	V9	IgG1, kappa	M0725 Culture supernatant	15 minutes heating – induced epitope retrieval (750 W) in 10 mmol/L citrate buffer, pH 6	1:30 in 0.02 M PBS, pH 7.2-7.6
Polyclonal Rabbit Anti-Glial Fibrillary Acidic protein (GFAP)	-	-	IS524	15 minutes heating – induced epitope retrieval (750 W) in 10 mmol/L citrate buffer, pH 6	1:30 in 0.02 M PBS, pH 7.2-7.6

Table 1: Antibodies used in the immunohistochemical investigation of BCAC

Histopathology and other laboratory findings

In the gross pathological examination, the tumour had creamy-colored nodular tissue that measured 16×14×5 cm with firm consistency and lobular appearance in the cut section. Some of nodules had thin capsules with calcified foci. Microscopic examination revealed a tumoural lesion with a multinodular pattern composed of basaloid cells that had round-to-oval nuclei with fine nucleoli and scant-to-moderate cytoplasm. Cells arranged in lobules, sheets, aggregates cords, trabeculae and membranous pattern. Hyaline Periodic Acid Schiff (PAS) positive materials with palisading and jigsaw puzzle patterns were observed. There were no more than six mitoses in the 10 High Power Field (HPF).

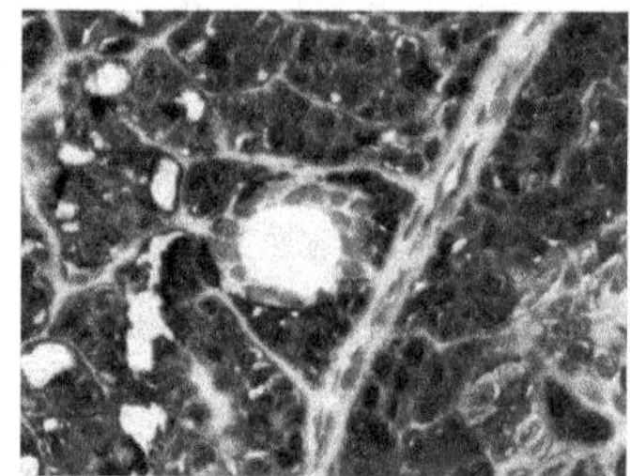

Figure 3: ASMA immunostaining positive in abluminal cells.

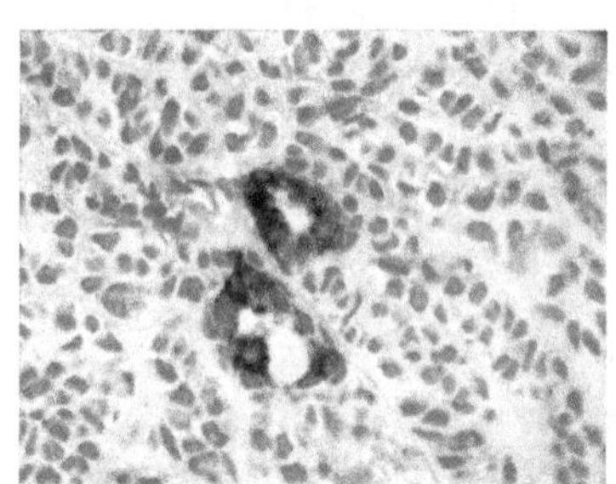

Figure 2: EMA immunostaining positive in luminal cell in areas of ductal differentiation

Cellular pleomorphism, necrosis, vascular and perineural invasion, and lymph node metastasis were absent. The primary diagnosis was low-grade basal cell adenocarcinoma. For ruling out other differential diagnoses, Immunohistochemistry (IHC) was performed. The tumoral cells were positive for CK AE1/3, SMA, S100 (moderately positive), EMA and CD117 (positive in luminal cells in areas of ductal differentiation), Vimentin (focally positive), and Ki67 (in 5 to 10% of the tumoral cells). CEA and GFAP were negative (Figures 2 and 3) (Table1).

Treatment

The tumor at the base of the skull and the deep portion of the parotid gland were resected, and suprahyoid dissection of the lymph nodes was performed, including the submandibular, submental, and upper third of the jugulodigastric nodes. Except marginal mandibular branch the facial nerve was preserved and post-operative irradiation were conducted.

Outcome and follow-up

At the one-year follow up, she had no recurrence of any of the features associated with bcac. Also, the metastasis workup revealed no sign of metastasis.

Discussion

Bcac is slow-growing, locally-destructive tumor. It was first defined as a malignant tumor of the salivary gland in 1991. The most important differential diagnosis for bcac is basal cell adenoma [1]. Both of them have similar histological appearances (basaloid pattern), but infiltrative growth is the distinguishing feature of bcac. Pathological criteria for the diagnosis of bcac include infiltrative growth with vascular or perineural invasion. Other features may include nuclear pleomorphism, necrosis, and mitotic activity [3,4]. In our patient, there were no more than six mitoses inthe 10 hpf. Cellular pleomorphism, necrosis, vascular and perineural invasion, and lymph-node metastasis were absent, but, clinically, it was a huge mass (10×15 cm) with wide extention and a history of multiple recurrences. Its invasion of the adjacent soft tissues was obvious during surgery. Ihc suggested bcac and ruled out a differential diagnosis. We believe that the diagnosis of bcac is clinicopathological, and sometimes it is very difficult to distinguish it from basal cell adenoma using only pathological criteria.

The rate of metastasis is low, but the rate of local recurrence is high. Metastasis occurs in less than 10% of cases, and only one case involving the lung has been reported [3,4]. Because of their biological behavior and their prognosis, bcacs should be classified as low-grade carcinomas. In our patient, a complete metastasis workup was performed, and there were no features of metastasis. There have been a few descriptions of facial paralysis or additional destruction of the salivary gland, but interesting findings in our patient's case were that the buccal branch of the facial nerve was weak and that the bcac extended up to the base of the skull, bulging into the parapharyngeal space. Many patients with bcac recognized after 7-10 years, but our patient had it for the long duration of about 30 years with five recurrences (may be denovo or transformation of basal cell adenoma). Most patients present with a solitary firm nodule between 1 and 3 cm that is slowly enlarging. The largest tumor described by Ellis et al. was 4 cm, but our patient's tumor was about10x15 cm. Local recurrence occurs in about one-third of the cases, and our patient had five recurrences over a 30-year period. Our case was unique with respect to its duration, the number of recurrences, and the size of the mass [5].

Bcac has four subtypes, i.e., solid, membranous, trabecular, and tubular. The solid areas of bcacs are composed of nonluminal cells, some of which contain tonofilaments and well-formed desmosomes; tubulo-trabecular differentiated into both luminal and nonluminal cells. Both growth patterns were associated with the formation of excess basal lamina, marginally and between nonluminal cells. The majority of these tumors are solid. They are characterized by islands and masses within the fibrous connective tissue stroma, the histological type of our patients bcac was membranous. The membranous type is actually the second most frequently-occurring type of bcac, accounting for about 20% of all occurrences. This type has thick, eosinophilic, periodic acid schiff positive hyaline laminae that surround and separate one tumor nest from another and a jigsaw puzzle formation (Figure 4). The trabecular type of bcac has anastomosing cords of basaloid epithelial cells that look like chinese characters [2,5].

Muller and Barnes conducted an extensive literature search in 1996, and they concluded that parotid is the most common salivary gland that is involved with BCAC (89% in the parotid, 10% in the submandibular gland, and 1% among the minor salivary glands). In our case, the parotid gland was involved. Most studies recommend wide loc al excision. Treatment for regional metastasis (neck) is done for significant lymphadenopathy on clinical or radiologic examination, and postoperative radiation is recommended for close surgical margins or following surgical excision of recurrent tumor [6-9].

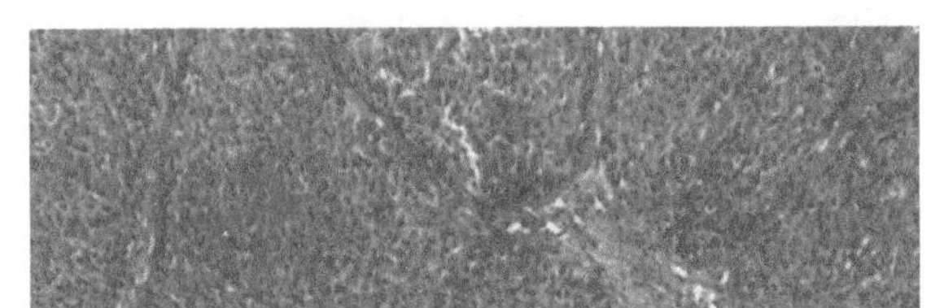

Figure 4: Lobules with jigsaw puzzle like pattern in Membranous BCAC

The surgical procedure we performed was resection of the tumor at the base of the skull with deep portion resection of the parotid gland with preservation of the facial nerve. At last we summarise at least 46 cases of parotid gland BCAC from 1990-2014 in two tables and compare them with our case (Tables 2 and 3).

Studies	Ellis et al. [5]	Muller et al. [10]	Kwang II [11]	Ikeda [12]	Golz et al. [13]
Cases and Sex	29	7(6 female and 1 male)	1(female)	1(female)	1(male)
Age	Adults with Peak incidence 6th decade	46-74	33	73	24
Location	Major salivary glands	Parotid gland(Except one case)	Left Parotid	Right Parotid	Left parotid
Size(mm)	Variable	Variable	20	50	30
common Histologic type	Solid	-	tubulotrabecular type	Solid and Tubular	
Manifestation	-	Parotid mass	Infraauricular mass	Parotid mass	Retroauricular abscess

Facial nerve status	-	Intact	Intact	Intact	Intact
Cervical lymphadenopathy	2	none	Negative	Negative	Negative
Local recurrences	7	2	Negative	Negative	Negative
Distant metastasis	1	1	Negative	Negative	Negative
Site of metastasis	Lung	-	-	-	-
Treatment	Parotidectomy	Local excision	Parotidectomy	Parotidectomy	Total
Follow up duration	Few months	30 month	24 months	24 months	30 months
Status after follow up	One case died	Tumor free	Tumor free	Tumor free	Tumor free

Table 2: Review of the literature

Studies	Keiichi Jingu [14]	Markanen et al.	Michael H Elvey [15]	Hamamoto [16]	Sarafraz et al.
Cases and Sex	4(2 female and 2 male)	1(male)	1(male)	1(female)	1(female)
Age	37-81	60	67	58	71
Location	3 cases right and 1 case in left Parotid gland	Bilateral Parotid gland	Parotid	Right parotid	Right parotid
Size(mm)	19-54 mm	Right:10 mm Left:6 mm	-	-	150 mm
Dominant Histologic type	-	Tubular	Solid	-	Membranous
Manifestation	Buccal swelling	Incidental in ultrasonography	Parotid mass Pain and swelling in his hand	Parotid mass	Parotid mass
Facial nerve status	Intact	Intact	Intact	Intact	Weakness in buccal branch
Cervical lymphadenopathy	1	Negative	Negative	Negative	Negative
Local recurrences	1	Negative	Negative	Negative	Negative
Distant metastasis	none	Negative	+	Negative	Negative
Site of metastasis	-	-	Second to 5th metacarpal	-	-
Treatment	Parotidectomy +radiotherapy	Parotidectomy	Parotidectomy +radiotherapy Distal forearm amputation	Superficial Parotidectomy +radiotherapy	Parotidectomy +radiotherapy
Follow up duration	3 Months	-	24 months	8 months	48 months
Status after follow up	No recurrence	-	No evidence of metastasis	Tumor free	No recurrence

Table 3: Review of the literature

References

1. Quddus MR, Henley JD, Affify AM, Dardick I, Gnepp DR (1999) Basal cell adenocarcinoma of the salivary gland: an ultrastructural and immunohistochemical study. Oral Surg Oral Med Oral Pathol Oral Radiol Endod 87: 485-492.
2. Sharma R, Saxena S, Bansal R (2007) Basal cell adenocarcinoma: Report of a case affecting the submandibular gland 11: 56-9.
3. Markkanen-Leppanen M, Makitie AA, Passador-Santos F, Leivo I, Hagström J (2010) Bilateral Basal cell adenocarcinoma of the parotid gland: in a recipient of kidney transplant. Clin Med Insights Pathol 3: 1-5.
4. Ward BK, Seethala RR, Barnes EL, Lai SY (2009) Basal cell adenocarcinoma of a hard palate minor salivary gland: case report and review of the literature. Head Neck Oncol 1: 41.
5. Ellis GL, Wiscovitch JG (1990) Basal cell adenocarcinomas of the major salivary glands. Oral Surg Oral Med Oral Pathol 69: 461-469.
6. Hirsch DL, Miles C, Dierks E (2007) Basal cell adenocarcinoma of the parotid gland: report of a case and review of the literature. J Oral Maxillofac Surg 65: 2385-2388.

7. Jayakrishnan A, Elmalah I, Hussain K, Odell EW (2003) Basal cell adenocarcinoma in minor salivary glands. Histopathology 42: 610-614.
8. Yu GY, Ubmuller J, Donath K (1998) Membranous basal cell adenoma of the salivary gland: a clinicopathologic study of 12 cases. Acta Otolaryngol 118: 588-593.
9. Parashar P, Baron E, Papadimitriou JC, Ord RA, Nikitakis NG (2007) Basal cell adenocarcinoma of the oral minor salivary glands: review of the literature and presentation of two cases. Oral Surg Oral Med Oral Pathol Oral Radiol Endod 103: 77-84.
10. Muller S, Barnes L (1996) Basal cell adenocarcinoma of the salivary glands. Report of seven cases and review of the literature. Cancer 78: 2471-2477.
11. Kim KI, Oh HE, Mun JS, Kim CH, Choi JS (1997) Basal cell adenocarcinoma of the salivary gland--a case report. J Korean Med Sci 12: 461-464.
12. Ikeda K, Watanabe M, Oshima T, Nakabayashi S, Kudo T, et al. (1998) A case of basal cell adenocarcinoma of the parotid gland. Tohoku J Exp Med 186: 51-59.
13. Golz A, Goldenberg D, Ben-Arie Y, Keren R, Netzer A, et al. (2000) Basal cell adenocarcinoma of the parotid gland presenting as a retroauricular abscess. Am J Otolaryngol 21: 421-426.
14. Jingu K, Hasegawa A, Mizo JE, Bessho H, Morikawa T, et al. (2010) Carbon ion radiotherapy for basal cell adenocarcinoma of the head and neck: preliminary report of six cases and review of the literature. Radiat Oncol 5: 89.
15. Michael H (2011) Metastasis of parotid basal cell adenocarcinoma to the hand a case report. Hand 6: 321-323.
16. Hamamoto M (2012) A case of basal cell adenocarcinoma of the parotid gland, practica oto rhino laryngological. 105: 441-446.

2

Benign but Aggressive Tumors of Infancy Report of Two Cases

Boutemeur S*, **Ramoul S, Azouani Y, Kabir A and Ferdjaoui A**

Department of Oral and Maxillo-facial Surgery, Mustapha Pacha Hospital, Algiers, Algeria

***Corresponding author:** Boutemeur S, Department of Oral and Maxillo-facial Surgery, Mustapha Pacha Hospital, Algiers, Algeria; E-mail: saidboutemeur@yahoo.fr

Abstract

Melanotic neuroectodermal tumour of infancy and Aggressive desmoid fibromatosis are histologically benign tumors but with aggressive behavior, it's occurring during the little infancy and are caracterised by Fast-growing, osteolysis and recurrence. The treatment is essentially surgical. Melanotic neuroectodermal tumour of infancy is a rare tumour which affects young children arising from neural crest with a black coloring. It grows rapidly and first touches the maxilla. We related the case of a three-month age male who presents a tumor in the right maxilla. The case have CT scan and histology feature. Aggressive desmoid fibromatosis is a benign tumor with locally infiltrative behavior and tendency to recur. We report a rare case involving the mandible arch of three years old girl with histopathological, immunohistochemical and imaging features. She underwent a large surgically resection of the arch of the mandible, there has been no recurrence three years after.

Keywords: Melanotic neuroectodermal; Desmoid fibromatosis; Benign; Aggressive; Infancy surgery

Introduction

Melanotic neuroectodermal tumour of infancy [1-4] is a benign rare tumour occurring during the first year of life with fast evolution and frequent recurrences.

It was described for the first time by Krombech in 1918 and since many cases was reported. It's affect jawbones but can affect other places like the skull, the epididymis and the brain. The maxillary bone is the most achieved with large bone destruction. The recurrence is seen within the first year after surgery and in some cases we can observe malignant transformation.

The word, "fibromatosis" is a generic term used to describe a group of benign fibroblastic lesions with similar microscopic features but with diverse biological behavior. They are classified as superficial and deep fibromatosis. They result from musculoaponeurotic structures disorders and usually described as an aggressive fibromatosis.

The computed tomography (CT) is the most contributory morphological examination and diagnostic support.

Case 1: Melanotic Neuroectodermal Tumour of Infancy

A three-month old male infant with a Melanotic neuroectodermal tumour of infancy developed in the right maxillary anterior region. He was admitted to the Hospital in because of a mass in the mouth with feeding disturbances. The mother had noticed the small mass as a black staining tumour sitting on the maxillary ridge when he was 30 days old. The mass appeared to be growing rapidly, and sucking and feeding were gradually impaired (Figure 1).

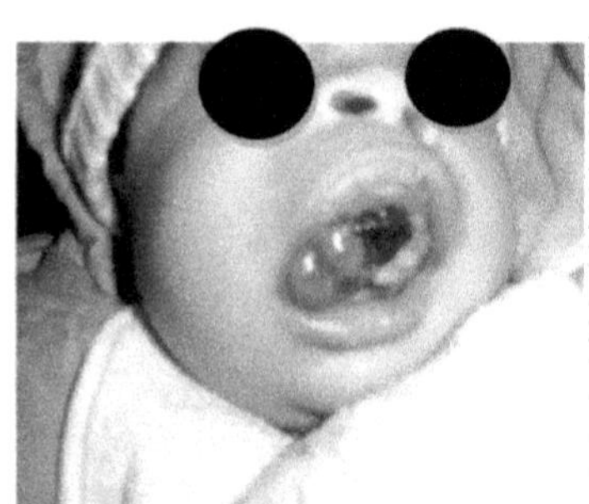

Figure 1: The mass appeared to be growing rapidly.

On physical examination, an obvious bulge in the right upper cheek was seen, but the overlying skin was intact. On Intraoral, a mass in the region of the right upper maxilla with a palate extending. There was ulceration on the mucosa with dark-coloured (Figure 2). The rest of the exam was normal (Figure 3-6).

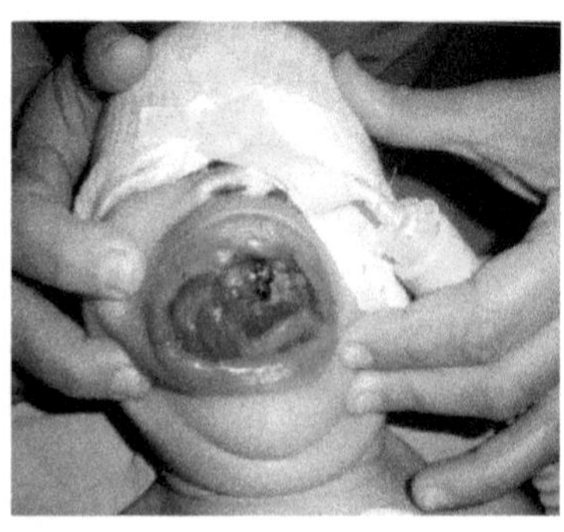

Figure 2: Ulceration on the mucosa with dark-coloured.

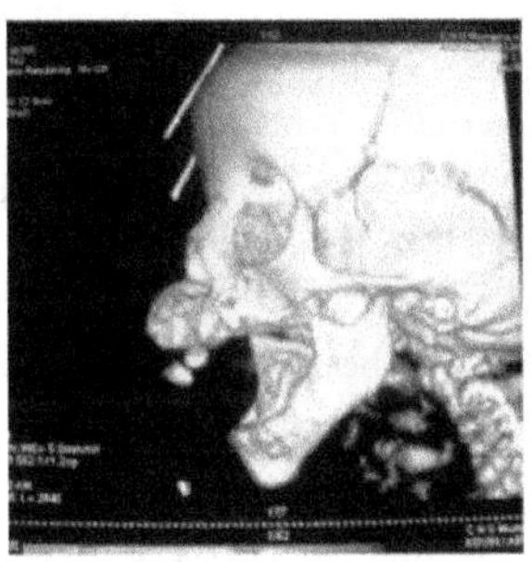
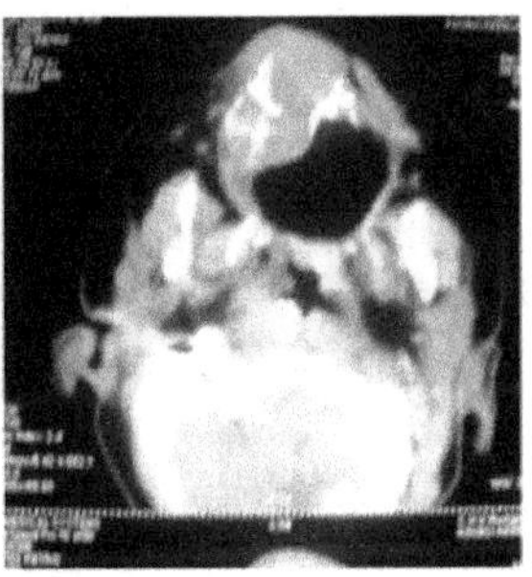

Figure 3: Radiographic CT scan studies revealed a large tumour with a large destruction of the right maxillary bones.

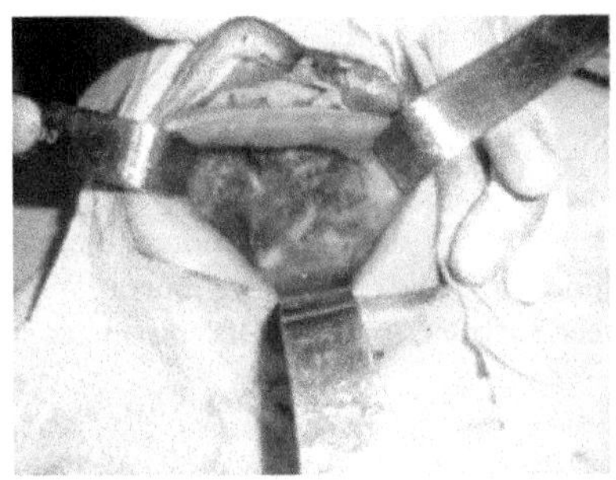

Figure 4: Biopsy revealed a Melanotic neuroectodermal tumour, the infant underwent surgery using an intraoral incision, it was totally resected without maxillectomy.

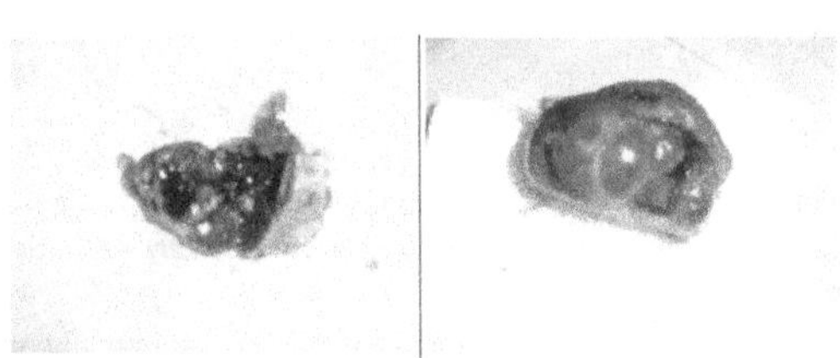

Figure 5: Surgical specimen, measuring 6 cm in its largest diameter, showing encapsulated, well circumscribed, and dark-coloured tissue.

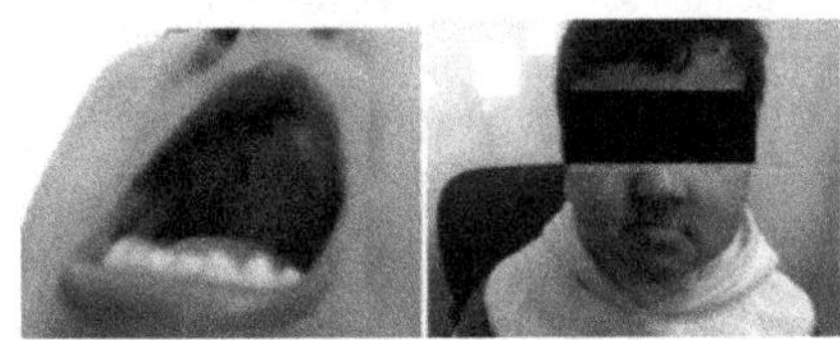

Figure 6: The postoperative period was uneventful and the infant was discharged. He is still being followed and shows no sign of recurrence during eight years.

Case 2: Agressive Desmoid Fibromatosis

A three-year old female infant presented with a swelling chin region. According to the mother, it was noticed past few weeks with a notion of trauma that preceded the onset of symptoms.

Clinical examination, the child was well nourished and moderately built it found a swelling of all the mandibular arch hard, deformed chin, extending to the oral floor, distending the chin skin and impeding food and elocution (Figures 7 and 8).

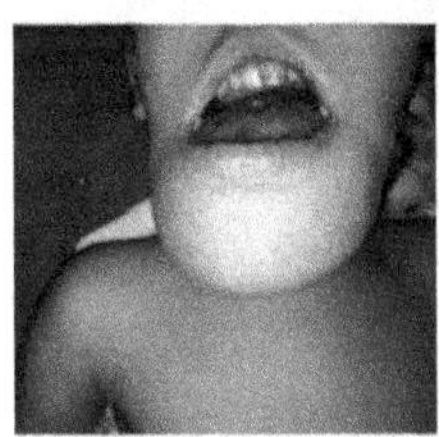
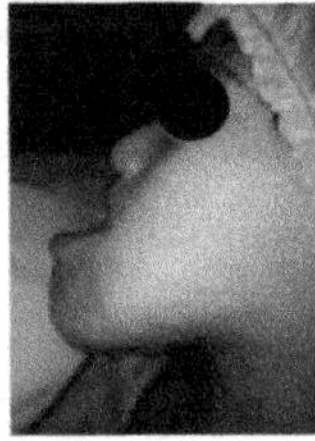

Figure 7: Traumatic ulceration was noted caused by teeth.

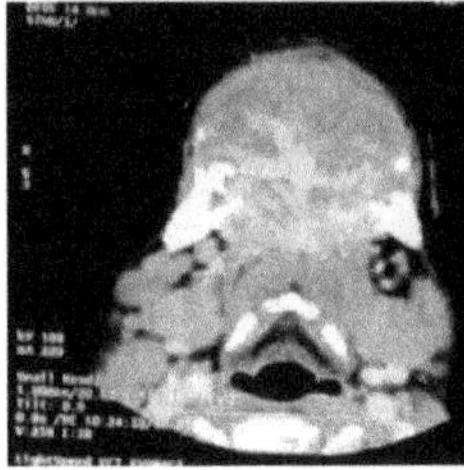
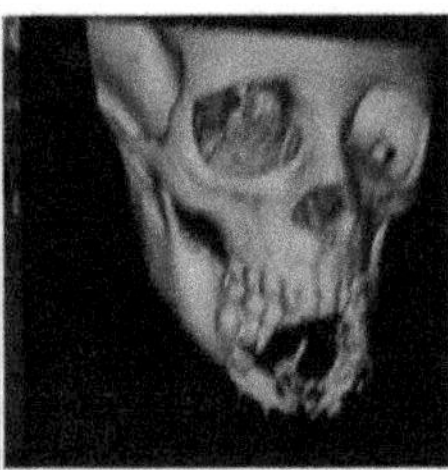

Figure 8: The CT scanner revealed a large bon destruction of the arch of the mandible.

A biopsy realised under a local anaesthesia revealed an aggressive fibromatosis desmoïde. The treatment was a large resection of all the mandibular arch through a cervical incision (Figure 9) with reestablishment of a continuity with a metallic arch (Figure 10).

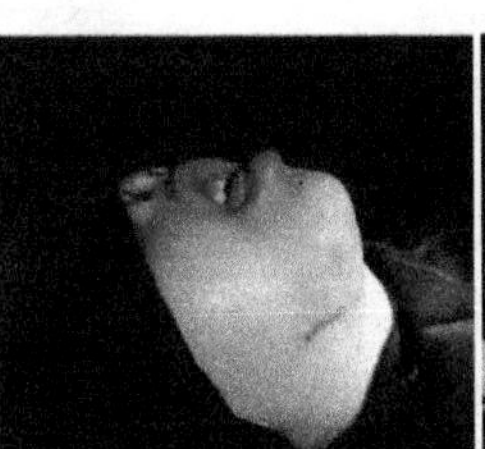
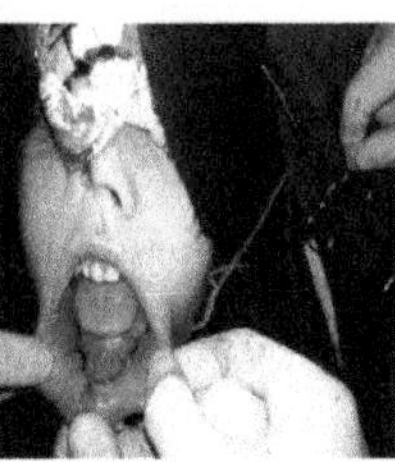

Figure 9: A large resection of all the mandibular arch through a cervical incision.

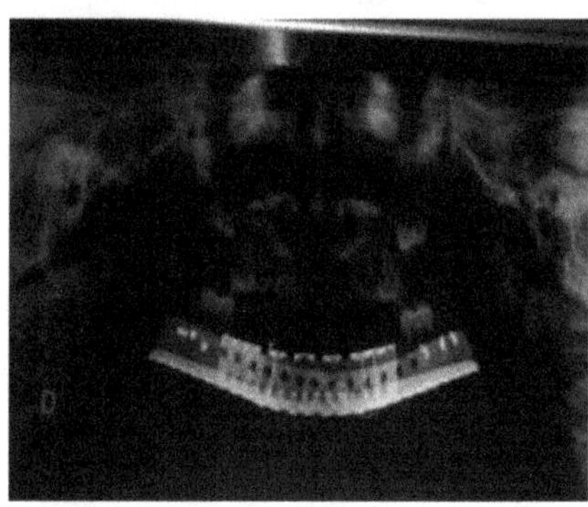

Figure 10: Re-establishment of a continuity with a metallic arch.

The immediate postoperative suites were good.

Microscopically a myofibroblastic proliferation of spindle cells active nucleus nucleolus immersed in a richly collagenous stroma. No mitotic activity (Figure 11).

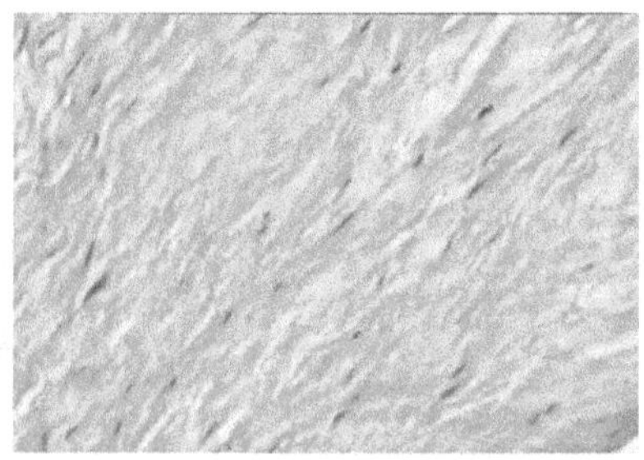

Figure 11: No mitotic activity.

Monitoring was marked by a dropping sutures and exposure of metallic arch.

The child is proposed for a reconstructive surgery.

Discussion

Melanotic neuroectodermal tumour of infancy (MNTI) is a benign rare tumour occurring during the first year with clinically and histological characteristic. Several theories for the origin of this tumour have been proposed. First by Krompecher [5] who called it congenital melanocarcinoma, the retinal anlage origin and the odontogenic origin gives a variety of terms like retinal anlage tumour, pigmented ameloblastoma, melanotic progonoma, congenital pigmented epulis and melanotic epithelial odontoma.

The report of a case with high urinary excretion of vanillylmandelic acid (VMA), suggesting a neural crest origin, which had been confirmed by, immunohistochemical [6] ,ultrastructural studies. They proposed the term as melanotic neuroectodermal tumour of infancy,which has been generally accepted.

MNTI frequently involves the maxilla but it has also been reported in the mandible cerebellum, brain, epididymis, skull, mediastinum and others region. This tumor affected more boys than girls and that it occurred most frequently within the first 06months of age. MNTIs are usually rapidly growing, expansive, and destructive recurrence has been noticed in the maxilla, and the recurrence rate has predominantly occurred during the first 4 months of age. Recurrence might be a consequence of incomplete enucleation of the primary tumour or might occur because of its multicentricity. A malignancy rate was reported and metastases have been described. At present, surgical resection with preservation of the function of adjacent structures and organs is the most often used procedure in most cases.

Chemotherapy and radiotherapy have been proposed to avoid mutilating operations.

The localisation of aggressive fibromatosis [7,8] in the jawbones is rare, presenting as infiltrative mass with unpredictable evolution. The young age and locoregional aggressiveness often suspected low-grade osteosarcoma. Factors triggering traumatic and hormonal may participate in the genesis of these tumours, the pathogenesis remains to be determined, there are several theories reported to explain the origin like a genetic predisposition hormonal by The Presence of estrogens receptors on tumour cells immunohistochemistry and cyto-genetics often redress the diagnostic.

According to the literature, surgery is the most common treatment of the head and neck localisation. However, particularly in children, alternative modes of therapy must be considered because of the high recurrence rate and to avoid mutilating operations, it's requiring cooperation between surgeons, pathologists and oncologists.

Conclusion

Melanotic neuroectodermal tumour of infancy and Aggressive desmoid fibromatosis, with its fast growing rate, could lead to the possibility of a malignant lesion with subsequent overtreatment. It has been considered as a benign neoplasm with high recurrence rate, Immunohistochemistry and computed tomography contributes to early diagnosis and careful follow-up after the complete surgical excision is required.

References

1. Fletcher (1995) Melanotic neuroectodermal tumour of infancy. Clinical pathology, immune cytochemical and flow cytometry study. Am J Surg Pathol 17: 566-573.
2. Kaya S, Unal OF, SaraÃ§ S, GedikoÄŸlu G (2000) Melanoticneuroectodermal tumor of infancy: Report of two cases and review of literature. Int J Pediatr Otorhinolaryngol 52: 169-172.
3. Heba S, Shagufta S, Khaled B, Abdulhafez AS (2008) Melanoticneuroectodermal tumour of infancy; review and case report. J Pediatr Surg 43: E25-E29.
4. Dilu NJ, Bobe A, Sokolo MR (1998) Progonome melanotique : A propos d'une volumineuse tumeur du nourisson. Rev Stomatol Chir Maxillofac 99: 103–105.
5. Krompecher E (1978) Zur histogenese und sonstiger Kiefergeschwulste. Beitr Pathol Anat 64: 165-197.
6. Barrett AW, Morgan M, Ramsay AD, Farthing PM, Newman L, et al (2002) A clinicopathologic and immunohistochemical analysis of melanotic neuroectodermal tumor of infancy. Oral Surg Oral Med Oral Pathol Oral Radiol Endod 93: 688-698.
7. Seper L, Bürger H, Vormoor J, Joos U, Kleinheinz J (2005) Agressive fibromatosis involving the mandible--case report and review of the literature. Oral Surg Oral Med Oral Pathol Oral Radiol Endod 99: 30-38.
8. Sharma A, Ngan BY, Sándor GK, Campisi P, Forte V (2008) Pediatric aggressive fibromatosis of the head and neck: A 20-year retrospective review. J Pediatr Surg 43: 1596-1604.

3

Case Report of Huge Esthesioneuroblastoma

Mouhannad Abdulber Fakoury*

Department of ENT, Dubai Hospital, Dubai, UAE

***Corresponding author:** Mouhannad Abdulber Fakoury, ENT Specialist, Dubai Hospital, Dubai, UAE; E-mail: mfakoury71@yahoo.com

Abstract

Esthesioneuroblastoma is a rare malignant tumor, account for only 1-5% of all malignant tumors of the paranasal sinuses; usually it presents with locally invasive disease, the delayed diagnosis of these tumors leads to tragic prognosis and bad results of surgery or conservative management. In this case, the diagnosis was too late in spite of followed up by medical doctors in deferent specialties; as a result it must be rules to avoid this problem like the mandatory of nasal endoscopy in all patients with nasal complaints (specially with refractory symptoms) and also radiologicinvestigations must be mandatory when epistaxis, nasal blockage, anosmia or headache does not respond to medical treatment.

Keywords: Esthesioneuroblastoma; Olfactory neuroblastoma; Epistaxis; CT; MRI

Introduction

Esthesioneuroblastoma is a rare malignant tumor, account for only 1-5% of all malignant tumors of the paranasal sinuses; usually it presents with locally invasive disease, the delayed diagnosis of these tumors leads to tragic prognosis and bad results of surgery or conservative management. In this case, the diagnosis was too late in spite of followed up by medical doctors in deferent specialties; as a result it must be rules to avoid this problem like the mandatory of nasal endoscopy in all patients with nasal complaints (specially with refractory symptoms) and also radiologic investigations must be mandatory when epistaxis, nasal blockage, anosmia or headache does not respond to medical treatment.

Case Report

Patient 50 year old, male came to ENT clinic with complaint of severe recurrent epistaxis 6 months ago, he underwent a lot of medications but without any improvement, recently he aggravated with right nasal obstruction, complete anosmia, right eyelids edema associated with epiphora, severe frontal headache unresponsive to pain killers and balance disorder without specific nervous signs.

By clinical examination there was huge mass filled completely right nasal cavity without any anatomical landmarks in the right nose. It was polypoid mass in shape, brown red color, soft fragile and associated with moderate bleeding when touch it. Examination of the left nasal cavity, mouth, ears, neck and cranial nerves were within normal limited.

Investigations

Computed tomography scan of paranasal sinuses done and it showed a huge nasal mass fills the right nasal cavity completely, invades bilateral all ethmoidal cells and destroys the cribriform plate to involve the brain (Figure 1).

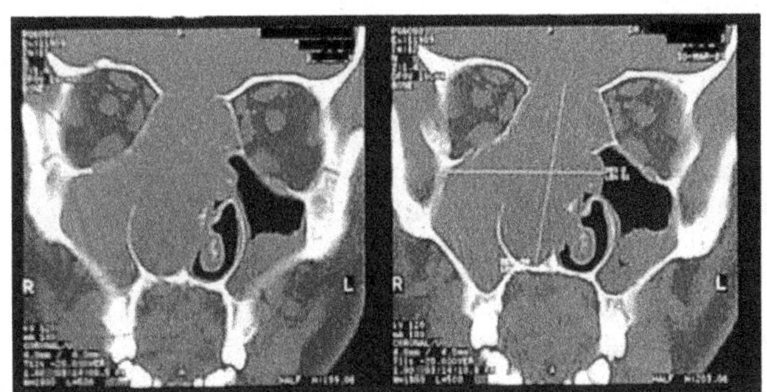

Figure 1: huge nasal mass fills the right nasal cavity completely, invades bilateral all ethmoidal cells and destroys the cribriform plate to involve the brain.

Magnetic resonance imaging of the head done and it showed that the mass invades frontal lobe of the brain, measures 4*5 cm in dimensions, push the midline of the brain to the left side, and associated with wide edema in right frontal lobe. Orbits and maxillary sinuses were intact (Figure 2).

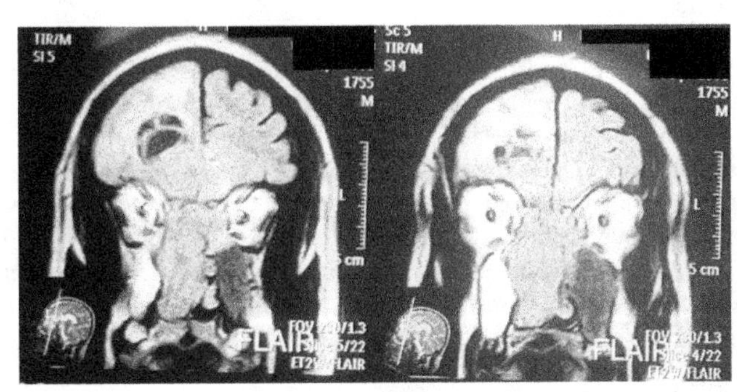

Figure 2: Orbits and maxillary sinuses were intact.

Surgical biopsy

Small surgical biopsy from the nasal cavity was taken under local anesthesia and histopathology result was Olfactory Neuroblastoma (Esthesioneuroblastoma).

General considerations

Esthesioneuroblastoma, first described by Berger et al. in 1924, [1] is an uncommon neoplasm that arises from olfactory epithelium high in the nasal vault and frequently invades the skull base, cranial vault, and orbit. Although esthesioneuroblastoma accounts for up to 3% of intranasal neoplasms in some series, fewer than 400 unique cases have been reported in the world literature. The recent apparent increase in incidence is at least in part attributable to improvements in diagnostic imaging and pathologic recognition of this relatively rare entity. Because of the limited number of subjects treated in different eras of medical and surgical practice, in addition to nonuniform treatment schemes and follow-up, management recommendations regarding these tumors have been based largely on anecdotal data and limited series.

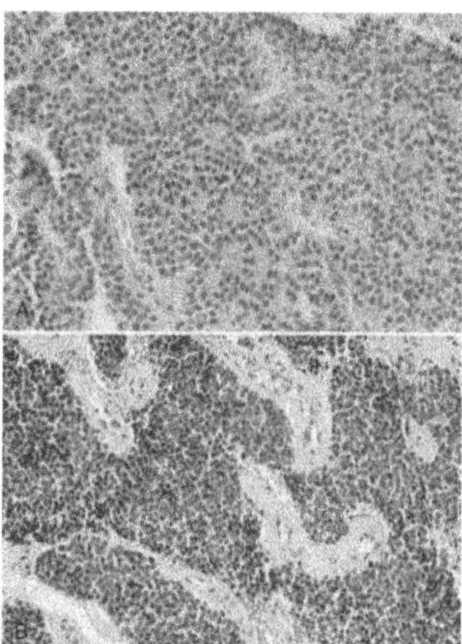

Figure 3: (A) Photomicrograph of an esthesioneuroblastoma showing a lobular arrangement of cells with round to oval nuclei and poorly defined cytoplasm, (B) Specimen from a higher grade tumor showing more cellularity with less tissue architecture.

Pathology

The morphologic, ultrastructural, and immunohistochemical features of esthesioneuroblastoma are similar to those of neuroblastoma of the adrenal glands and sympathetic nervous system. Light microscopy reveals a lobular architecture with sheets of cells in a dense neurofibrillary background. Individual cells have round to oval nuclei with scant, poorly defined cytoplasm. Occasionally, olfactory rosettes or pseudorosettes are present. A grading system based on histology has been proposed as a prognostic tool but has achieved varying success (Table 1 and Figure 3) [2].

Grade	I	II	III	IV
Cytoarchitecture	Lobular	Lobular	+/−	+/−
Mitotic rate	0	Low	Moderate	High
Nuclear pleomorphism	Absent	Slight	Moderate	Marked
Rosettes	+/−	+/−	True rosettes	None
Necrosis	Absent	Absent	Mild	Extensive

Table 1: Hyams' Histologic Grading System for Esthesioneuroblastoma.

Ultrastructurally, dense membrane-bound neurosecretory granules are seen along with neurofilaments and microtubules. On immunohistochemical staining, most esthesioneuroblastomas are positive for neuron-specific enolase (NSE), neurofilament, synaptophysin, chromogranin, and Leu-7 and variably positive for S-100. Although similar to neuroblastoma histologically, correlated coexpression of NSE and cytokeratin points to an epithelial rather than neural crest origin of these tumors [3].

Staging

Several staging systems, including Hymans, Kadish, and TNM systems, have been proposed as a guide to choosing treatment modalities. Tumor staging is an important guide for prognosis and therapy.

Kadish et al. were the first to propose a staging classification for esthesioneuroblastoma (ENB) [4]. ENBs were divided into 3 categories: groups A, B, and C. Group A is limited to tumors of the nasal fossa; in group B, extension is to the paranasal sinuses; and group C is defined as extension beyond the paranasal sinuses and nasal cavity.

Some authors have noted that effectively stratifying patients with the Kadish system can be difficult. Recognizing these inadequacies, Morita et al. in 1993 published a revised Kadish system that redefined stage C (consisting of local disease spreading beyond the paranasal sinuses) and included a stage D (distant metastasis) [5].

In 1992, Dulguerov and Calceterra proposed a classification based on the tumor, node, metastasis (TNM) system, which is predicated on CT and MRI findings that can be identified before treatment [6]. Although this classification system has gained popularity, attempts have been made to further modify the Kadish system for ENB.

The TNM classification is as follows:

T1 - Tumor involving the nasal cavity and/or paranasal sinuses (excluding sphenoid), sparing the most superior ethmoidal cells

T2 - Tumor involving the nasal cavity and/or paranasal sinuses (including the sphenoid), with extension to or erosion of the cribriform plate

T3 - Tumor extending into the orbit or protruding into the anterior cranial fossa, without dural invasion

T4 - Tumor involving the brain

N0 - No cervical lymph node metastasis

N1 - Any form of cervical lymph node metastasis

M0 - No metastasis

M1 - Distant metastases present

In our case, pt. was in stage C regarding Kadish staging system and T4N0M0 in TNM classification. The patient was informed that the prognosis is unsecured, the treatment of choice is surgery to resolve or reduce the symptoms, the recurrence is possible, and postoperative radiotherapy is important to reduce the recurrence.

Operation

Surgery was performed in combined approaches: 1. Cranial approach (by Neurosurgeon) (Figure 4) and 2. Intranasal endoscopic sinus surgery (by ENT surgeon). The neurosurgery was performed by Bifrontal approach and removal of the cerebral component of tumor which was consisted of cystic and solid components with moderate vascularity and then pericranial flap was used to close the defect in the skull base.

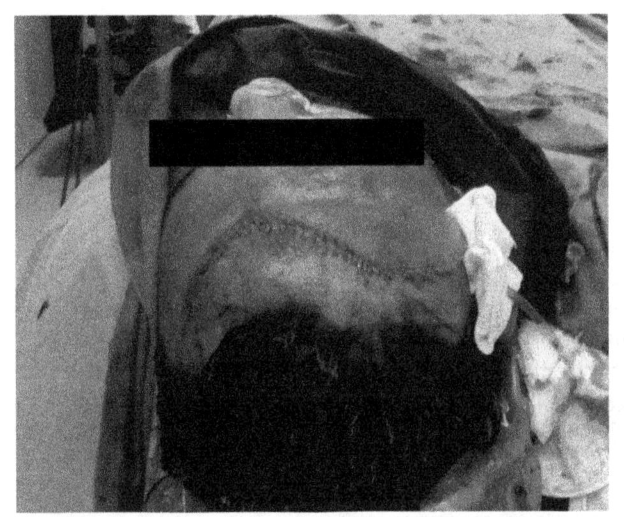

Figure 4: Post operation - Bifrontal approach flap.

Intranasal endoscopic sinus surgery performed and it was possible due to the tumor concentrated in the central part of the nasal cavity without erosion of bony structures of the maxillary sinus or orbits, the density in Rt. maxillary sinus was fluid density in MRI (not tumor tissue) and the lamina papyracea in both sides were intact.

The intranasal surgery done by removal of all nasal component of tumor by shaver and create one cavity between the orbits in the upper part of nasal cavity, detection and clean the skull base and tumor's bed, contact with the pericranial flap which previously repaired by neurosurgeon, too thick mucus was sucked from the Rt. maxillary sinus and support defect's closure in the skull base by muscular fascia and nasal packs.

Post-operation histopathology

Histopathology was done for cerebral component witch removed by an en-bloc resection technique and it measured 4.0*4.5 cm in size but the nasal component was removed by micro electric surgical Debrider, so no histopathology for nasal component.

Follow up

Patient underwent post-operative adjuvant radiotherapy, standard techniques include external megavoltage beam with 5500 cGy dose. Regular monthly follow up done until 8 months, and it was without any recurrence or complications. After that the follow up was not available.

Conclusion

Diagnosis in this case was too late – despite of the patient previously was seen and treated by several doctors from various specialties - as a result nasal endoscopy must be mandatory in all patients with nasal complaints (specially with unresponded cases). Epistaxis is not always benign symptom and may be it hides underlying disaster, so investigations must be mandatory when epistaxis does not respond to medical treatment. In this case there was history of exposure to Irradiated Uranium and Nuclear Weapons in the war, may be explain the etiology of this tumor, but there is no previous studies about that, may be this form a good idea for new studies and research.

References

1. Berger L, Luc H, Richard A (1924) Lesthesioneuroepitheliomeolfactif. Bull Assoc Franc Etude Cancer 13: 410-421.
2. Hyams VJ (1988) Tumors of the upper respiratory tract and ear. In Hyams VJ, Batsakis JG, and Michaels L (eds): Atlas of Tumor Pathology, Second Series, Fascicle 25. Washington DC: Armed Forces Institute of Pathology 240-248.
3. Banerjee AK, Sharma BS, Vashishta RK (1992) Intracranial olfactory neuroblastoma: Evidence for olfactory epithelial origin. J Clin Pathol 45: 299-302.
4. Kadish S, Goodman M, Wang CC (1976) Olfactory neuroblastoma. A clinical analysis of 17 cases. Cancer 37: 1571-1576.
5. Morita A, Ebersold MJ, Olsen KD, Foote RL, Lewis JE, et al. (1992) Esthesioneuroblastoma: Prognosis and management. Neurosurgery 32:706-714.
6. Dulguerov P, Calcaterra T (1992) Esthesioneuroblastoma the UCLA experience 1970-1990. Laryngoscope 102: 843-849.

Cervical Schwannoma- A Case Report

Jyotiranjan Das[1*], Jayant saha[2], Shantanu Dutta[2] and Ajay manickam[1]

[1]*Department of ENT, RG Kar Medical College, Kolkata, India*

[2]*ILS Hospitals, Dumdum, West Bengal, India*

***Corresponding author:** Jyotiranjan Das, RG Kar Medical College, Kolkata, India; E-mail: jdbegins007@gmail.com

Abstract

Schwannomas are benign, slow-growing, encapsulated tumours deriving from the peri neural cells located in the nerve sheath. They can arise from any peripheral, cranial or autonomic nerves, and show a predilection for the head and neck region. Extra cranial Head and Neck schwannomas are rare tumours. They may produce secondary symptoms like nasal obstruction, dysphagia, and hoarseness of voice depending upon the location of the tumour. The preoperative diagnosis is difficult. Although preoperative imaging or fine needle aspiration cytology may help to reveal diagnosis, they are inadequate. The definitive diagnosis is made by histopathological examinations.

Keywords: Para pharyngeal space; Schwannoma; Benign tumour; Magnetic resonance image; Trans cervical

Introduction

Schwannomas are benign, solitary and well-differentiated tumours originating from Schwann cell [1]. Nearly 45% of all schwannomas occur in the head and neck area, where they may originate from any of the peripheral, cranial or autonomic nerves [2]. These benign tumours occur regardless of age or sex and are painless, insidious and slow growing [3]. So, they are of long duration at the time of the presentation and rarely show a rapid course [4]. Malignant transformation is very rare. The nerve of origin is not identified in around 10 to 40% of schwannomas [5]. Among the cranial nerves, schwannomas can arise from the glossopharyngeal, accessory, and hypoglossal nerves, while the most common type is acoustic neuroma differentiating from the vestibulocochlear nerve. The most commonly affected regions are the temporal bone, lateral neck (Para pharyngeal space), and paranasal sinuses [6].

It may present as a lump in neck with dysphagia, pain. Patients with malignant tumours are more likely to present with a rapidly growing neck mass, pain, trismus, otalgia, or cranial nerve deficits.

We present a case of neck mass without any of above features which after surgery on histopathological examination shows schwannoma. It was considered in differential diagnosis of other mass in Para pharyngeal mass like metastatic cervical nodes, paragangliomas, branchial cysts, lymphomas, neurofibromas.

Case Report

A 37 year lady came to outpatient department of a tertiary care hospital with a swelling in left side of neck for last one year. It was slow in onset and gradually progressive in nature. There was no complain of breathing difficulty, change of voice, pain or difficulty in swallowing or pain in ear.

On general examination, patient was moderately built. Vitals were stable. There was no pallor, icterus, clubbing or edema. There was no palpable neck node or enlarged gland.

On local examination, a nonpulsatile oval shaped 3.5 × 2.5 cm swelling in left side of neck (Figure 1) in supraclavicular area with ill-defined margins. It was nontender, firm in consistency, mobile. It was getting more prominent on moving the neck against resistance.

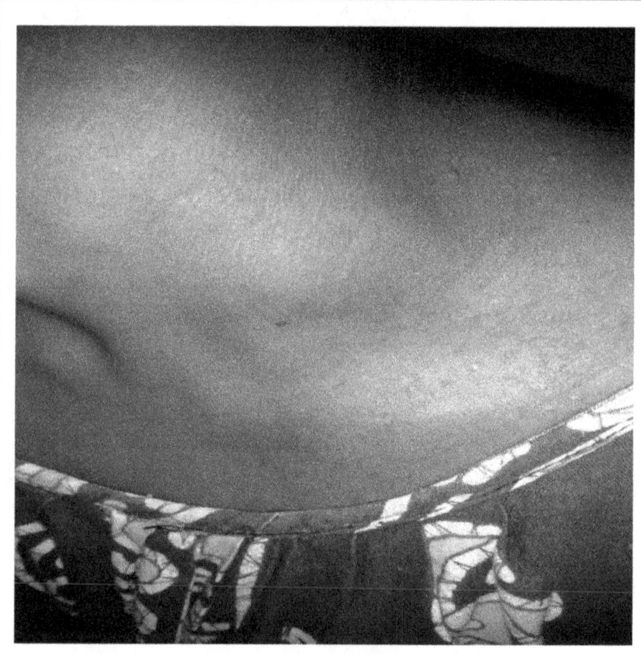

Figure 1: Swelling in left side of neck.

Local examination larynx by indirect laryngoscopy was normal. Ear, nose, oral cavity examination were within normal limit. Systemic examination was normal. FNAC was done which showed spindle cell tumour.

Magnetic resonance imaging revealed left sided soft tissue tumour in (Figure 2) both T1 and T2 images. Mass was excised by trans cervical approach (Figures 3 and 4) under general anaesthesia and sent for histopathological examination which showed schwannoma.

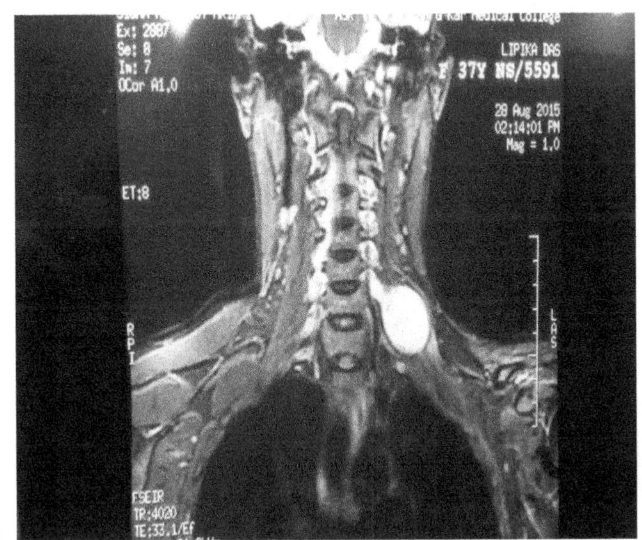

Figure 2: MRI image showing soft tissue swelling.

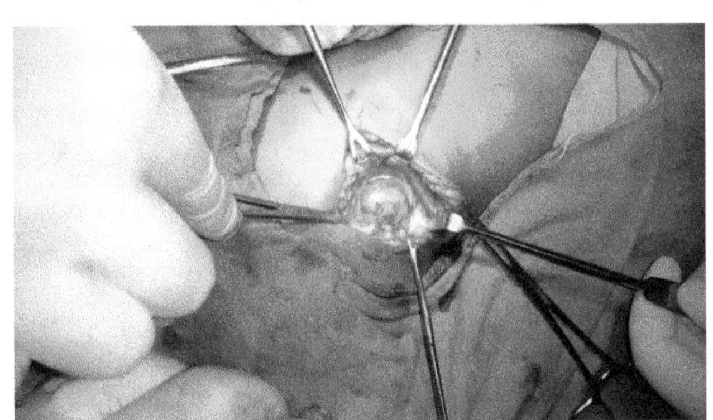

Figure 3: Trans cervical approach.

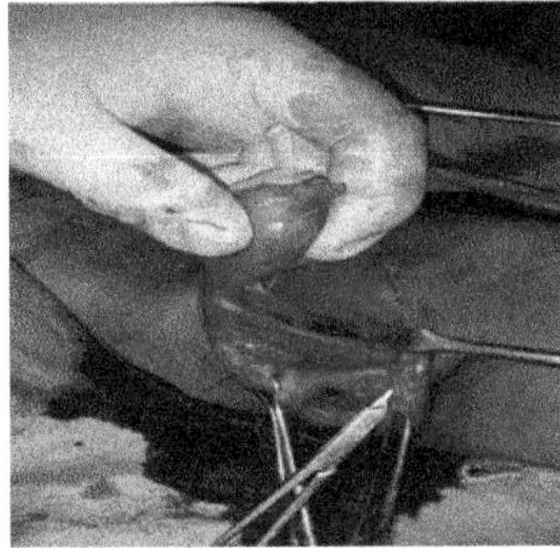

Figure 4: Excison of mass by tanscervical approach.

Postoperative recovery was uneventful. On gross examination of mass, it was encapsulated oval shape with 3.5 × 2.5 cm size, firm with smooth surface (Figure 5).

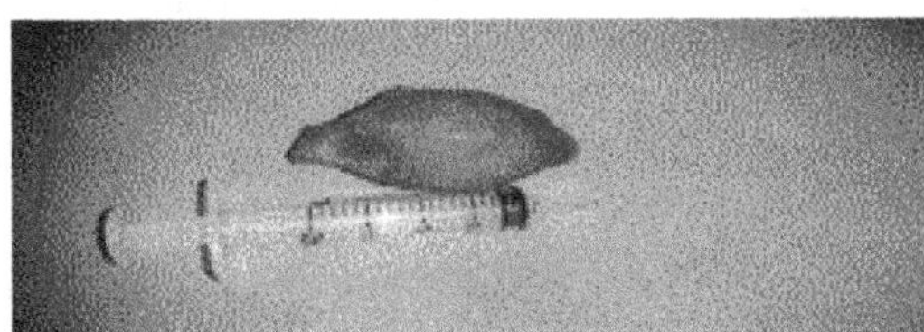

Figure 5: Gross appearance of mass.

Histopathological report showed verrocay bodies which confirmed it to be schwannoma (Figure 6). Patient was followed up for six months and there was no recurrence.

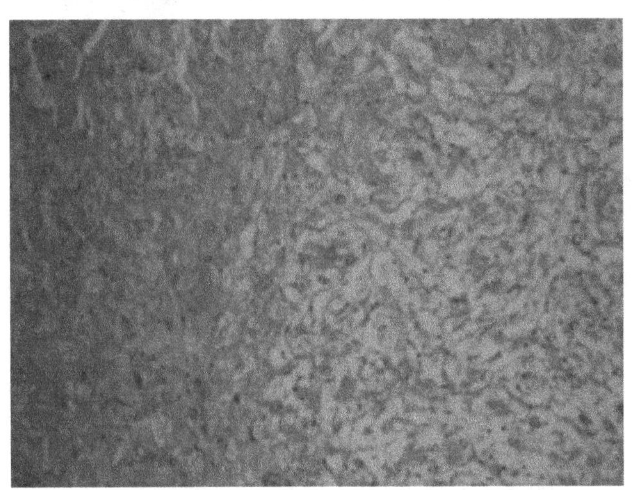

Figure 6: Histopthological image of schwannoma.

Discussion

Neurogenic tumours arise from the neural crest which differentiates into the Schwann cells and the sympathicoblasts. The Schwann cells give rise to neurofibroma and neurilemmoma (Schwannoma). A schwannoma is a slow growing solitary and encapsulated tumour attached to a nerve. Degenerative changes such as cystic alterations and haemorrhagic necrosis are seen in schwannoma 1 whereas such changes are not seen in neurofibroma. Schwannoma may arise from any cranial or spinal nerve that has a sheath i.e., any motor or sensory nerve other than the optic and the olfactory nerves which do not have the Schwann cell sheath. Schwannoma was first established as a pathological entity by Verocay in 1908 who later called it neurinoma in 1910. Later the term neurilemmoma 3 was coined by Stout in 1935. Para pharyngeal space is the site of schwannoma in head and neck region accounting for 25-40% of all reported patients. The first case of neurilemmomma within the Para pharyngeal space was reported in 1933 by Figi. Other sites in the head and neck like submandibular space, paranasal sinuses, cheek and, oral cavity are rare.

The size of the tumour may vary from few mm to over 24 cms. The clinical signs and symptoms vary according to the anatomic site of the tumour in the head and neck. Majority of the patients present with a painless mass and pain may be present only in few cases. Other symptoms may be difficulty in breathing(nose), dysphagia(pharynx), epistaxis (PNS), hoarseness (larynx)or only a swelling in the neck(Para pharyngeal space). The swelling is freely mobile in soft tissues, but when it is connected to a large nerve or trunk there is restriction of the movements, even primary nerve of origin may be entirely encompassed within the tumour. The schwannoma may arise at any age and there is no gender or race [7]. It has been reported that in the nose and paranasal sinuses, maxillary branches of trigeminal nerve, intranasal nerve and branches of autonomic nervous system may be the site of origin. In the neck, the schwannoma has been divided into medial and lateral group. Medial group arises from the last four cranial nerves and cervical sympathetic chain. Lateral group arises from the cervical nerve trunk, cervical plexus and the brachial plexus. Schwannoma may also originate from vagus nerve, sympathetic chain or the glossopharyngeal nerve [7]. A case has been presented in submandibular region which shows atypical site of origin [8].

The preoperative diagnosis of schwannoma in the head neck region is difficult. Most of the investigations like FNAC, CT or Magnetic resonance Imaging (MRI) are generally done. MRI possesses many advantages and has excellent soft tissue contrast, three dimensional modelling. On the other hand, CT is useful where bone is involved like pteryrgoid plates or bone of posterior wall of maxillary sinus [9].

Treatment is surgical excision, trans cervical approach (for post styloid compartment) [9]. The tumour is radio resistant and the possibility of the malignant change of the benign tumour is extremely rare. Radiotherapy should be reserved for palliation only in cases of inoperable tumours [7].

Histopathologically it has typical presentation. Diagnostic features include a fibrous capsule, hyaline vessels, cellular (Antoni A) and loose textured (Antoni B) areas, Verocay bodies (opposing rows of spindle nuclei separated by anucleate rows of eosinophilic processes). Retrogressive changes are common in large, old tumours, and include "degenerative nuclear atypia," vascular sclerosis and haemorrhage as well as occasional micronecroses. Micro cyst formation, some with a pseudo epithelial lining of plump Schwann cells may also be seen [10].

Conclusion

Cervical schwannomas, which most often present as asymptomatic unilateral neck masses, are rare tumours. The preoperative diagnosis may be difficult and it is often not made until the time of surgery. The definitive diagnosis relies on clinical suspicion and histopathological confirmation. In the treatment of head and neck schwannomas, complete surgical excision with appropriate approaches is efficient. It is important bearing in mind possible vagal or sympathetic chain injury. Local recurrence is extremely rare.

References

1. Rootman J, Goldberg C, Robertson W (1982) Primary orbital schwannomas. Br J Ophthalmol 66: 194-204.
2. Gupta T, Brassfiel R, Strong E, Hajdu S (1969) Benign solitary schwannoma (neurilemmoma). Cancer 24: 355-366.
3. Diaz DD, Kennedy KS, Parker GS, White VJ (1991) Schwannoma of the submandibular gland. Head Neck 13: 239-242.
4. Dhupar V, Yadav S, Dhupar A, Akkara F (2012) Cavernous hemangioma--uncommon presentation in zygomatic bone. J Craniofac Surg 23: 607-609.
5. Gallo WJ, Moss M, Shapiro DN, Gaul JV (1977) Neurilemoma: review of the literature and report of five cases. J Oral Surg 35: 235-236.
6. Piscioli F, Antolini M, Pusiol T, Dalrì P, Lo Bello MD, et al. (1986) Malignant schwannoma of the submandibular gland. A case report. ORL J Otorhinolaryngol Relat Spec 48: 156-161.
7. Garg MK, Garg U, Aggrawal D, Rana P (2013) Schwannoma of Neck, the Journal of Mahatma Gandhi Institute of Medical Sciences 18: 74-77.
8. Gaffar A, Fikret C, Fatmagul KC (2014) Schwannoma of the submandibular gland: a case report, Journal of Medical Case Reports 8: 231.
9. Michael G, George GB, Martin JB, Ray C, Hibbert J, et al. (2011) Scott brown's otorhinolaryngology, head and neck surgery, Ann R Coll Surg Engl 93: 559.
10. Kurtkaya-Yapicier O, Scheithauer B, Woodruff JM (2003) The
11. pathobiologic spectrum of Schwannomas. Histol Histopathol 18: 925-934.

5

Combined Evaluation of FDG-PET/CT and CT Imaging Characteristics of Cervical Lymph Nodes to Increase the Interpretation Accuracy for Nodal Metastatic Involvement in Head and Neck Cancer

Richard A Marshall M.D [1], Peter M Som M.D[1], Livnat Uliel M.D., M.Sc [1*], Eric Genden M.D [2], Michael Buckstein M.D., PhD [3], Vishal Gupta M.D [3], Brett Miles, DDS, M.D [2], Neetha Gandikota M.D [1], Idoia Corcuera-Solano M.D [1], Krzysztof Misiukiewicz M.D [4], Andrew G. Sikora M.D., PhD [2,5,6] and Lale Kostakoglu M.D, MPH [1]

[1]*Department of Radiology, The Mount Sinai Medical Center, One Gustave L. Levy Place, New York, USA*

[2]*Department of Otolaryngology, The Mount Sinai Medical Center, One Gustave L. Levy Place, New York, USA*

[3]*Department of Radiation Oncology, The Mount Sinai Medical Center, One Gustave L. Levy Place, New York, USA*

[4]*Department of Hematology and Medical Oncology, The Mount Sinai Medical Center, One Gustave L. Levy Place, New York, USA*

[5]*The Tisch Cancer Institute, One Gustave L. Levy Place, Icahn Building, New York, USA*

[6]*Department of Otolaryngology – Head and Neck Surgery, Baylor College of Medicine, Houston, TX, USA*

***Corresponding author:** Livnat Uliel, Department of Radiology, The Mount Sinai Medical Center, One Gustave L. Levy Place, New York, USA;
E-mail: livnat.uliel@mountsinai.org

Abstract

Rationale and objectives: Accurate staging of regional lymph nodes in patient with head and neck squamous cell carcinoma (HNSCC) has important therapeutic and prognostic implications. The objective of this study was to assess qualitative and quantitative imaging characteristics of cervical lymph nodes on FDG PET/CT and contrast enhanced CT (CECT), either alone or in cross-modality combinations, for more accurate diagnosis of nodal metastatic involvement in HNSCC patients who had hypermetabolic cervical lymph nodes on PET/CT imaging.

Materials and methods: Lymph nodes were evaluated using quantitative PET/CT parameters (SUVmax, SUVmean, metabolic tumor volume, total lesion glycolysis) and qualitative and quantitative CT parameters (shape, margin, focal hypoattenuation, fatty hilum, short axis, long axis, volume, eccentricity factor). A subset analysis was performed on FDG-avid lymph nodes that lacked imaging findings suggestive of extracapsular spread or necrosis. Statistical outcomes included sensitivity, specificity, accuracy, positive likelihood ratio, and odds ratio.

Results: In the full cohort (174 nodes), the most malignancy specific parameters were ill-defined margin and focal hypoattenuation, and the most accurate variables included SUVmax, SUVmean, ill-defined margin, short axis, and focal hypoattenuation. On multivariate analysis, ill-defined margin, short axis measurement, and SUVmax independently predicted nodal metastasis.

In the subgroup of smaller lymph nodes without ill-defined margin or focal hypoattenuation (100 nodes), round shape was among the most accurate and specific criteria for malignancy. Cross-modality combination criteria with SUVmax and shape, eccentricity factor, or long to short axis ratio resulted in statistically significant improvements in specificity and accuracy for lymph node metastasis.

Conclusion: A combined evaluation strategy using individual PET/CT and CECT characteristics in cross modality combinations, particularly SUVmax with round shape on axial imaging or with loss of eccentricity, can improve diagnostic accuracy of malignant nodal involvement in the evaluation of indeterminate cervical lymph nodes for malignancy.

Keywords: Head and neck squamous cell carcinoma; FDG PET/CT; Malignant lymphadenopathy; CT

Introduction

In patients with head and neck cancer, cervical lymph node metastasis is one of the most important predictors of poor prognosis and thus, significantly impacts management decisions and ultimately clinical outcomes [1,2]. Given the significant morbidity and cost of unwarranted treatment of histologically negative necks, it is imperative for clinicians to accurately diagnose malignant nodal involvement. Alternatively, undertreating involved lymph nodes can lead to disease progression and shortened survival.

With the recognition of the importance of modern imaging modalities, the American Joint Committee on Cancer recommends clinical staging including both physical examination and imaging modalities [3]. The National Comprehensive Cancer Network (NCCN) recommends CT and/or MRI with contrast as part of the initial workup of newly diagnosed head and neck cancer. In the NCCN guidelines PET/CT imaging should be considered in the more advanced stages of certain head and neck primary tumors [1].

Basic CECT or contrast enhanced MRI, are used to evaluate lymph nodes based on size, contrast enhancement patterns, morphological characteristics (including shape and margins) and distribution [4]. Central necrosis, suggested by focal hypoattenuation on CECT or by T2 hyperintensity on MRI, and extracapsular spread, suggested by irregular margins, are the most accurate and specific markers for metastatic involvement, and affected nodes are generally considered to harbor metastasis irrespective of size [4-6]. Size and abnormalities in nodal architecture such as round shape, clustering, and absence of fatty hilum, are considered less reliable criteria in clinical practice [6,7]. Advanced imaging techniques including diffusion weighted MRI and CT or MRI dynamic perfusion imaging are less used in clinical practice.

PET/CT assesses both metabolic and anatomic parameters of the lymph nodes. PET/CT has gained acceptance in the evaluation of cervical nodes by providing improved sensitivity and accuracy compared to other imaging modalities including US, CT and MRI [8-11]. However, concerns remain regarding the non-specific nature of FDG uptake, which results in false positive readings. Recent publications comparing hybrid PET/magnetic resonance imaging (PET/MR) and PET/CT demonstrated equivalent or slight superiority of PET/MR in the imaging workup of patients with head and neck cancer, however additional data is needed to establish the role of PET/MR as preferred imaging modality or problem solving tool [12,13].

The diagnostic benefit of interpretation the PET/CT in correlation with the CECT, is well established; however, it remains challenging for imaging experts to differentiate between benign reactive changes and metastatic disease in FDG-avid lymph nodes that lack one or more highly specific criteria for malignancy [2,14]. Research is now directed toward finding optimal diagnostic algorithms for these indeterminate nodes. Initial reports of diagnostic gains when analyzing PET/CT and CECT examinations together are promising [8, 9]; however, there remains a need for the development of a reliable combination analysis for distinguishing reactive hyperplasia from metastatic disease in equivocal FDG-avid cervical lymph nodes.

We hypothesized that nodal assessment of imaging characteristics and measurable parameters in cross-modality combinations, would improve reader specificity and diagnostic accuracy for lymph node metastasis, particularly for those lymph nodes which did not have highly specific imaging features of metastatic involvement. Our objective was to describe clinically useful metrics derived from PET/CT and CECT, used alone or in combinations, for more accurate diagnosis of the histopathological nature of cervical lymph nodes in patients with HNSCC and FDG-avid cervical lymph nodes.

Methods

Patients

The Institutional Review Board approved this study and patient informed consent was waived based on the retrospective design in compliance with the Health Insurance Portability and Accountability Act. The objective of this study was to assess qualitative and quantitative imaging characteristics of cervical lymph nodes on FDG PET/CT and CECT, either alone or in cross-modality combinations, for more accurate diagnosis of nodal metastatic involvement in HNSCC patients who had hypermetabolic cervical lymph nodes on PET/CT imaging.

From a database of 1,744 patients who underwent both PET/CT and CECT between March 2006 and November 2012, 131 patients with HNSCC fulfilled the eligibility criteria either at staging or restaging (Table 1). Eligibility criteria included diagnosis of HNSCC either at staging or restaging, minimum 18 years of age, whole body PET/CT and CECT of the neck obtained simultaneously or within 4 weeks of each other with no intervening therapy, and the availability of either histopathology or long-term follow up of at least 12 months for confirmation of imaging findings. The interval between the last treatment and imaging was at least 3 months in the restaging group. Exclusion criteria included known granulomatous disease, HIV positive serology, active infection, diabetes with blood glucose level over 220 mg/dl, and patients on oral prednisone.

Imaging protocols

The PET/CT protocol included a whole-body FDG PET⁄CT obtained 60 min after injection of 10-15 mCi 18-FDG. The associated CT of the PET/CT study was acquired either with or without intravenous iopamidol (8-detector, 120 kVp, auto mAs of up to 380).

The dedicated multidetector CECT of the neck was acquired with the following protocol: 90 mL of intravenous iopamidol (Isovue-370); 30 seconds delay; 140 kVp, automatic current-time product (auto mAs) of up to 380 mAs. The term PET/CT is used for all PET/CT studies, with or without intravenous contrast.

Image interpretation

PET/CT and neck CECT were evaluated independently by a nuclear medicine physician (LK) and a neuroradiologist (PS), respectively, each reader with more than 30 years experience. The readers were blinded to each other's interpretation and to other clinical information except the patient's primary diagnosis and the time of imaging with respect to therapy.

Qualitative analyses

For CECT studies, lymph nodes were evaluated for round shape (defined as a loss of the reniform nodal shape) (yes/no), margin irregularity (defined as ill-defined contour or infiltration of adjacent tissues) (yes/no), focal hypoattenuation (yes/no), and fatty hilum (yes/no).

For PET/CT studies, a positive lesion was defined as increased FDG uptake incompatible with normal anatomical or physiological variants compared to a contralateral normal appearing site or adjacent background tissue when the contralateral site was involved by disease.

For statistical evaluation of reader performance, both the PET/CT and CECT readers evaluated nodes for metastasis using a five-point qualitative scale of reader confidence (1=Benign, 2=Probably Benign, 3=Equivocal, 4=Probably Malignant, 5=Malignant). Data were subsequently dichotomized as negative (scores 1-2) and positive (3-5) for end-point analyses.

Quantitative analyses

CECT quantitative parameters included short axis (SA) (mm), long axis (LA) (mm), short / long axis ratio, eccentricity factor (EF), and volume. CECT images were processed using OncoQuant imaging software via PACS reading platform (GE Healthcare, Wisconsin, USA) which used a semi-automated three-dimensional technique to calculate volumetric measurements. After the longest diameter of each cervical lymph node was manually measured on a transverse plane, the software automatically separated the node from surrounding anatomic structures and defined a region of interest that tightly enclosed the node. Once segmentation was completed, nodes were revaluated by the neuroradiologist and, if needed, manual corrections were made. Subsequently, computer software analyzed each axial image and produced unidimensional and volumetric measurements. The EF (EF $= \sqrt{1-(SA/LA)^2}$) was calculated using the resulting parameters [15].

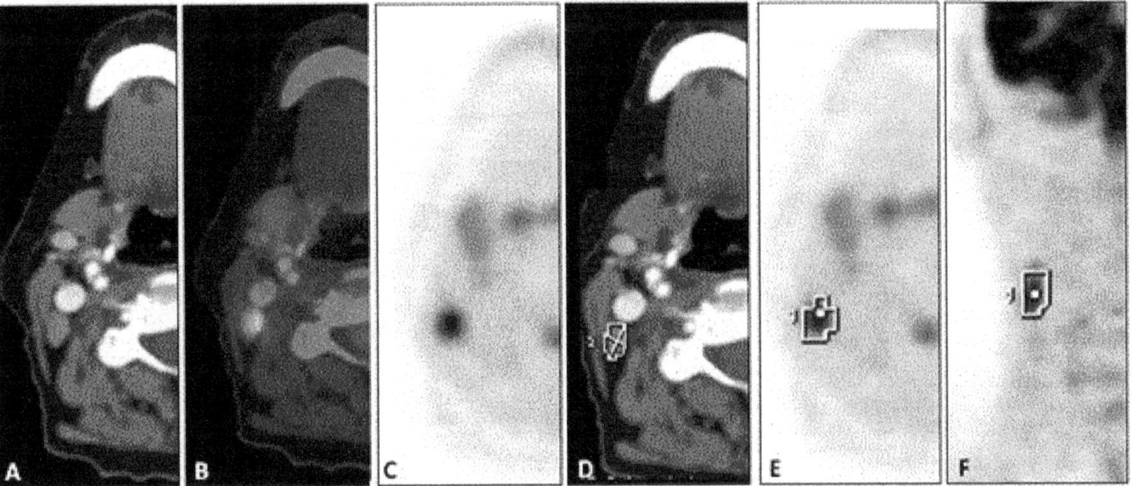

Figure 1: 61 year old woman with SCC of the tongue. (A) axial CECT image of the neck demonstrates level IIB lymph node, with rounded shape, no ill-defined margin or focal hypoattenuation (B) axial fused PET/CT image and (C) axial PET image show increased FDG uptake in the lymph node. (D) segmentation of the lymph node on the CECT study, the SA was measured 6 mm and the LA 11 mm, the volume 1480 mm2 and the average density 55 HU. Segmentation of the lymph node on the PET/CT study in the axial plane (E) and coronal plane (F), the volumetric analysis revealed SUVmax of 5.1, SUVmean of 3.1, Volume 2140 mm3 and TLG 6669.5.

PET/CT quantitative parameters included maximum standardized uptake value (SUVmax)(g/mL), SUVmean (g/mL), metabolic tumor volume (MTV)(mL), and total lesion glycolysis (TLG)(g)(TLG = MTV X SUVmean). Each lymph node was also segmented in three-dimensions using PETVCAR software via AW workstation platform (GE Healthcare, Wisconsin, USA). The automated segmentation technique defined nodal borders using a fixed threshold of 42% of maximal activity within the tumor (SUVmax) [16]. All tissue with activity greater than that percentage was included within the tumor volume. The 3D segmentation of each node was reviewed by a radiologist, and if needed, minor manual adjustments were made to completely avoid physiological sites (Figure 1).

Surgery and histopathology

All positive findings on either PET/CT or CECT were confirmed by biopsy within 6 weeks of initial positive imaging result (n=137) or serial clinical and imaging follow up of ≥ 12 months (n=37) (median 17 months) as reference standard.

In patients without histopathology data, final diagnosis was considered benign if the node was stable for ≥ 12 months of clinical and radiographic follow-up when there was no therapy administration, or if the node decreased in size in the absence of intervening therapy. For image-histopathology correlation, images were analyzed on a level-by-level basis based on 6 cervical node levels, bilaterally.

Statistical analysis

Statistics were analyzed using IBM SPSS statistical software (version 20; SPSS, Inc. Chicago, Ill). Receiver Operator Curves (ROC) were generated, and area under the curve (AUC) and optimal cutoffs by Youden criteria were compared using nonparametric methods [17].

2X2 tables were created against our reference standard to calculate sensitivity, specificity, accuracy, positive likelihood ratio, and odds ratio, and significance was determined using chi-squared analyses ($p<0.05$, 2-sided). Multivariate analyses were performed using binomial logistic regression.

These analyses were performed on the full data set, as well as on a subset of lymph nodes without findings suggestive of extracapsular spread or necrosis (ill-defined margins or central hypoattenuation, respectively) in order to characterize the most discriminative characteristics for malignancy in difficult to evaluate nodes without these highly specific criteria. The PET/CT and the CECT derived variables were combined sequentially to maximize specificity, and these combinations were evaluated using relative positive likelihood ratios (rLR+) as described by Macaskill et al. [18]. If the rLR+ was greater than 1 and its 95% confidence interval did not contain 1, the combined test was considered significantly more accurate in identifying metastasis.

Results

A total of 174 lymph nodes from 114 patients were analyzed. Patient and lymph node characteristics are summarized in Table 1.

Evaluation of FDG -avid lymph nodes in the entire cohort

Specificity, sensitivity and accuracy data at optimal cutoffs are summarized in Table 2. In univariate analysis, the variables most specific for malignancy were ill-defined margin (97%) and focal hypoattenuation (94%), and the variable most sensitive for malignancy was the absence of fatty hilum (95%). The most accurate tests included in a descending order were SUVmax, SUVmean, ill-defined margin, focal hypoattenuation, and short axis. On multivariate analysis, only ill-defined margin, short axis, and SUVmax were found to independently predict nodal metastasis (Table 2).

Patient, Primary Cancer, and Lymph Node Characteristics		
Variable	n	%
Patient:		
Count	114	
Age, years		
Median (Mean, Range)	61 (62, 27-90)	
Sex, M/F	71/43	
Primary Site		
Oral Cavity	52	46
Pharynx	40	35
Larynx	15	13
Hypopharynx	1	1
Unknown	6	5
Lymph Node:		
Count (Malignant/Total)	87/174	50
Level		
I	33	19
II	104	60
III	27	16
IV	6	3
V	4	2
Lymph Node Identified at		
Staging	114	66
Restaging	60	34

Table 1: Patient, primary cancer, and lymph node characteristics.

Across all possible cutoffs, the best performing quantitative PET/CT and CECT variables by ROC analysis (AUC) were SUVmax (0.87), SUVmean (0.87), and short axis (0.85). Short axis performed significantly greater in the detection of nodal metastasis than long axis (0.78) (p=0.02; 95% CI 0.009 – 0.124), but did not perform statistically greater than volume (p=0.081; 95% CI -0.006 – 0.105). SUVmax performed significantly greater in the detection of nodal metastasis than MTV (0.64) (p<0.001; 95% CI 0.13–0.34).

Evaluation of lymph nodes without focal hypoattenuation or ill-defined margin

In the subgroup analysis including lymph nodes without imaging findings suggestive of necrosis or extracapsular spread , which were borderline by size criteria, (n=100, 20 malignant), the individual criteria found to have the greatest overall accuracy at optimal cutoffs in univariate analysis included in descending order; round shape, SUVmean (cutoff=2.4), and SUVmax (cutoff=3.9) (Table 3). EF (cutoff=0.8) and long/short axis ratio (cutoff=1.6), performed identically on this data set. On multivariate binomial logistic regression of significant univariate, nonderivative variables, only SUVmax (>3.9), and short axis measurement independently predicted nodal metastasis.

A node was 1.9 times more likely to be malignant using SUVmax (cutoff 3.9) together with either EF or long axis/short axis ratio (relative LR+1.9; 95% CI 1.1-3.3; p=0.031) versus using SUVmax alone (relative LR+1.9; 95% CI 1.1-3.3; p=0.031), increasing the specificity for malignancy from 73% (SUVmax>3.9 alone) to 89% (SUVmax with either EF or long/short axis). The combination of SUVmax with reader defined shape improved specificity from 73% to 94%, but was not significantly better than SUVmax alone (relative LR+2.3; 95% CI 0.96–5.68; p=0.063). SUVmax with short axis (>6.5mm) did not produce a significant rLR+ improvements (rLR+1.39; 95% CI 0.97–1.99; p=0.076). Short axis combined with shape did not improve the results compared to shape alone (rLR+1.4; 95% CI 0.9–2.2; p=0.162).

Across all possible cutoffs, the best performing quantitative PET/CT and CECT variables by ROC analysis (AUC) were SUVmean (0.83), SUVmax (0.83), and short axis measurement (0.79). The AUC for SUVmax was not statistically superior to short axis measurement (p=0.54; 95% CI -0.082–0.157). In addition, the AUC for the combination of SUVmax with short axis (0.84) was not significantly greater than SUVmax alone (p=0.693; 95% CI -0.055–0.082).

Discussion

In this study, we demonstrated that the use of cross-modality combinations of lymph node imaging characteristics, particularly SUVmax combined with round shape (subjective roundness or long/short axis ratio or EF), significantly improved diagnostic accuracy for predicting malignancy in smaller FDG-avid lymph nodes with no imaging findings strongly suggestive of malignancy, such as extracapsular spread or necrosis. Other groups have reported synergistic gains in diagnostic accuracy when the overall assessments for malignancy on PET/CT and CT were combined [8,9]. These studies, however, are limited by the use of combinations of multiple parameters to define malignancy on each imaging modality, with any of several individual positive variables such as shape, size, necrosis or clustering, being sufficient for definition of metastasis.

In the present paper, we reinforced that while certain parameters in isolation (e.g. ill-defined margins and focal hypoattenuation) are highly specific for the diagnosis of metastasis, other parameters in isolation, such as axial size, are not sufficient in borderline nodes. We further report that in those lymph nodes without highly specific findings for malignant involvement, cross modality combinations of criteria, specifically SUVmax >3.9 associated with a measure of node "roundness" (long/short axis ratio >1.6cm, or EF <0.8), are highly specific for nodal metastatic disease. Although the combination of these imaging characteristics demonstrated relatively high specificity (89%), the sensitivity was lower (65%). We believe that analysis of these parameters using both CECT and PET/CT, after further validation, may serve to enhance reader accuracy and confidence in identification of metastasis in difficult to evaluate FDG-avid cervical lymph nodes.

Detection of Malignant Lymph Node by Individual Criteria									
	Optimal Cutoffs							All Cutoffs	
All Nodes	Cutoff	Sens. (%)	Spec. (%)	Acc (%)	O.R.	95% CI	p-value	AUC	p-value
Univariate:									
PET/CT:									
PET/CT Reader	-	94	43	68	12.1	4.5 - 32.9	< 0.001	-	-
SUVmax	4.1	87	72	79	17.1	7.8 - 37.8	< 0.001	0.87	<0.001
SUVmean	2.4	89	70	79	19.2	8.4 - 44.1	< 0.001	0.87	<0.001
MTV	3,405	43	91	67	7.3	3.1 - 17.0	< 0.001	0.64	<0.001
TLG	6,928	67	84	75	10.3	5.0 - 21.4	< 0.001	0.81	<0.001
CECT:									
CT Reader	-	87	84	86	36	15.4 - 84.5	< 0.001	-	-
Shape (round)	-	66	77	72	6.6	3.3 - 12.9	< 0.001	-	-
Focal Hypoattenuation	-	61	94	78	25.6	9.4 - 69.5	< 0.001	-	-
Ill-Defined Margin	-	61	97	79	43.6	12.8 - 149.3	< 0.001	-	-
Absence of Fatty Hilum	-	95	21	58	5.4	1.7 - 16.7	0.001	-	-
Long Axis	14.5	61	84	72	8.1	4.0 - 16.6	< 0.001	0.78	<0.001
Short Axis	8.5	71	82	76	11	5.4 - 22.5	< 0.001	0.85	<0.001
Long / Short Axis	1.6	82	63	72	7.6	3.8 - 15.3	< 0.001	0.75	<0.001
EF	0.8	82	63	72	7.6	3.8 - 15.3	< 0.001	0.75	<0.001
Volume	854	76	69	72	7	3.6 - 13.8	< 0.001	0.79	<0.001
Multivariate:									
Ill-Defined Margin	-	-	-	-	22.5	4.6-110.7	<0.001	-	-
Short Axis	-	-	-	-	1.6	1.2-2.2	0.001	-	-
SUVmax	-	-	-	-	1.4	1.1-1.8	0.019	-	-

Table 2: Detection of malignant lymph node by individual criteria.

Evaluation of FDG-avid lymph nodes in the entire cohort

Imaging findings suggestive of necrosis and extracapsular spread are considered specific characteristics for cervical nodal metastasis in HNSCC with reported specificity of 94-100% [5, 19, 20] and 98% [5], respectively. Nonetheless, no consensus exists on their relative value in FDG-avid nodes when metabolic parameters, such as SUVmax, are concurrently available. In the present study, we report high specificity for ill-defined margin and focal hypoattenuation as predictors of nodal metastasis of 97% and 94%, respectively.

In clinical practice, size cutoffs remain one of the most commonly used criteria for identification of abnormal lymph nodes; however, debate remains over the optimal use of short axis measurement as compared to long axis. Within nodes with increased FDG uptake, we report significantly greater accuracy for metastasis using short axis as compared to long axis as well as at optimal cutoffs of 8.5mm and 14.5mm, respectively. This is in line with increasing data that suggests that short axis may be a more reliable marker for malignancy than long axis [19, 22]. These findings, however, are not reflected in current TNM guidelines for head and neck which recommend long axis ("greatest dimension") as the only recommended size based criteria for nodal staging [3]. With further study and validation, these findings may support revision of current staging paradigms to reflect increased diagnostic reliability of short axis versus long axis.

Detection of Malignant Lymph Node by Individual Criteria											
Excluding LN with focal hypoattenuation or ill-defined margin											
										All Cutoffs	
	Cutoff	Sens. (%)	Spec. (%)	LR+	LR-	Acc (%)	O.R.	95% CI of O.R.	p-value	AUC	p-value
Univariate:											
PET/CT:											
PET/CT Reader	-	85	45	1.55	0.33	53	4.6	1.3 - 17.1	0.014	-	-
SUVmax	3.9	85	73	3.09	0.21	75	14.9	4.0 - 56.0	< 0.001	0.83	<0.001
SUVmean	2.4	85	74	3.24	0.2	76	15.9	4.2 - 59.9	< 0.001	0.83	<0.001
MTV	3,435	20	90	2	0.89	76	2.3	0.6 - 8.4	0.218	0.45	0.467
TLG	3,417	90	44	1.6	0.23	53	7	1.5 - 32.2	0.005	0.68	0.014
CECT:											
CT Reader	-	45	90	4.5	0.61	81	7.4	2.3 - 23.1	< 0.001	-	-
Shape(round)	-	45	83	2.57	0.67	75	3.9	1.3 - 11.1	< 0.001	-	-
Absence of Fatty Hilum	-	85	23	1.1	0.67	35	1.6	0.4 - 6.3	0.461	-	-
Long Axis	14.5	30	86	2.18	0.81	75	2.7	0.9 - 8.5	0.084	0.6	0.173
Short Axis	6.5	90	59	2.18	0.17	65	12.8	2.8 - 59.0	< 0.001	0.79	<0.001
Long / Short Axis	1.6	80	64	2.21	0.31	67	7	2.1 - 23.0	< 0.001	0.75	<0.001
EF	0.8	80	64	2.21	0.31	67	7	2.1 - 23.0	< 0.001	0.75	<0.001
Volume	788	70	66	2.07	0.45	67	4.6	1.6 - 13.3	0.003	0.66	0.026
Combination Variables:											
SUVmax + Shape	-	45	94	7.2	0.59	84	12.3	3.5 - 43.4	< 0.001	-	-
SUVmax + Long/Short ratio	-	65	89	5.78	0.39	84	14.7	4.6 - 46.3	< 0.001	-	-
SUVmax + EF	-	65	89	5.78	0.39	84	14.7	4.6 - 46.3	< 0.001	-	-
SUVmax + Volume	-	55	88	4.4	0.51	81	8.6	2.8 - 25.8	< 0.001	-	-
SUVmax + Short Axis	-	75	83	4.29	0.3	81	14.1	4.4 - 45.3	< 0.001	-	-
SA + Shape	-	40	89	3.56	0.68	79	5.3	1.7 - 16.3	0.002	-	-
Multivariate:											
SUVmax	-	-	-	-		-	1.5	1.0-2.1	0.038		
Short Axis	-	-	-	-		-	1.4	1.0-1.9	0.047		

Table 3: Detection of malignant lymph node by individual criteria.

In our analysis, we examined the role of several less well studied metrics such as MTV and three dimensional nodal volume. In our analysis, MTV performed statistically inferior to SUVmax, and volume, and though not statistically significant, trended towards inferiority compared to short axis (p=0.081). Thus presently we cannot recommend these as reliable metrics in isolation for determination of metastasis.

Evaluation of lymph nodes without focal hypoattenuation or ill-defined margin

While in the full cohort of lymph nodes, shape was not among the most accurate characteristics, in our subset of nodes without findings on imaging suggestive of extracapsular spread or necrosis, round shape was one of the most specific variables for lymph node metastasis of any criteria tested. Shape has traditionally been considered for node discrimination only in borderline nodes by size criteria [7], and the stand alone diagnostic value of shape has been questioned with reports of marginal incremental accuracy and specificity [7, 19]. In this study, we illustrated that in the absence of imaging findings suggestive of extracapsular spread or necrosis, shape should perhaps be considered as a stronger indicator of malignancy than short or long axis measurements based on the higher specificity at optimally defined cutoffs. Our data support continued evaluation of shape as criteria for determining malignancy, with initial preference over more widely accepted and utilized size criteria, to be used specifically in difficult to define FDG-avid nodes.

The sequential combination of SUVmax (>3.9) with a measurement of "roundness", EF (<0.8) or long axis/short axis ratio (<1.6), were the only combination variables that resulted in statistically significant improvement in the likelihood that a node truly harbors metastasis. SUVmax with reader defined round shape was the most specific combination variable for metastasis (94%); however, the combination was not significantly better than SUVmax alone (p=0.063). This data may suggest that some measure of roundness (reader defined node shape or long/short axis ratio or EF) in combination with SUVmax may be highly specific for metastasis in lymph nodes without ill-defined margin or focal hypoattenuation. These combined criteria for defining malignancy have not yet been addressed in the literature. We believe these findings warrant further investigation of roundness in combination with SUVmax for validation and description of appropriate cutoffs for use in clinical practice.

The use of size and SUVmax together has been considered as a means of improving diagnostic accuracy using cutoff based criteria. In the present study, across all cutoffs (ROC analysis), we found no statistically significant improvement using SUVmax with short axis versus SUVmax alone; however, at optimal cutoffs of SUVmax >3.9 and short axis >6.5mm, the improvement over SUVmax alone trended towards significance (p=0.076). Matsubara et al [21] suggests using a measure of length to discriminate malignancy in nodes with increased FDG uptake. They report that long axis is significantly greater in PET/CT identified FDG-avid true positive nodes as compared to false positive nodes. Similar to our study; however, Matsubara et al. calculated no significant improvement for either long axis or short axis over performance of SUVmax alone, though their results trend towards significance. Though inconclusive, and providing little in terms of concrete recommendations, together, these findings suggest there may be a role for using SUVmax with a measure of axial length to better identify borderline FDG-avid lymph nodes.

Limitations

As with any retrospective analysis, inherent diagnostic and treatment biases may confound results. Nonetheless, the histopathological nature of the majority of the abnormal lymph nodes (137/174) was determined by either fine needle aspiration (FNA), core biopsy or excisional biopsy. Our data include lymph nodes with potentially micrometastasis or lymph nodes with metastatic involvement that do not appear hypermetabolic on PET/CT. However the purpose of this study was to identify parameters useful in clinical practice to improve assessment of FDG-avid lymph nodes in HNSCC patients.

Although only part of the PET/CT examinations were acquired with intravenous contrast, which may give advantage to the PET/CT reader over studies without contrast, all of the patients also underwent thin slice CECT of the neck which was reviewed separately by blinded expert reader. Moreover the analysis of the PET/CT derived parameters was not affected by the presence or absence of contrast. Therefore we do not think that including these two imaging PET/CT protocols had substantial impact on the results.

The computer-assisted generation of select parameters may be incongruous with manually acquired measurements and difficult to replicate in the closely approximated anatomy of the neck. However, validation of our statistically valid results based on SUVmax and size measurements, can be tested without the need for the automated software used for this study.

Conclusions

In summary, the combinatorial analysis of anatomical and functional imaging parameters illustrates the incremental gains in specificity that are achievable when cross-modality combinations of imaging features are used to discriminate malignancy in indeterminate cervical lymph nodes. Our findings highlight the value of highly specific CECT criteria, such as ill-defined margin and focal hypoattenuation, as an initial step in the evaluation of any FDG-avid lymph node. In borderline lymph nodes without these highly specific findings, the sequential combination of functional and anatomic criteria, such as SUVmax plus an indicator of node roundness on axial CECT slices may also be highly specific for metastatic nodal involvement. Together, these findings address the incremental value, and optimal use, of PET/CT and CECT criteria, used alone or in combination, for the evaluation of cervical lymph nodes for malignancy in HNSCC.

References

1. National Comprehensive Cancer Network. Clinical Guidelines in Oncology: Head and Neck Cancers. Version 1.2012.
2. Leibel SA, Scott CB, Mohiuddin M, Marcial VA, Coia LR, et al. (1991) The effect of local-regional control on distant metastatic dissemination in carcinoma of the head and neck: results of an analysis from the RTOG head and neck database. Int J Radiat Oncol Biol Phys 3: 549-556.
3. Edge SB (2010) American Joint Committee on Cancer. AJCC cancer staging manual. (7th ed.), Springer, New York.
4. Hoang JK, Vanka J, Ludwig BJ, Glastonbury CM (2013) Evaluation of cervical lymph nodes in head and neck cancer with CT and MRI: tips, traps and a systematic approach. AJR 200: 17-25.
5. Rodrigues RS, Bozza FA, Christian PE, Hoffman JM, Butterfield RI, et al. (2009) Comparison of whole-body PET/CT, dedicated high-resolution head and neck PET/CT, and contrast-enhanced CT in preoperative staging of clinically M0 squamous cell carcinoma of the head and neck. J Nucl Med 8: 1205-1213.
6. Nakamura T and Sumi M (2007) Nodal imaging in the neck: recent advances in US, CT and MR imaging of metastatic nodes. Eur Radiol 5: 1235-1241.
7. Saindane AM (2013) Pitfalls in the staging of cervical lymph node metastasis. Neuroimaging Clin N Am 1: 147-166.
8. Lee SH, Huh SH, Jin SM, Rho YS, Yoon DY, et al. (2012) Diagnostic value of only 18Ffluorodeocyglucosepositron emission tomography/computed tomography-positive lymph nodes in head and neck squamous cell carcinoma. Otolaryngol Head Neck Surg 4: 692-698.
9. Yoon DY, Hwang HS, Chang SK, Rho YS, Ahn HY, et al. (2009) CT, MR, US,18F-FDG PET/CT, and their combined use for the assessment of cervical lymph node metastases in squamous cell carcinoma of the head and neck. Eur Radiol 3: 634-642.
10. Sadick M, Schoenberg SO, Hoermann K, Sadick H (2012) Current oncologic concepts and emerging techniques for imaging of head and

neck squamous cell cancer. GMS Curr Top Otorhinolaryngol Head Neck Surg 11: 8-9.

11. Roh JL, Park JP, Kim JS, Lee JH, Cho KJ, et al. (2014) 18F Fluorodeoxyglucose PET/CT in head and neck squamous cell carcinoma with negative neck palpation findings: A prospective study. Radiology 1: 153-161.
12. Kuhn FP, Hullner M, Mader CE, Kastrinidis N, Huber GF, et al. (2014) Contrastenhanced PET/MR imaging versus contrast-enhanced PET/CT in head and neck cancer: how much MR information is needed?. J Nucl Med 55: 551-558.
13. Queiroz MA, Hullner M, Kuhn F, Huber G, Meerwein C, et al. (2014) PET/MRI and PET/CT in follow-up of head and neck cancer patients. Eur J Nucl Med Mol Imaging 41: 1066-1075.
14. Al-Ibraheem A, Buck A, Krause BJ, Scheidhauer K, Schwaiger M (2009) Clinical Applications of FDG PET and PET/CT in Head and Neck Cancer. J Oncol 2009: 208725-208729.
15. Schwartz LH, Colville JA, Ginsberg MS, Wang L, Mazumdar M, et al. (2006) Measuring tumor response and shape change on CT: esophageal cancer as a paradigm. Ann Oncol 6: 1018-1023.
16. Erdi YE, Mawlawi O, Larson SM, Imbriaco M, Yeung H, et al. (1997) Segmentation of lung lesion volume by adaptive positron emission tomography image thresholding. Cancer 12: 2505-2509.
17. DeLong ER, DeLong DM, Clarke-Pearson DL. (1988) Comparing the areas under two or more correlated receiver operating characteristic curves: a nonparametric approach. Biometrics 3: 837-845.
18. Macaskill P, Walter SD, Irwig L, Franco EL (2002) Assessing the gain in diagnostic performance when combining two diagnostic tests. Stat Med 17: 2527-2546.
19. van den Brekel MW, Stel HV, Castelijns JA, Nauta JJ, van der Waal I, et al. (1990) Cervical lymph node metastasis: assessment of radiologic criteria. Radiology 2: 379-384.
20. Kaji AV, Mohuchy T, Swartz JD (1997) Imaging of cervical lymphadenopathy. Semin Ultrasound CT MR 3: 220-249.
21. Matsubara R, Kawano S, Chikui T, Kiyosue T, Goto Y, et al. (2012) Clinical significance of combined assessment of the maximum standardized uptake value of F-18 FDG PET with nodal size in the diagnosis of cervical lymph node metastasis of oral squamous cell carcinoma. Acad Radiol 6: 708-717.
22. Sumi M, Ohki M, Nakamura T (2001) Comparison of sonography and CT for differentiating benign from malignant cervical lymph nodes in patients with squamous cell carcinoma of the head and neck. Am J Roentgenol 4: 1019-1024.

Correlation Between Serum and Salivary House Dust Mite Specific Immunoglobulins in Allergic Rhinitis (AR) Patients and Non-Allergic Rhinitis Matched Controls

Sethu T Subha[1*], Loy Heng She[2], Wong Shew Fung[3], Davendralingam Sinniah[4], Valuyeetham Kamaru Ambu[5]

[1]*Department of Surgery/ENT, Faculty of Medicine & Health Sciences, University Putra Malaysia, Malaysia*

[2]*Canberra Hospital, Yamba drive, Garran, Australia*

[3]*Department of Pathology, International Medical University, Malaysia*

[4]*Department of Paediatrics, International Medical University, Clinical School Seremban, Malaysia*

[5]*Department of ENT, Hospital Tuanku Jaafar Seremban, Ministry of Health Malaysia, Seremban, Malaysia*

[*]**Corresponding author:** Sethu T Subha, MS, Department of Surgery/ENT, Faculty of Medicine and Health Sciences, University Putra Malaysia, 43400, Serdang, Malaysia; E-mail: subhast2@yahoo.com

Abstract

Background and objectives: Allergic rhinitis (AR) is characterised by inflammation of the nasal mucosa associated with IgE mediated immune response to specific allergens. Studies have shown that the most commonly implicated aeroallergens in AR are house dust mites. *Dermatophagoides pteronyssinus* (Dp), *Dermatophagoides farinae* (Df) and *Blomia tropicalis* (Bt) are the three most common mite species in Malaysia. Previous studies have reported the presence of high IgE and non-IgE antibodies in both serum and saliva samples of AR patients, but the correlation between them is not clear. The objective of this study was to determine the levels and correlation of mite specific IgE and IgA against *D. farinae* and *B. tropicalis* in serum and salivary samples of AR patients and non-allergic rhinitis matched controls.

Methods: A total of 205 adults were studied, they included 103 with AR and 102 healthy controls matched for age and gender. Among the 103 AR patients, 20 had concomitant asthma. Indirect ELISA was used to measure the levels of serum and salivary IgE and IgA respectively.

Results: Correlation between the serum and salivary antibody levels was analysed using Spearman correlation test, while the differences between groups were analysed using Mann-Whitney test and Kruskal Wallis test. Serum IgE and IgA levels against *D. farinae* and *B. tropicalis* were higher in AR patients. Salivary IgA against *D. farinae* and salivary IgE against *B. tropicalis* were significantly higher in AR patients. Serum and salivary IgE levels were positively correlated with serum and salivary IgA levels in AR subjects against both mite species. There was no significant difference in antibodies levels between asthmatic AR and non-asthmatic AR to both mite species in serum and saliva samples. Antibodies levels were not correlated with severity of signs and symptoms in AR patients.

Conclusion: The presence of high IgA level in saliva might be a potential investigation tool to test for allergic rhinitis when blood sampling is not an option.

Keywords: Allergic rhinitis; *Dermatophagoides pteronyssinus*; *Dermatophagoides farina*; *Blomia tropicalis*; Serum immunoglobulins; Salivary immunoglobulins

Introduction

Allergic rhinitis is clinically characterised by watery runny nose with two or more of the following symptoms such as sneezing, nasal obstruction and nasal itching [1]. Allergic rhinitis is estimated to affect 20% of the population in the USA and Europe [2] and in some other countries it can affect up to 50% of the population [3]. Nevertheless, the prevalence of this condition is increasing over time. Allergic rhinitis often co-exists with asthma and it increases the risk for asthma exacerbations. In a study done in Malaysia, it revealed that 28.8% of the adult rhinitis patients had concomitant history of asthma [4]. The prevalence of allergic rhinitis in asthmatic patients is as high as 80-90% [5]. There are many allergens found in the environment that can cause allergic rhinitis such as house dust mites, cockroach, cat or dog's dander, pollens, food and also mould spores. According to the Allergy Centre of Malaysia, house dust mite is the most common allergen which causes 85% of all allergic rhinitis cases [6]. The most common house dust mite species found worldwide include *Dermatophagoides pteronyssinus*, *Dermatophagoides farinae* and *Euroglyphus maynei* [7]. In Malaysia, Blomia tropicalis was found to be the most densely populated species followed by *D. pteronyssinus* [8]. Malaysia is located at tropical region, thus the risk of exposure to house dust mites is a major concern. Nonetheless, house dust mites are also well-known to induce other atopic diseases such as asthma, atopic conjunctivitis and atopic dermatitis [9]. Allergic rhinitis is a response ultimately mediated by IgE but studies have shown that allergens derived from house dust mite are potential immunogens that are recognised not only by IgE but also IgA and IgG subclasses in allergic individuals [10]. Several studies have reported that serum IgA and IgG levels were significantly increased in allergic patients [10,11]. A previous study has managed to detect a 928.4% mean augmentation of IgE in saliva of allergic patients compared to healthy subjects [12]. Similar findings were also reported for IgA and IgG in saliva samples [10,13]. Kitani et al. demonstrated that mite-specific IgA in serum and sputum samples were higher in mite-sensitive patients than in normal controls [11]. Although many studies have been done on allergic rhinitis but the idea of association between serum and salivary immunoglobulins in these patients is still vague. One of the studies has managed to detect a correlation between IgE levels of salivary and nasal symptoms in allergic rhino-conjunctivitis patients [14], whereas in the other study, remarkable increase of salivary IgE in allergic syndromes was reported [12]. Moreover high IgA levels were detected in serum and sputum samples in allergic patients. All these evidences lead to the idea of using salivary antibodies in the diagnosis of allergic rhinitis when blood samples are not available in any circumstances.

Methodology

The institutional ethical Committees approved this descriptive comparative study. Informed consent was obtained from the patients as well as all the control subjects. A total of 103 allergic rhinitis patients with and without mild to moderate asthma who attended the otolaryngology outpatient clinic was recruited. The inclusion criteria included male and female patients from three major ethnic groups who aged from 18-65 years old. Besides that, allergic rhinitis was diagnosed clinically according to ARIA guidelines.

Patients were allowed to clarify any of their concern before giving consent. Finally, a detailed history taking and endoscopic nasal examination on those who agreed to participate were performed by a qualified physician. Patients who are pregnant or lactating, have a previous history of anaphylaxis and severe chronic obstructive pulmonary disease (COPD) were excluded from this study. Besides that, 102 of gender and age matched healthy controls who consented to participate in this study were also recruited. The matched healthy controls must not have history of asthma, allergic rhinitis, skin allergies, anaphylaxis and COPD.

A data collection sheet was prepared to record the patient's demographic and epidemiological data. The clinical history and physical examination findings were also recorded by a qualified physician. Based on ARIA 2008 updated guidelines, the patients were categorised into intermittent or persistent, mild to moderate-severe according to the severity of their symptoms and how badly it affected their lifestyle.

Collection of blood and saliva

After demographic data collection and physical examination, 5 mL of blood was withdrawn from median cubital vein of each subject. The blood was transferred into IMPROVACUTER® Blood Collection Tube without additive (Improve, China) and allowed to clot for 30 min at room temperature. The samples were then kept in a cooler box while transferred from the clinic to the laboratory. The serum was collected after centrifugation at 3000 rpm at 4°C for 10 min using a refrigerated centrifuge (Sigma, USA). The serum was stored in -20°C freezer until further uses.

Subject was instructed to pool his/her saliva in the mouth and allowed the saliva to drool down through a straw into a sputum container (Gongdong, China). This step was repeated until approximately 5 mL of sample was collected. The supernatant was collected after centrifuging the saliva at 5000 rpm at 4°C for 15 min. The supernatant was stored in -20°C freezer until further immunological assay.

Culturing and harvesting of house dust mites

The live mites (*Dermatophagoides farinae* and *Blomia tropicalis*) were cultured and maintained in fish flasks (TetraMin Crisps, Germany) at 25°C and 75% relative humidity. The cultures were checked regularly under a stereomicroscope (Nikon, Japan) to ensure maximal growth and to prevent any contamination. Routine sampling (once a week) of the mites from the culture flasks for cross-contamination was performed by clearing and placing the mites on a drop of Hoyer's medium on a microscope slide.

Live mites were harvested using the floatation technique. The floating layer of mites and faecal pellets were filtered through filter paper of 10 μm pore size (Whatman, England) with multiple rinses of ultrapure water in order to remove the residual salt. The mites and faecal pellets were air-dried and were either placed into 1.5 mL microcentrifuge tube (Eppendorf, Germany) to be stored at -80°C freezer for further use or proceed to homogenising process.

The protein concentration of the mite extract was quantified using Quick Start™ Bradford assay (Bio-Rad Laboratories, Hercules, CA) according to manufacturer's protocol.

Quantification of mite specific immunoglobulins

Mite specific serum and salivary IgE and IgA were determined using indirect ELISA method. Immunolon-2HB Removable strips (Sigma-Aldrich Corporation, USA) were coated with crude mite extract prepared earlier in coating buffer at concentration of 0.1 μg/μL (50 μL) per well overnight at 4°C.

Data analysis

Statistical analysis was performed using IBM® SPSS® Statistics version 20 (IBM cooperation, US). Since the antibody levels were not distributed normally, therefore non-parametric test was used to analyse the data. Correlation between the serum and salivary antibody levels were analysed using Spearman correlation test, whereas the differences between groups were analysed using Mann-Whitney test and Kruskal Wallis test.

Results

Concentration of crude mite extracts

The concentrations of mite extracts were determined using Bradford assay. *D. farinae* and *B. tropicalis* were found to have concentration 15.4 and 1.74 μg/μL respectively.

Subject data

The demographic and clinical characteristics of the recruited subjects are shown in Table 1. A total of 103 allergic rhinitis patients with mean age of 37.70 years (Standard deviation, SD=13.62) were successfully recruited based on their clinical signs and symptoms. Besides that, 102 of age and gender matched healthy control subjects were also recruited. The majority of the patients (n=35, 33.98%) fell into the youngest age group (18-26 years), a steady increase of number of patients were observed as the age increased from age groups 27-53 except for the oldest age group . Of all the allergic rhinitis patients, 66% of them were female and 34% were male. Malay (~ 44%) patients made up the most for the recruited cohort, followed by Indian (~ 37%), Chinese (~ 17%) and others (~ 2%). Most of the allergic rhinitis patients were on antihistamines (82.5%) and nasal steroids (74.8%) (Table 1).

	Groups	
Characteristics	**Allergic Rhinitis**	**Control**
Number of subjects, n	103	102
Gender (M:F)	34: 66	35: 65
Age, years	37.70 ± 13.62	38.36 ± 13.63
(Mean ± SD)		
Asthma	19.00%	
Clinical symptoms		
Sniffling, nasal block	74.80%	
Throat clearing		
Allergic shiners	31.10%	
Nasal crease	19.40%	
Nasal examination		
Mucosal swelling	78.20%	
Pale thin secretions	60.80%	
Other abnormalities	60.80%	
Cobble stone appearance	42.60%	
Post nasal drip	34.30%	
Rhonchi	2.00%	
ARIA classification		
Persistent moderate-severe	49.51%	
Intermittent moderate-severe	29.13%	
Intermittent mild	14.56%	
Persistent mild	6.80%	
Medication history		
Antihistamines	82.50%	
Nasal steroids	74.80%	
Nasal decongestants	5.80%	
Steroid inhaler	3.90%	
Leukotriene antagonist	2.90%	

Table 1: Demographic data and clinical characteristics of the recruited subjects.

Patients mainly suffered from sneezing (95.1%) followed by nasal discharge (84.5%), nasal block (79.6%), nasal itching (73.8%) and eye symptoms (72.8%). Among the 103 allergic rhinitis patients, 20 of them were diagnosed with asthma. Additionally, 74.8% of the allergic rhinitis patients showed signs of sniffling or throat clearing during clinic visit. Most of the patients were found to have mucosal swelling (78.2%) and pale thin secretions (60.8%) during ear, nose and throat examination (Table 1).

About half of the patients (~ 50%) were having persistent moderate-severe symptoms, followed by intermittent moderate-severe (~ 29%), intermittent mild (14%) and persistent mild (7%) as shown in Table 1.

The most common allergenic triggers recalled by the majority of the patients were dust (72.82%) and temperature change (59.22%). Furthermore, food (15.33%), strong smell (8.74%), smoke (2.91%), trauma (2.91%) and pet's dander (0.91%) were other allergenic triggers that affected minority of the patients.

Looking at the impact of daily activities due to allergic rhinitis by life style factors listed in ARIA 2008 guidelines, the majority of the patients agreed that the symptoms were troublesome (73.70%). In addition to that, more than half of the patients complained that allergic rhinitis lead to impairment to their daily activities (63.20%), work or school performance (61.10%) and sleep disturbances (51.60%).

Sensitisation profiles to *D. farinae* and *B. tropicalis* of the recruited subjects

The sensitisation rate of allergic rhinitis patients and control subjects to *D. farinae* and *B. tropicalis* in serum and saliva samples are summarized in Table 2. ELISA results of the allergic rhinitis patients revealed higher sensitisation to *B. tropicalis* (23.5%) than to *D. farinae* (20.6%). Similar sensitisation rates were observed for *B. tropicalis* (13.9%) and *D. farinae* (5.9%) determined using saliva samples. However, this was the opposite for the control serum (*D. farinae*: 5.8% versus *B. tropicalis*: 2.0%) and salivary (*D. farinae*: 13.0% versus *B. tropicalis*: 9.0%) samples. All subjects in both groups had serum and salivary IgA above cut-off points to *D. farinae* and *B. tropicalis*.

		Groups		
	Allergic rhinitis		**Controls**	
	Df	**Bt**	**Df**	**Bt**
Serum IgE	20.60%	23.50%	5.80%	2.00%
Salivary IgE	5.90%	13.90%	13.00%	9.00%
Serum IgA	100.00%	100.00%	100.00%	100.00%
Salivary IgA	100.00%	100.00%	100.00%	100.00%

Table 2: Sensitisation rates of the recruited subjects against D. farinae and *B. tropicalis*, Df - *D. farina*, Bt - *B. tropicalis*, Cut-off point Df IgE=0.0716*, Cut-off point Df IgA=0.0463*, Cut-off point Bt IgE=0.0580*, Cut-off point Bt IgA=0.0438*, *Mean ± 3 Standard Deviations.

IgE levels against *D. farinae* and *B. tropicalis*

Levels of serum IgE against *D. farinae* extract were significantly higher in allergic rhinitis patients (OD geometric mean [gm]: 0.0552) than control subjects (OD gm: 0.0288; $p<0.01$). Similarly, this was also observed for the levels of serum IgE against B. tropicalis (OD gm: 0.0413 versus 0.0171; p<0.01). The levels of mite-specific salivary IgE were higher in allergic rhinitis patients compared with control subjects. However, the results were only significant for B. tropicalis (OD gm: 0.0426 versus 0.0382; p<0.05) but not for *D. farinae* (OD gm: 0.0414 versus 0.0407; p>0.05) (Table 3).

	Groups			
Antibodies	**Allergic (N=103)**		**Control (N=102)**	
	Mean rank	**Mean ± SD**	**Mean rank**	**Mean ± SD**
			(OD)	**(OD)**
Serum anti-Df IgE	140.12**	0.063 ± 0.049	63.50**	0.037 ± 0.057
Salivary anti-Df IgE	105.71	0.045 ± 0.026	96.25	0.051 ± 0.046
Serum anti-Df IgA	111.44*	0.970 ± 0.400	92.47*	0.840 ± 0.400
Salivary anti-Df IgA	123.22**	2.200 ± 0.500	74.54**	1.780 ± 0.390
Serum anti-Bt IgE	145.36	0.048 ± 0.036	58.21**	0.019 ± 0.012
Salivary anti-Bt IgE	109.50*	0.045 ± 0.016	92.42*	0.041 ± 0.016
Serum anti-Bt IgA	113.77**	0.520 ± 0.350	90.11**	0.390 ± 0.230
Saliva anti-Bt IgA	92.53	1.140 ± 0.490	105.68	1.250 ± 0.490

Table 3: Mean rank and mean of different antibodies in allergic rhinitis patients and control subjects against *D. farinae* and *B. tropicalis* (Mann Whitney U Test), *Mean rank difference was significant at the 0.05 level (2-tailed), **Mean rank difference was significant at the 0.01 level (2-tailed), OD=Optical density.

The correlation of antibodies level between *D. farinae* and *B. tropicalis* in allergic rhinitis and control subjects are shown in Table 4. When analysing correlation of IgE levels between *D. farinae* and *B. tropicalis* in allergic rhinitis patients, the levels of serum anti-*D. farinae* IgE showed weak positive correlation with serum anti-*B. tropicalis* IgE (r=0.254; p<0.05). However, there was no correlation found for saliva IgE samples.

Whereas in control subjects, serum anti-*D. farinae* IgE was weakly correlated with serum anti-*B. tropicalis* IgE (r=0.458; p<0.01) and moderately correlated for saliva samples (r=0.520; p<0.01) (Table 4).

Correlation between different antibodies to *D. farinae* and *B. tropicalis* in patients and control subjects were also determined (Table 5). It was found that serum IgE levels were weakly and positively correlated to IgA for both allergens in allergic rhinitis (Df: r=0.247, p< 0.05; Bt: r=0.331, p<0.01) and control subjects (Df: r=0.294, p<0.01; Bt: r=0.423, p<0.01). Similarly, correlation between salivary IgE and IgA also shared the same findings in allergic rhinitis (Df: r=0.434, p<0.01; Bt: r=0.488, p<0.01) and control subjects (Df: r=0.207, p<0.05; Bt: r=0.375, p<0.01).

The correlation between serum and salivary antibodies against *D. farinae* and *B. tropicalis* in allergic rhinitis and control subjects are summarized in Table 6. There were no correlations between serum and salivary IgE levels against *D. farinae* (r=-0.009; p>0.05) and *B. tropicalis* (r=0.010; p>0.05) in allergic rhinitis patients. However, a weak correlation was found between serum and salivary IgE levels against *D. farinae* (r=0.346; p<0.01) but not for *B. tropicalis* (r=0.154; p>0.05) in control subjects.

Levels of serum IgA against *D. farinae* and *B. tropicalis* were significantly higher in allergic rhinitis patients (OD gm: 0.8913 and OD gm: 0.4339, respectively) than control subjects (OD gm: 0.7289, p<0.05 and OD gm: 0.3320, p<0.01 respectively). Likewise, salivary IgA levels against *D. farinae* were significantly higher in patients (OD gm: 2.1349) compared with control subjects (OD gm: 1.7184, p<0.01). There was no difference between salivary IgA levels against B. tropicalis in allergic patients (OD gm: 1.0356) and control subjects (OD gm: 1.1505, p>0.05).

Correlation of serum and salivary IgA levels between *D. farinae* and *B. tropicalis* in patients and control subjects are shown in Table 4. There was a strong positive correlation between levels of serum IgA against *D. farinae* and *B. tropicalis* in allergic rhinitis patients (r=0.810; p<0.01) and control subjects (r=0.782; p<0.01). Furthermore, the correlations found in salivary IgA against *D. farinae* and *B. tropicalis* in patients (r=0.698; p<0.01) and control subjects (r=0.568; p<0.01) were moderately positive.

					D. farinae			
	Allergic rhinitis				**Controls**			
	Serum		**Saliva**		**Serum**		**Saliva**	
	IgE	**IgA**	**IgE**	**IgA**	**IgE**	**IgA**	**IgE**	**IgA**
	r=0.254*	r=0.810*	r=0.122	r=0.698*	r=0.458*	r=0.782*	r=0.520*	r=0.568*
B. tropicalis	p<0.05	p<0.01	p>0.05	p<0.01	p<0.01	p<0.01	p<0.01	p<0.01

Table 4: Spearman correlation of antibodies levels between *D. farinae* and *B. tropicalis* in allergic rhinitis patients and control subjects, *Mean rank difference was significant at the 0.05 level (2-tailed), **Mean rank difference was significant at the 0.01 level (2-tailed).

There were weak and positive correlations between serum and salivary IgA against B. tropicalis in both allergic rhinitis patients (r=0.280; p<0.01) and control subjects (r=0.257; p<0.05). On the other hand, there were no correlations between serum and salivary IgA against *D. farinae* in both patient and control groups (Table 6).

IgE & IgA	Correlation (r)	
	Patients	Controls
Anti-Df IgE vs Anti-Df IgA	0.247*	0.294**
Sal- Anti-Df IgE vs Sal- Anti-Df IgA	0.434**	0.207*
Anti-Bt IgE vs Anti-Bt IgA	0.331**	0.423**
Sal- Anti-Bt IgE vs Sal- Anti-Bt IgA	0.488**	0.375**

Table 5: Spearman correlation for serum and salivary (Sal-) IgE and IgA against *D. farinae* and *B. tropicalis* in allergic rhinitis patients and control subjects, *Correlation was significant at the 0.05 level (2-tailed), **Correlation was significant at the 0.01 level (2-tailed).

IgE and IgA levels of asthmatic allergic rhinitis patients

A subset of allergic rhinitis patients with asthma (N=20) was used for the comparison of the difference in mite-specific antibodies levels with patients who were suffering allergic rhinitis alone. There were no differences in serum and salivary IgE and IgA levels between the two subsets against *D. farinae* and *B. tropicalis.* There was also no correlation between serum and salivary mite-specific antibodies in the asthmatic subset.

	Allergic rhinitis (serum)				Control (serum)			
	IgE		IgA		IgE		IgA	
	Anti-Df	Anti-Bt	Anti-Df	Anti-Bt	Anti-Df	Anti-Bt	Anti-Df	Anti-Bt
	r=0.009	r=0.010						
Saliva	p>0.05	p>0.05	p>0.05	p<0.01	p<0.01	p>0.05	p>0.05	p<0.01

Table 6: Spearman correlation between serum and salivary IgA and IgE levels against *D. farinae* and *B. tropicalis* in allergic rhinitis patients and control subjects, *Correlation was significant at the 0.05 level (2-tailed).

Interpretation of clinical signs and symptoms of allergic rhinitis patients

Serum and salivary antibodies levels against *D. farinae* and *B. tropicalis* between different severity levels of the clinical signs and symptoms were analysed. It was found that there were no significant differences between antibodies levels in different severity levels for nasal discharge, sneezing, nasal block and nasal itching. There were no differences in serum and salivary IgE and IgA levels against both mite species between different ARIA subgroups. Additionally, no correlation was found between antibodies levels and ARIA subgroups.

Discussion

The knowledge regarding allergen specific antibodies level especially IgE subclass was well-known to be associated with the manifestation of atopic diseases. Although many articles have confirmed that mite-specific serum IgE has increased remarkably in patients that were sensitised to house dust mites, the presence of salivary IgE antibody and other subclass such as IgA was less studied, not to mention about the relationship between serum and salivary antibodies or among antibody isotypes. Furthermore, as the prevalence of allergic diseases especially allergic rhinitis is on the rise, symptomatic treatment will not be the best solution to effectively halt the progress of this disease. Studies in the field of atopic diseases were more commonly done for younger age groups such as infants and children as compared to adults.

In the current study, house dust mite specific antibodies levels were assessed in allergic rhinitis patients of young adult to middle aged groups. The majority of the allergic rhinitis patients fell into the youngest age group (18-26 years) and lesser patients in the older age groups. In our study, dust appeared to be the predominant trigger among allergic rhinitis patients. A previous study in Malaysia showed that house dust mites accounted for 70% of the positive skin prick test which again confirmed that it was the most commonly implicated aeroallergen [15]. Besides that, several studies that looked into the house dust mite fauna in Malaysia and Singapore homes found that *B. tropicalis* was the most prevalent species followed by *D. pteronyssinus* [8,16]. Furthermore, regarding the sensitisation profiles of Malaysian and Singaporean subjects, Yeoh et al. (2003) concluded that dual sensitisation to both *D. pteronyssinus* and *B. tropicalis* were common in the general populations [17]. Although the current study was conducted on a different Dermatophagoides species, sensitisation to *B. tropicalis* was still found to be higher compared with *D. farinae* which again confirmed that Malaysian are sensitised more to Blomia species than Dermatophagoides species.

Patients who were suffering from allergic rhinitis had significant higher serum IgE levels against *D. farinae* and *B. tropicalis* compared with control subjects. Besides that, IgE level in saliva was found to be higher in allergic rhinitis patients which suggested that IgE might be produced locally at the oral mucosa or passively transferred from serum or nasal secretions. However, this was only true in patients that were sensitised to *B. tropicalis* but not *D. farinae.* This result favours the finding from one of the previous study which showed increased salivary and tear IgE levels in allergic group [14].

In the current study, serum IgA levels to both species were higher in allergic rhinitis patients as compared with control subjects. This is also true for salivary IgA against *D. farinae* but not *B. tropicalis.* A few studies reported similar results where IgA levels were higher in allergic patients compared with non-allergic subjects [11,13]. Furthermore, in the present study detection rate for IgA level was higher compared with IgE and the positive correlation between both antibodies were also recorded. Possible explanation for those findings can be due to better stimulation of specific IgA by the allergen or probably reflecting a persistent antigenic stimulation of the respiratory mucosa. Despite of the similar results from previous studies, there are actually few studies that reported contrasting results. Ludviksson et al. found that the correlation of lower IgA and increase allergy manifestation is stronger at age of 2 but this association is no longer present after 2 years of follow-up [18] which suggested that levels of IgA also depend on the maturation of immune system. Thus, the role of non-IgE antibodies in pathogenesis of allergic diseases and their interaction with the immune system remains to be studied.

A weak but significant correlation was observed between serum and salivary IgA levels against *B. tropicalis* species in the current study. This corresponded to the results found in a cohort study that studied the serum and salivary immunoglobulins in pre-school children [18]. These findings probably suggest that secretory immune responses were also stimulated together with systemic immune responses in allergic subjects during the course of disease. However, this correlation is not found in patients sensitised to *D. farinae*. A difference in the sensitisation rates for both species was noted in allergic rhinitis patients. Therefore, this might account for the positive findings in the correlation between serum and salivary antibodies of *B. tropicalis* but not *D. farinae*. On the other hand, regarding IgE subclass, no correlation was found between serum and salivary antibodies. In addition to that, positive moderate to strong correlation between anti-D. farinae antibodies and anti-*B. tropicalis* antibodies were noted in the present study. These perhaps indicated that the allergenic cross-reactivity between both species was present to some extent.

Among the 103 allergic rhinitis patients, about 20% of the patients were found to be concomitantly affected by asthma. Since the relationship between allergic rhinitis and asthma is prominent, it is also interesting to find out whether patients who suffered from allergic rhinitis alone and those affected by both diseases has any difference in their antibodies level.

When patients with allergic rhinitis and asthma were studied separately, surprisingly, there were no differences regarding serum and salivary IgE and IgA levels against *D. farinae* and *B. tropicalis* in asthmatic and non-asthmatic rhinitis. Furthermore, no correlation was found between serum and salivary specific antibodies in asthmatic and non-asthmatic rhinitis patients. Possible explanation that accounted for these findings might be the relative small sample size of patients having allergic rhinitis and concomitant asthma.

When the patients in the current study were categorised according to ARIA guidelines, it was found that most patients were in the persistent moderate-severe category. There were no significant difference between the antibodies level and the severity of the signs and symptoms. Additionally, no correlation was found between severity of signs and symptoms and antibodies levels. There were also no differences in regards of the antibodies levels and the number of lifestyle factors affected. Most of our study subjects were on antihistamines and nasal steroids which might also account for the negative findings. Nonetheless, none of the patients were on systemic steroids.

Conclusion

The potential relationship between serum and salivary antibodies proposed that salivary IgA might be a useful tool to monitor levels of IgA during allergen-specific immunotherapeutic procedures when serum is not readily available.

Limitations of Current Study

Both allergic rhinitis patients and controls should be screened for their allergenic profiles using skin prick test prior to recruitment, so that same amount of patients that are allergic to each species can be selected accordingly to make valid comparison regarding the correlation of serum and salivary antibodies. Furthermore, patients on medication are not advisable to be recruited as their clinical signs and symptoms may be suppressed, thus interfering with the outcome of the results.

References

1. Bousquet J, Khaltaev N, Cruz AA, Denburg J, Fokkens WJ, et al. (2008) Allergic Rhinitis and its Impact on Asthma (ARIA) 2008 update (in collaboration with the World Health Organization, GA(2)LEN and AllerGen). Allergy 63 Suppl 86: 8-160.
2. Ozdoganoglu T, Songu M (2012) The burden of allergic rhinitis and asthma. Ther Adv Respir 2: 11-23.
3. Nihlén U, Greiff L, Montnémery P, Löfdahl CG, Johannisson A, et al. (2006) Incidence and remission of self-reported allergic rhinitis symptoms in adults. Allergy 61: 1299-1304.
4. Asha'ari ZA, Yusof S, Ismail R, Che Hussin CM (2010) Clinical features of allergic rhinitis and skin prick test analysis based on the ARIA classification: a preliminary study in Malaysia. Ann Acad Med Singapore 39: 619-624.
5. Leynaert B, Neukirch F, Demoly P, Bousquet J (2000) Epidemiologic evidence for asthma and rhinitis comorbidity. J Allergy Clin Immunol 106: S201-S205.
6. Manmohan Y (2009) Rhinitis.
7. Solarz K (2009) Indoor mites and forensic acarology. Exp Appl Acarol 49: 135-142.
8. Mariana A, Ho TM, Sofian-Azirun M, Wong AL (2000) House dust mite fauna in the Klang Valley, Malaysia. Southeast Asian J Trop Med Public Health 31: 712-721.
9. Nadchatram M (2005) House dust mites, our intimate associates. Trop Biomed 22: 23-37.
10. Miranda DO, Silva DA, Fernandes JF, Queiros MG, Chiba HF, et al. (2011) Serum and salivary IgE, IgA, and IgG4 antibodies to Dermatophagoides pteronyssinus and its major allergens, Der p1 and Der p2, in allergic and nonallergic children. Clin Dev Immunol : 302739.
11. Kitani S, Ito K, Miyamoto T (1985) IgG, IgA, and IgM antibodies to mite in sera and sputa from asthmatic patients. Ann Allergy 55: 612-620.
12. Negretti F, Casetta P (1990) Remarkable increases of salivary IgE levels in allergic syndromes. Int Arch Allergy Appl Immunol 92: 103-104.
13. Böttcher MF, Häggström P, Björkstén B, Jenmalm MC (2002) Total and allergen-specific immunoglobulin A levels in saliva in relation to the development of allergy in infants up to 2 years of age. Clin Exp Allergy 32: 1293-1298.
14. Mimura T, Usui T, Mori M, Aixinjueluo W, Funatsu H, et al. (2010) Immunochromatographic assay for measurement of total IgE in tears, nasal mucus, and saliva of patients with allergic rhinoconjunctivitis. J Asthma 47: 1153-1160.
15. Gendeh BS, Mujahid SH, Murad S, Rizal M (2004) Atopic sensitization of children with rhinitis in Malaysia. Med J Malaysia 59: 522-529.
16. Chew FT, Lim SH, Goh DY, Lee BW (1999) Sensitization to local dust-mite fauna in Singapore. Allergy 54: 1150-1159.
17. Yeoh SM, Kuo IC, Wang DY, Liam CK, Sam CK, et al. (2003) Sensitization profiles of Malaysian and Singaporean subjects to allergens from Dermatophagoides pteronyssinus and Blomia tropicalis. Int Arch Allergy Immunol 132: 215-220.
18. Lúdvíksson BR, Arason GJ, Thorarensen O, Ardal B, Valdimarsson H (2005) Allergic diseases and asthma in relation to serum immunoglobulins and salivary immunoglobulin A in pre-school children: a follow-up community-based study. Clin Exp Allergy 35: 64-69.

7

Deciphering Tinnitus from the Shoulders of Giants: A Kuhnian Shift may be Required

Sylvester Fernandes*

Department of Health Sciences, Newcastle University, Australia

***Corresponding author:** Dr. Sylvester Fernandes, 46 Fairfax Road, Warners Bay, NSW 228, Australia; E-mail: mdsfe@yahoo.com.au

Abstract

The mechanism contributing to the causation of tinnitus continues to evade us. It is unlikely that our current thinking is progressing in the right direction. The literature on the subject is mounting but with no real insights. Perhaps we are all barking up the wrong tree!

The objective of this paper is to introduce, if possible, a paradigm shift that may produce a different trend in thinking and hopefully change our direction and lines of research.

This is attempted by employing the basic technique of logical thinking aided by modern computer logic and also incorporating neuroscience, artificial intelligence, psychology and philosophy. It is admitted that this hypothesis is subject to confirmational empiricism.

Keywords: Subjective tinnitus; Tinnitus mechanisms

Introduction

Idiopathic tinnitus is a conscious "phantom" noise, with the descriptive interpretation provided by the sufferer and hence investigators have been misled in ascribing tinnitus to the ear. As a result, a significant effort has been expended over the years in explaining the exact site of the anatomical pathology in the ears [1,2]. Understandably such attempts have been futile.

There is little doubt now that tinnitus is a conscious central percept [3-6] and is not perceived during sleep or anesthesia. Some literature [7-12] suggests a peripheral initiator (hearing loss) to explain the plasticity incentive for the central states. And in the presence of normal hearing, an ultra-high frequency loss [13] and a "hidden hearing loss" [14] is offered to explain the central changes. Ironically the latter possibilities and the absence of any loss whatsoever can only suggest that the tinnitus may originate centrally.

Tinnitus has several similarities with pain and the neuroses and possibly addiction [15-20]. These are essentially heuristic behaviors for a three-dimensional world which had survival value for our ancestors and will be referred to as "tinnitus similars" in this argument.

These "tinnitus similars", like tinnitus, occupy the attention by way of (negative) automatic thoughts. Such "tinnitus similars" have:

1. Reiterative qualities
2. no immediate impending threats
3. similar aggravating factors
4. may be associated with each other [35]
5. Imaging identifies similar regions [21-26]
6. similar treatments may help
7. also occur in lower species.

Such "tinnitus similars" may have the same pathological mental state.

Known Characteristics of Tinnitus

The qualia (subjective qualitative experience) of the tinnitus are private and privileged only to the sufferer. As this is not publicly observable, it does not occupy a physical space for it to be accessible to our current methods of detection. The clinical inferences have behavioral and mainly distress manifestation overtones. Although attempted, the exact qualia are difficult for others to appreciate, and this explains the existence of the various tinnitus matching tests that inhabit the audiology template with no consistent inferences. Even musicians often have difficulty locking their tinnitus into these tests [27].

The point is made at this stage that tinnitus, like thoughts, feelings etc occupies the consciousness domain, being private and individual.

This paper aims to address the symptom of the phantom sound manifestation only. The distress manifestation of tinnitus are fairly well explained by invoking limbic connections [28,29].

Hearing and Tinnitus may have Separate Pathways

At this stage of our knowledge, it is admitted that this is subject to confirmational empiricism. The following pointers however may suffice to suggest the plausibility that the hearing and tinnitus pathways may be separate:

1. Tinnitus can occur in the presence of normal hearing, indicating that separate pathways are highly probable. A single path will necessarily create problems, allowing only hearing or only tinnitus. Also, if hearing and tinnitus had a common path, absence of one would necessarily summon the other into action. This is not supported

by the empirical evidence. The Heller and Bergman and other studies lend support to this co-occurrence [30-32].

2. Only some patients with hearing loss develop tinnitus [3,33]. If all individuals with hearing loss developed tinnitus, only a single path may allow such. But as not all individuals with hearing loss develop tinnitus, separate paths are more likely.

3. Even the documented reorganization of the central auditory components with hearing loss [7-12] does not explain [5] the non occurrence of tinnitus in the many other hearing loss patients (with the such expected reorganization), and hence further supporting separate paths.

4. Absence of both hearing as well as tinnitus is plausible with separate paths. Absence of hearing allows the tinnitus path uninterrupted access to conscious 'attention' but only if other more pressing attention occupiers are not in competition, in which case tinnitus also loses. Similarly in the absence of a hearing loss, the occurrence of tinnitus may be explained by the presence of a "tinnitus similar" facilitator [34,35].

5. Somatosensory tinnitus occurs in the absence of a hearing loss, further contributing to the plausibility of dual paths.

6. If ototoxic drugs and excessive noise damage the hearing pathway and contribute to a hearing loss then it is unlikely that tinnitus will travel the same functionally damaged path to produce the sensation of sound. Yet tinnitus thrives in the presence of a hearing loss. Hence another (undamaged) path for tinnitus is more likely.

In summary, tinnitus is independent of a hearing loss, thus throwing serious doubt on the available theories [34] which attempt to explain tinnitus in the presence of a hearing loss, attributing central changes to sensory deprivation [7-12,36,37]. It is possible that the various documentations (excitatory and inhibitory, neural plasticity, neuromodulation, neuroprotection etc.) provided may be co-related occurrences (compensatory) rather than causations. It appears that ultimately the explanations may lie at the final conscious 'attention' level, access being only available via separate paths.

In some individuals, genetic synaptic pruning by the relevant caspases results in destruction of the tinnitus path and this contributes to the unavailability of the tinnitus path in the presence of a hearing loss in later life. It is also possible that the hearing path may be similarly destroyed early, thus contributing to a congenital genetic hearing loss. These latter individuals may still complain of tinnitus.

With the available theories, it is assumed that a hearing loss is present. Then various mechanisms are recruited with the final inference being "constitutes a reasonable candidate mechanism leading to the sensation of tinnitus".

But exactly how this occurs is not explained. It is also not explained why these changes could not be attributable to the tinnitus itself. Some studies refute such mechanisms [5,6].

It is proposed here that tinnitus does not start de novo, but is the clear "winner" in the presence of a hearing loss, at the conscious 'attention' level in the attention game.

In cases where tinnitus occurs in the absence of a hearing loss (from 250 Hz to 8 KHz), the credibility of the audiology of such studies is questioned and the loss of ultra high frequency losses (10-20 KHz) is recruited to explain the theories. But it must be remembered that even if one case of tinnitus occurs without any hearing loss [38,39], then these theories become untenable.

An innate tinnitus, possibly evolutionary (see below), incorporating all the hearing frequencies is proposed here. Competitively therefore, the "dead" frequencies will gain prominence in the symptomatic tinnitus. This appears to be the empirical audiological fact [40,41]. This also explains why tinnitus is best masked by incorporating the "dead" frequencies.

The two paths are in very close proximity that may not be discernible to our current methods of detection. As both paths have the same outcome, which is the perception of sound, this proximity is most likely. Also evolution tends to engineer a close fit between functionality and economy of structure and this arrangement certainly satisfies our argument.

The difficulty in hearing experienced in the presence of tinnitus is indicative of the proximity of these paths and the tendency to be mutually interfering (ephaptic transmission) at subcortical levels. This may also explain the masking of tinnitus by noise.

The masking noise tends to crowd out the tinnitus path, causing the generation of tinnitus to break down and this contributes to residual inhibition, before tinnitus can find its way back, on cessation of the masking noise.

Sensation along the hearing path is initiated by sound at the ear and finally perceived consciously by the brain. Tinnitus (and "tinnitus similar") may initiate at a "reiterative (nagging) center" (the site with the "halting problem", see below) in the subcortex and finally be perceived consciously, attention allowing, by the brain.

Electromagnetic provocation (electroconvulsive therapy, vagal stimulation, transcranial magnetic stimulation) [42], can be expected to interfere with the "reiterative center" and cause disruption of its activity, atleast momentarily and hence contribute to the transient therapeutic efficacy in these conditions (tinnitus et similar).

The brain is a massively parallel processor (see below) and in this regard, the concept of a "reiterative center" should not relate its function to a single distinct part but to several localizable parts to include emotional, cognitive, attentional and memory components. The current functional MRIs bear testimony to this fact.

These established Hebbian connections are further reinforced with the advance of symptomatic tinnitus.

Conscious and Subconscious Components

Tinnitus is a mental state [43] which triggers further mental states involving the limbic and autonomic nervous systems.

Initially the limbic system turn-on is initiated by the cortex (reached possibly via the ventral parts of the thalamus) and then relegated to the subcortex (possibly the medial and dorsal parts of thalamus). Once such links are established, it appears that cortical control is lost and difficult to regain as is evidenced by the significant failures of the counselling therapies.

At any moment 'attention' occupies the focus of consciousness, although a state of "fringe consciousness" which is a latent awareness of the background, to which we can shift attention when needed, lurks. This absolute attention workspace may be occupied by one of several options to include sense data, thoughts, tinnitus etc. and the competition for this workspace is like radio channels competing for a narrow frequency band with a "winner take all" equilibrium [44]. It may be at this level that tinnitus loses to hearing, in hearing individuals, and in the absence of hearing, tinnitus tends to thrive. The reiterative propensity of the "tinnitus et similar" allows them an added mathematical probability advantage of 'winning' in the attention game. The 'attention' workspace is also biased towards emotion laden stimuli [45] which further advantages tinnitus which has a definite emotional salience.

Counselling aids the patient to take control of this space and oust the negative intruders by introducing positive thoughts ("voluntary" top-down attention) and as this space is limited, this can work. Sound therapy also works ("reflexive" bottom-up attention) by attempting to occupy this space. The concept of space is employed here to facilitate our human comprehension, although another (nonmetapysical) dimension may be involved.

As tinnitus is absent during sleep and anesthesia, the subjective experience of tinnitus lies in the realm of phenomenal consciousness. Consciousness thus provides us the key to our inquiry.

Tinnitus, like pain, is a broad term and encompasses several subjective qualities in different patients. It is also possible that anxiety and depression also have different subjective qualities. Further excavation in this regard is required.

Functional MRIs tend to localize areas of activation in tinnitus [46]. Exactly how this translates into tinnitus at the conscious level is not explained. The currently identified shortcomings of these imaging techniques include reverse inferences [5] and pre-emptive blood flow (in anticipation). To date these studies have provided inconsistent and contradictory results and "a vague picture of the neuronal correlates of tinnitus" [47].

Because consciousness is essentially subjective, it is an entity, objective science will never be able to explain according to McGinn [48] who argues that there must be a physical truth about consciousness, but it is conceptually impossible for humans to grasp.

What we can Learn from Computers

Neurons only fire when their inputs reach a certain threshold. The available theories ignore [35,36] this fundamental concept. Hence, as neurons have threshold firing only, tinnitus is most likely to be a "halting problem" as mentioned below.

Computers use the von Neumann architecture, employing memory to contain both data and a program for operating on the data. The human brain possibly also uses memory to store and manipulate emotions, ideas, sensations, etc. and employs parallel connectome processing at the subcortex level. The tinnitus sound (and "tinnitus similar") is also available at the subcortical level to draw upon, depending upon the Hebbian connections established for access to the conscious 'attention' level.

The senses employ a form of multi-layer nets in perception. Such nets are also good at pattern recognition. Each layer finds patterns in the layer below it and it is this ability to create the internal representations from the external world that is finally perceived [49]. In tinnitus such a layer of neurons may be subject to a "halting problem".

Incidentally artificial neural nets which employ multi-layer nets also utilize the technique of back propagation of errors. Backpropagation approximates the non-linear relationship between the input and the output by adjusting the weighting values internally. Such a technique may also be employed in the hindbrain for the phenomena of 'homeostasis' (regulation of body temperature, respiration, etc.) where a fixed output is desired irrespective of the variability of the inputs.

Computer scientists are able to build such machines that mimic human abilities and still not understand the mechanism of those abilities.

As such, the mechanism of the "halting problem" of the Turing machine (a mathematical concept) remains an enigma.

It is important to be wary of computational models [50,51]. Such models are usually capable of handling only the known input variables, parameters, constraints, usually with limited interactive processing and interdependent manipulation. Also unlike in biological systems, this processing is essentially bottom-up, without cortical control and eventually is subject to automatic generalization. In other words, computational models can sometimes err seriously.

Does Evolution Contribute?

It is proposed that tinnitus may be an evolutionary incident, initiating in earlier times as "siren" hearing, to warn the organism to be on guard constantly for predators. The "siren" sound creates an atmosphere of present-centeredness which may have adaptive value for the organism by forcing the recruitment of a broad network of task-related neural resources. The triggered limbic and autonomic events may be such responses. Habituation will not occur as this noise is centrally induced. Prior to the long period of evolution of the basic tasks required of an auditory system, to include acoustic feature discrimination, sound source localization, frequency analysis, and auditory scene analysis, this "siren" hearing may have had survival value. As tinnitus is lost during sleep, such organisms had to ensure safe quarters during sleep. Such a natural "siren" may be comparable in computer terms to the "halting problem" of the Turing machine. As evolution proceeded, and possibly to reduce energy consumption, "alarm" (normal) hearing evolved with cortical representation. "Siren" hearing was relegated to the subcortex with access to conscious attention. In our argument this provides an abductive (inference to the best explanation) advantage. Due to the eons of time involved, this of course cannot be subjected to falsifiability. This concept may also bear an evolutionary similarity to saccadic vision [52] (employed for tracking moving prey or predators by our ancestors). This inference also helps to support the concept of separate paths for hearing and tinnitus, having evolved at different times for different needs.

In the Heller and Bergman study [29], 94% of 80 normal individuals experienced tinnitus in quiet surroundings. Considering such a high proportion which is also available in other similar studies [30,31] including one with a placebo suggestion [31], the possibility that tinnitus may lie in our evolved cognitive architecture cannot be ruled out.

The animal models support that tinnitus exists in retrohuman species, at least as far back as rodents [53]. If the occurrence of neuroses in animals is extrapolated as a "tinnitus similar" to tinnitus itself, this further supports our argument.

Further, as per our argument, tinnitus similar being an adaptive evolutionary behaviour, the oft-noted association of such with the "fight or flight" autonomic response is easily explained.

Thus it appears that animals can experience tinnitus but the human characteristics of language and narrative; the tendency to attribute causes to events in the world; and perhaps the ability to experience emotions like awe make tinnitus a concern for some individuals.

Some Considerations of the Current Literature on Tinnitus

In the elucidation of tinnitus, it may benefit to visualize a three stage model:

1. Stimulus
2. Mechanism
3. Effect (tinnitus percept)

In general, if the first two are known we can predict the effect (percept). If the last two are known we can retrodict the stimulus (cause). If the first and last are known we can provide the mechanism (explanation).

However, when only one is known we need a hypothesis, which when confirmed by experimentation leads to a theory.

In the tinnitus literature, no such visualization process is in evidence to date. Only the effect (tinnitus in this case) is known. Fragmented mechanisms to explain the experimentally obtained facts are provided. Hence statements like, "Thus, correlations between brain activity and/or connectivity and tinnitus can tentatively be turned into causal relationships" [54] are necessarily incomplete.

Further the authors by their own admission appear to "tentatively" confound correlations with causes. There are basic problems:

1. Correlations are patterns, occurrences, or changes that vary in relation to each other. Is this variation proven here?

2. Although inferences from correlations assert a predictable relationship between variables, they do not account for it; thus they are less powerful than causal inferences.

3. Can the brain activity and/or connectivity signify two or other more different, even opposite things i.e may be even attempts to nullify the tinnitus?

4. Is tinnitus responsible for the brain activity and/or connectivity rather than the other way around?

5. Is there a basis for thinking that the relationship is anything other than a mere coincidence?

6. Could tinnitus itself have multiple causes? Are we looking for one cause only?

Further, the fact that a particular mechanism leads from the first to the last (tinnitus) provides no confirmation that it is the only mechanism that could produce that outcome. It also does not confirm that such is the mechanism that actually produced that result in reality.

Nevertheless the plausible relevance/irrelevance of some literature to this hypothesis is mentioned:

The Neurophysiological model of tinnitus [55]

The Jastreboff Neurophysiological model does not provide a mechanism for the generation of the acoustic component of tinnitus and attempts a dissociation approach (tinnitus retraining therapy) at alleviating the symptoms and distress caused by tinnitus. This is not at odds with the "voluntary" top-down attention (education) and the "reflexive" bottom-up attention (sound therapy) to crowd out the 'attention space', as indicated in this hypothesis.

Cognitive model of tinnitus [56]

As mentioned above, this hypothesis only attempts to deal with the acoustic component of tinnitus. However, if an evolutionary basis for tinnitus is accepted, the cognitive component of tinnitus is essentially the remnant of the type 1 error (false positive) response which is etched into our constitution, and which was the more reliable interpretation necessary for the survival of our ancestors when a predator clue emerged. Imagine an ancestor interpreting an unfamiliar sound as nonthreatening (false negative or type 2 response). Not many such interpreters would survive and reproduce. Having got out of (the perceived) harm's way pronto, the ancestor is now subject to (negative) thinking to involve the identity of the supposed predator (fear) and methods of deceit/escape etc. Persistence of this thinking fosters anxiety and depression. A hypervigilance state thus established may reduce the cognitive capacity needed to perform tasks that require voluntary, conscious, effortful, and strategic control.

Extinction of this basic response is the aim of Cognitive Behavioural Therapy (CBT).

Three neural networks model (eg attention, distress, memory) [54]

This paper points to the limitation of functional imaging studies in identifying specific neuronal correlates of tinnitus (attention, distress, memory). Brain stimulation is offered as able to identify the neuronal correlates of the various clinical aspects of tinnitus. It should be obvious that the evolutionary hypothesis suggested above is not at odds with this view. However it must be remembered that the tinnitus response is a "joint effort" by the whole patient (mind and body) to react to a perceived threat and is best investigated holistically.

Extra/leminiscal model of tinnitus [57]

Apart from imparting a conceptual viability to dual pathways, the extra/leminiscal (somatosensory) characteristic is not of relevance to this hypothesis for several reasons:

- The separate tinnitus path concept in this hypothesis is not exclusory of any particular type of tinnitus.
- The paths for hearing and tinnitus are entirely separate except ephaptically in this hypothesis.
- Being an evolutionary phenomenon, there is no age restrictions to the path.

Moller et al. introduced the concept of the non-classical pathways in 1992, as occurring only in children and only in some forms of tinnitus and autism. To date neither a overarching (commonality) reason or cause to account for such connectivity, and only in some of these individuals, has not been provided. Considering that it occurs only in "some cases", it is more likely than not, that such paths may only be an incidental finding and not specifically destined.

'Hidden hearing loss' contribution to tinnitus [14]

In the quest for a hearing loss to lend credence to the 'auditory deprivation for central plasticity' hypothesis, unreliable audiometry elsewhere, very high frequency loss and 'hidden hearing loss' have all been summoned. It is profitable to note that in the King-Kopetzky Syndrome (KKS), a normal audiogram is also obtained. However in these patients who actually complain of a hearing disability, no imploration for a 'hidden hearing loss' is made. The term Auditory Processing Disorder (APD) is also used here, which ascribes a mechanistic cause but no evidence to support this term is provided. If brain stem imaging studies in this disorder (not available yet) also reveal the same findings as that in tinnitus then it may be possible that the such findings could be related to the auditory processing mechanism and not necessarily directly to tinnitus. If the findings are not similar, then the 'hidden hearing loss' gets closer to biting the dust. Incidentally in KKS, it is proposed that a combination of psychological, social, and biological factors lead to the experience of 'hearing difficulties' and the 'impairment' may not be auditory. It may be purely psychological or psychologically 'amplified' [58]. Psychological reverberations also abound in tinnitus.

Also the Schaette et al. paper attempts to translate hearing loss findings from the mice peripheral system to the human brain stem. In the paper this is further conflated with tinnitus.

Ultimately whilst Schaette et al. attempt to provide a hearing loss cause for tinnitus, this hypothesis maintains that a hearing loss only helps to uncover tinnitus at the consciousness level. Another way of looking at this would be that if tinnitus is considered genetic then hearing loss may only provide an epigenetic footing.

Schaette et al., posit a "hidden hearing loss" in tinnitus.

In the Heller and Bergman study, 94% of 80 normal individuals experienced tinnitus in quiet surroundings. Such a high proportion is also available in other similar studies including one with a placebo suggestion.

Extrapolating the Schaette et al., postulate, 94% of individuals in the Heller and Bergman study may have a "hidden hearing loss". Such an eventuality is clearly untrue and absurd.

However, both the above assertions could be true, if it is held that an intermittent and spontaneous hearing loss can occur, but only under the Heller and Bergman study conditions. Again, clearly this is another absurdity.

Taken together these studies only serve to indicate that a hearing loss is not required for tinnitus.

What predictions can be made by this hypothesis?

1. Being an evolutionary phenomenon, tinnitus may only succumb to psychotherapy in some cases

2. The most effective therapy is Cognitive Behavior Therapy. So efforts at better methods of such delivery need to be addressed.

3. Drug therapy must aim at cognition-altering or attention- altering medication without affecting reason /consciousness.

Conclusion

A credible mechanism for tinnitus must conclusively explain how tinnitus occurs in the absence of a hearing loss. It must also explain why tinnitus only occurs in some but not all cases of hearing loss.

It is proposed here that hearing and tinnitus occupy separate proximate paths competing for conscious 'attention'. The identification of the exact mechanism of this "winner takes all attention" at the conscious level is essential for further progress. Thus the suggested "Kuhnian shift" demands a search at the consciousness level.

In other words the most important question about tinnitus may be the one we don't yet know how to ask.

References

1. Eggermont JJ (1990) On the pathophysiology of tinnitus; a review and a peripheral model. Hear Res 48: 111-123.
2. Hazell JW, Jastreboff PJ (1990) Tinnitus. I: Auditory mechanisms: a model for tinnitus and hearing impairment. J Otolaryngol 19: 1-5.
3. Eggermont JJ, Roberts LE (2004) The neuroscience of tinnitus. Trends Neurosci 27: 676-682.
4. Eggermont JJ (2003) Central tinnitus. Auris Nasus Larynx 30 Suppl: S7-12.
5. Langers DR, de Kleine E, van Dijk P (2012) Tinnitus does not require macroscopic tonotopic map reorganization. Front Syst Neurosci 6: 2.
6. Adjamian P, Hall DA, Palmer AR3, Allan TW3, Langers DR2 (2014) Neuroanatomical abnormalities in chronic tinnitus in the human brain. Neurosci Biobehav Rev 45: 119-133.
7. Rajan R (2001) Plasticity of excitation and inhibition in the receptive field of primary auditory cortical neurons after limited receptor organ damage. Cereb Cortex 11: 171-182.
8. Rajan R, Irvine DR (1998) Neuronal responses across cortical field A1 in plasticity induced by peripheral auditory organ damage. Audiol Neurootol 3: 123-144.
9. Burrone J, Murthy VN (2003) Synaptic gain control and homeostasis. Curr Opin Neurobiol 13: 560-567.
10. Schaette R, Kempter R (2006) Development of tinnitus-related neuronal hyperactivity through homeostatic plasticity after hearing loss: a computational model. Eur. J. Neurosci. 23: 3124–3138.
11. Norena AJ (2011) An integrative model of tinnitus based on a central gain controlling neural sensitivity. Neurosci Biobehav Rev 35: 1089-1109.
12. Irvine DR, Rajan R, Brown M (2001) Injury- and use-related plasticity in adult auditory cortex. Audiol Neurootol 6: 192-195.
13. Kim DK, Park SN, Kim HM, Son HR, Kim NG, et al. (2011) Prevalence and significance of high-frequency hearing loss in subjectively normal-hearing patients with tinnitus. Ann Otol Rhinol Laryngol 120: 523-528.
14. Schaette R, McAlpine D (2011) Tinnitus with a normal audiogram: physiological evidence for hidden hearing loss and computational model. J Neurosci 31: 13452-13457.
15. Møller AR (2007) Tinnitus and pain. Prog Brain Res 166: 47-53.
16. Flor H, Nikolajsen L, Staehelin Jensen T (2006) Phantom limb pain: a case of maladaptive CNS plasticity? Nat Rev Neurosci 7: 873-881.
17. King T, Vera-Portocarrero L, Gutierrez T, Vanderah TW, Dussor G, et al. (2009) Unmasking the tonic-aversive state in neuropathic pain. Nat Neurosci 12: 1364-1366.
18. Folmer RL, Griest SE, Martin WH (2001) Chronic tinnitus as phantom auditory pain. Otolaryngol Head Neck Surg 124: 394-400.
19. Koob GF (2000) Neurobiology of addiction. Toward the development of new therapies. Ann N Y Acad Sci 909: 170-185.
20. Simpson RB, Nedzelski JM, Barber HO, Thomas MR (1988) Psychiatric diagnoses in patients with psychogenic dizziness or severe tinnitus. J Otolaryngol 17: 325-330.
21. Mühlau M, Rauschecker JP, Oestreicher E, Gaser C, Röttinger M, et al. (2006) Structural brain changes in tinnitus. Cereb Cortex 16: 1283-1288.
22. Drevets WC, Price JL, Simpson JR Jr, Todd RD, Reich T, et al. (1997) Subgenual prefrontal cortex abnormalities in mood disorders. Nature 386: 824-827.
23. Mayberg HS, Lozano AM, Vet V (2005) Deep brain stimulation for treatment-resistant depression. Neuron 45: 651–660.

24. Ploghaus A, Becerra L, Borras C, Borsook D (2003) Neural circuitry underlying pain modulation: expectation, hypnosis, placebo. Trends Cogn Sci 7: 197-200.

25. Melcher JR, Levine RA, Bergevin C, Norris B (2009) The auditory midbrain of people with tinnitus: abnormal sound-evoked activity revisited. Hear Res 257: 63-74.

26. Schneider P, Andermann M, Wengenroth M, Goebel R, Flor H, et al. (2009) Reduced volume of Heschl's gyrus in tinnitus. Neuroimage 45: 927-939.

27. Jansen EJ, Helleman HW, Dreschler WA, de Laat JA (2009) Noise induced hearing loss and other hearing complaints among musicians of symphony orchestras. Int Arch Occup Environ Health 82: 153-164.

28. Cacace AT (2004) The Limbic System and Tinnitus in Tinnitus: Theory and Management.

29. Jastreboff PJ, Hazell JW (1993) A neurophysiological approach to tinnitus: clinical implications. Br J Audiol 27: 7-17.

30. Heller MF, Bergman M (1953) Tinnitus aurium in normally hearing persons. Ann Otol Rhinol Laryngol 62: 73-83.

31. Tucker DA, Phillips SL, Ruth RA, Clayton WA, Royster E, et al. (2005) The effect of silence on tinnitus perception. Otolaryngol Head Neck Surg 132: 20-24.

32. Del Bo L, Forti S, Ambrosetti U, Costanzo S, Mauro D, et al. (2008) Tinnitus aurium in persons with normal hearing: 55 years later. Otolaryngol Head Neck Surg 139: 391-394.

33. Hoffman HJ, Reed GW (2004) Epidemiology of tinnitus. Tinnitus: Theory and Management.

34. Han BI, Lee HW, Kim TY, Lim JS, Shin KS (2009) Tinnitus: characteristics, causes, mechanisms, and treatments. J Clin Neurol 5: 11-19.

35. Malakouti S, Mahmoudian M, Alifattahi N, Salehi M (2011) Comorbidity of chronic tinnitus and mental disorders. Int Tinnitus J 16: 118-122.

36. Dominguez M, Becker S, Bruce I, Read H (2006) A spiking neuron model of cortical correlates of sensorineural hearing loss: Spontaneous firing, synchrony, and tinnitus. Neural Comput 18: 2942-2958.

37. Chrostowski M, Yang L, Wilson HR, Bruce IC, Becker S (2011) Can homeostatic plasticity in deafferented primary auditory cortex lead to travelling waves of excitation? J Comput Neurosci 30: 279-299.

38. Shim HJ, Kim SK, Park CH, Lee SH, Yoon SW, et al. (2009) Hearing abilities at ultra-high frequency in patients with tinnitus. Clin Exp Otorhinolaryngol 2: 169-174.

39. Rauschecker JP, Leaver AM, Mühlau M (2010) Tuning out the noise: limbic-auditory interactions in tinnitus. Neuron 66: 819-826.

40. Meikle MB, Vernon J, Johnson RM (1984) The perceived severity of tinnitus. Some observations concerning a large population of tinnitus clinic patients. Otolaryngol Head Neck Surg 92: 689-696.

41. Norena A, Micheyl C, Chéry-Croze S, Collet L (2002) Psychoacoustic characterization of the tinnitus spectrum: Implications for the underlying mechanisms of tinnitus. Audiol Neurootol 7: 358–369

42. De Ridder D, Vanneste S, Engineer ND, Micheal P, Kilgard MP (2014) Safety and Efficacy of Vagus Nerve Stimulation Paired With Tones for the Treatment of Tinnitus: A Case Series. Neuromodulation: Technology at the Neural Interface 17: 170–179.

43. Putnam H (1967) The Nature of Mental States. Pittsburgh University Press, USA.

44. Baars BJ, Franklin S, Ramsoy TZ (2013) Global workspace dynamics: cortical "binding and propagation" enables conscious contents. Front Psychol 4: 200.

45. Lang PJ, Davis M (2006) Emotion, motivation, and the brain: reflex foundations in animal and human research. Prog Brain Res 156: 3-29.

46. Arnold W, Bartenstein P, Oestreicher E, Römer W, Schwaiger M (1996) Focal metabolic activation in the predominant left auditory cortex in patients suffering from tinnitus: a PET study with [18F]deoxyglucose. ORL J Otorhinolaryngol Relat Spec 58: 195-199.

47. Schecklmann M, Lehner A, Poeppl TB, Kreuzer PM, Rupprecht R, et al. (2013) Auditory cortex is implicated in tinnitus distress: a voxel-based morphometry study. Brain Struct Funct 218: 1061-1070.

48. McGinn C (1989) Can We Solve the Mind-Body Problem? Mind 98: 349-366.

49. Harvey RL, DiCaprio PN, Heinemann KG (1991) A Neural Network Architecture for General Image Recognition. The Lincoln Laboratory Journal volume 4: 189 -207.

50. Schaette R, Kempter R (2012) Computational models of neurophysiological correlates of tinnitus. Front Syst Neurosci 6: 34.

51. Bystritsky AA, Nierenberg JD, Feusner M (2012) Rabinovich Computational non-linear dynamical psychiatry: A new methodological paradigm for diagnosis and course of illness. Journal of Psychiatric Research Volume 46: 428-435.

52. Krauzlis RJ (2008) Eye movements. Fundamental Neuroscience, (3rd edn), Elesevier, Amsterdam, Netherlands.

53. Kaltenbach JA (2011) Tinnitus: Models and mechanisms. Hear Res 276: 52-60.

54. Langguth B, Schecklmann M, Lehner A, Landgrebe M, Poeppl TB, et al. (2012) Neuroimaging and neuromodulation: complementary approaches for identifying the neuronal correlates of tinnitus. Front Syst Neurosci 6: 15.

55. Jastreboff PJ (1990) Phantom auditory perception (tinnitus): mechanisms of generation and perception. Neurosci Res 8: 221-254.

56. McKenna L, Handscomb L, Hoare DJ, Hall DA (2014) A scientific cognitive-behavioral model of tinnitus: novel conceptualizations of tinnitus distress. Front Neurol 5: 196.

57. Møller AR, Moller MB, Yokota M (1992) Some forms of tinnitus may involve the extralemniscal auditory pathway. Laryngoscope 102: 1165-1171.

58. Zhao F, Stephens D (2007) A critical review of King-Kopetzky syndrome: Hearing difficulties, but normal hearing? Audiological Medicine 5: 119-124.

8

Delayed Distant Metastasis of Tonsillar Squamous Cell Carcinoma Origin

Hermann Simo[1], Louis De Las Casas[2], Vasuki Anandan[2], Michal Preis[3] and Reginald Baugh[4*]

[1]*The University of Toledo College of Medicine & Life Sciences, The University of Toledo Medical Center, Toledo, OH 43614, USA*
[2]*Department of Pathology, The University of Toledo Medical Center, The University of Toledo Medical Center, Toledo, OH 43614, USA*
[3]*Department of Otolaryngology, Maimonides Medical Center, The University of Toledo Medical Center, Toledo, OH 43614, USA*
[4]*Department of Surgery, Division of Otolaryngology, Head & Neck Surgery, University of Toledo Medical Center, The University of Toledo Medical Center Toledo, OH 43614, USA*

Abstract

Introduction: The incidence of distant metastases from head and neck Squamous Cell Carcinoma (SCC) is reportedly low; reports of distant metastases from tonsil carcinoma are rare. 85% of distant metastases of SCC in head and neck cancers usually become apparent within two years of primary diagnosis, but can take up to five years before diagnosis.

Background: Metastases from tonsillar cancers are uncommon, with less than 1% reported to go to subcutaneous tissues. Metastases are reported to occur within 1-48 months after initial treatment.

Methods and results: A case report is presented of a patient seen with an isolated temporal scalp Squamous Cell Carcinoma (SCC) lesion 8 years after treatment for a tonsillar SCC and negative annual PET scans thereafter. The comparative immunehistochemical study and in situ hybridization done between the scalp tumor and the previous tonsil tumor eight years earlier, showed similarities, thus suggesting a metastasis from the tonsil tumor.

Conclusions: A tonsillar SCC metastasis presenting as a temporal scalp lesion 8 years after primary tumor treatment and locoregional control achievement is a uniquely rare event. The case highlights the need for a method to identify and track tumor cell lineage, and the need for better understanding of cancer stem cells role in head and neck SCC.

Keywords: Distant metastasis; Oral pharyngeal cancer; Stem cell; Squamous cell carcinoma; Tonsillar cancer

Introduction

Primary cutaneous squamous cell carcinoma tumors often arise from the overlying epidermis or display an epidermal connection, the epidermis will show in-situ component or dysplasia, and the tumors will be located more superficially. In contrast squamous cell carcinoma tumors originating from a metastasis lack connection with the epidermis and the overlying epidermis will lack an in-situ component or dysplasia and they are often located in the deeper dermis or subcutaneous fat. Once we know that the tumor is a metastatic squamous cell carcinoma, the next question we need to address is whether the metastasis is originating from the primary head and neck cancer, or is it a nodal presentation of a yet unknown primary tumor?

We report a rare presentation of delayed distant metastasis of tonsillar squamous cell carcinoma to the temporal scalp, eight years after the primary tumor was treated and loco-regional control was achieved. Comparative immunehistochemical stain and in situ hybridization between the current tumor and the previous tumor eight years earlier showed similarities.

In light of patients clinical history of previous tonsilar carcinoma, combined with the facts that the current tumor has a similar morphology as the previous tonsilar tumor, immunohistochemical and In-situ hybridization studies (P16 and high risk HPV) of both tumors had similar pattern; we felt confident concluding that we were dealing with a metastasis from the previous tonsil SCC tumor as opposed to a metastasis of a yet unknown primary.

This occurrence highlights the importance for identifying cancer stem cell lineage and the need for better methods and tools for testing and detection of sub-pathological distant metastases.

Case Report

A sixty-five year old male was referred to our Otolaryngology clinic for follow-up after being diagnosed with subcutaneous squamous cell carcinoma of the right temporal scalp at an outside facility.

The patient was originally diagnosed in 2003 with a 3cm keratinizing, moderately to poorly differentiated squamous cell carcinoma of the left tonsil, which had spread to the left neck (Figure 1). He underwent radical tonsillectomy and left radical neck dissection. Two lymph nodes were positive, 4.5 cm maximal diameter, with extra nodal extension; the internal jugular vein and sternocleidomastoid muscle were free of tumor. Following surgery he received radiation therapy (6580cgy). Locoregional control was achieved.

Annual PET scans were negative for local recurrence or metastasis until 2012 when an uptake was noted in the right temporal scalp; this uptake was interpreted as an infected sebaceous cyst.

The lesion gradually grew, and in September 2012, started secreting a clear, sometimes blood-stained discharge. The lesion was biopsied and the pathological report showed subcutaneous squamous cell carcinoma

***Corresponding author:** Reginald F. Baugh, Department of Surgery, Division of Otolaryngology, The University of Toledo Medical Center, States3000 Arlington Avenue, Toledo, OH 43614, USA; E-mail: Reginald.Baugh@utoledo.edu

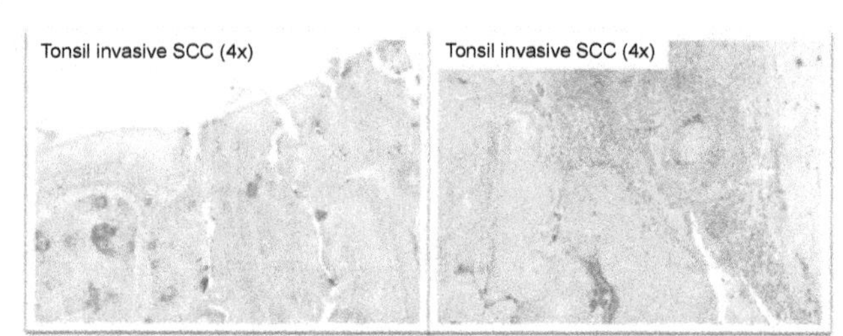

Figure 1: Tonsil Invasive squamous cell carcinoma with hematoxylin and eosin stain.

involving all surgical margins; consistent with metastasis (Figure 2). The patient was referred to our care, we completed a wide local excision with 2cm circumferential margin, the deep margin was superficial to the temporalis fascia by 3mm; the temporalis fascia was not involved but was removed as part of the specimen as an extra measure of protection. The pathology report showed SCC of similar histology as the primary tonsil tumor; a comparative immunohistochemical stain of p16 and high-risk HPV in situ hybridization between the current tumor and the previous tumor eight years ago showed similarities, further supporting a distant metastasis from the original tonsil tumor (Figure 3). Both original tumor and supporting metastasis stained negative for high-risk HPV.

Discussion

The detection of a delayed distant metastasis in head and neck SCC poses a challenge to the physician: first of all is it a primary cutaneous tumor or a metastatic tumor? Secondly is it a metastasis originating from the primary head and neck cancer, or is it a nodal presentation of a yet unknown primary tumor?

The tonsil is the most common primary site for carcinoma of the oropharynx. The incidence of distant metastasis for oropharyngeal cancer varies extensively in the literature, ranging between 4%-31% in clinical studies [1-5]. Metastases to the skin are extremely rare, occurring in 1-2% of patients with head and neck SCC [6,7]. They are often associated with oral cavity cancers and have been reported to account between 10-15% of all distant metastatic lesions [2,5-9]. The incidence of metastasis is influenced by various factors including location of primary tumor, initial staging, histological differentiation and adequacy of loco-regional control at the primary site [1-5]. The occurrence of skin metastases after treatment of head and neck SCC has been reported to be extremely rare, developing in less than 0.8% of patients with oropharyngeal head and neck SCC; with a time of occurrence between 1-36 months after initial treatment [10].

Tumors with advanced loco-regional extension at the primary site carry an increased risk for distant metastatic spread [11]. Patients having achieved loco-regional control at the primary site are considered cured of the cancer. When they later develop distant metastases; it poses a challenge to the physician- were these occult distant metastases present at the time of loco-regional treatment? What processes lead them to develop into clinically apparent disease?

For hematologic and lymphatic spread to occur so long after the primary tumor was treated with curative intent is quite intriguing and unlikely. In our case, the fact that no enlarged lymph nodes were palpated and the PET scan did not show any lymph node involvement leads to think of a hematogenous spread. Hematogenous spread would suggest that the circulating cancer cells used the blood to migrate from the primary site, then, hibernated for eight years before they began growing in the scalp to give rise to a cancer. Lymphatic spread would seem even less likely with the cancer cells passing through the regional lymph nodes to then enter the bloodstream to spread to the scalp. Even if these implausible events were to occur, metastases do not typically reproduce the entire spectrum of cancer subpopulations within the primary cancer. In fact, if it were not for the similarity in immunohistochemical staining as the primary tumor, this metastasis would have been mistaken for a second primary tumor. What triggered the development of cancer eight years after the primary remains speculative; however, recent studies in cancer biology have linked Cancer Stem Cells (CSC) to tumor recurrence and metastatic spread in head and neck squamous cell carcinoma [12]. These recent discoveries make cancer stem cells the most plausible and promising etiologic factor in our case.

Occult metastases could originate from cancer stem cells. Cancer Stem Cells (CSC) can either arise from normal stem cells or from mutated progenitor cells; and thus they possess characteristics similar to normal stem cells, specifically the ability to give rise to all cell types found in a particular cancer sample [13,14]. Therefore, due to their ability to generate tumors through the stem cell processes of self-renewal and differentiation into multiple cell types, these cancer stem cells have been proposed to persist in tumors as a distinct population and to cause relapse and metastasis by giving rise to new tumors [14,15]. Normal adult stem cells are usually dormant undifferentiated cells that reside among differentiated cells in an organ or tissue. When the need arises; they divide and differentiate to replace the surrounding differentiated cells. During the differentiation process, they are not immune from mutation and could well give rise to a mutated cell that

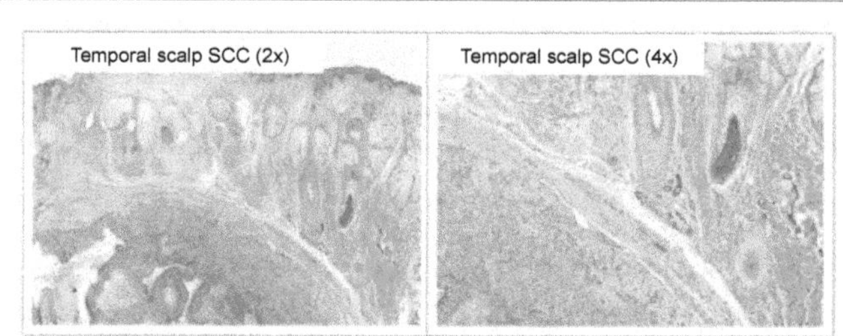

Figure 2: Temporal skin squamous cell carcinoma with hematoxylin and eosin stain.

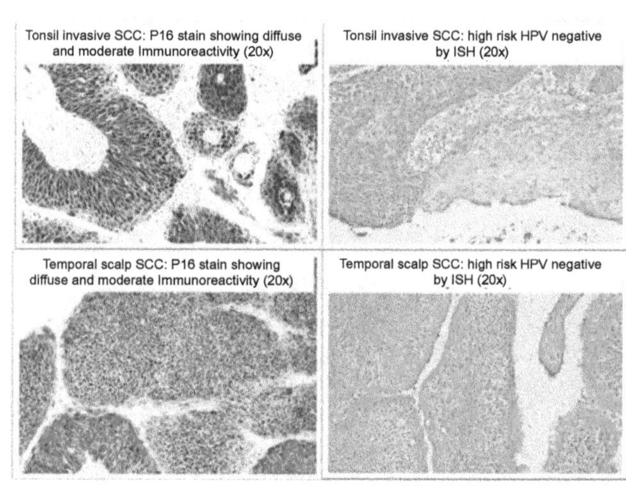

Figure 3: Temporal skin squamous cell carcinoma with hematoxylin and eosin stain.

becomes cancerous, a stem cell cancer. A stem cell cancer arising within a stem cell population can lead to the appearance of tumor cells at any time. Uniquely, CSC can give rise to all the malignant subpopulations within a cancer, truly reproducing the entire primary cancer.

A stem cell whether be normal or cancerous, has to have the built-in ability to better withstand pressure (chemical or physical) from the environment than its counterpart differentiated cells if its primary purpose is to regenerate cells that have been destroyed, otherwise there will be no regeneration if these stem cells were easily negatively affected by environmental factors. This ability to withstand pressure from the environment can make cancer stem cells less vulnerable or more resistant even to therapies used against tumors. Conventional therapies have been successful at targeting differentiated, rapid growing cells, but not so much for slow growing cells such as CSC. Because of their slow growing nature, CSC could evade these therapies and regenerate tumors or metastases with time. This approach could explain recurrence and delayed metastases after therapy and/or loco regional control have been achieved. Furthermore, some markers like CD133 found on CSC have been showed to give these cells the ability to resist radiotherapy further allowing CSC to persist despite therapy [14].

A critical step in metastasis is the ability for tumor cells to migrate away from the primary tumor; normal stem cells have been known to facilitate that process in order to generate or replace cells. Similarly, cancer stem cells are capable of using the same mechanism to generate metastases [12]. Studies are currently underway focusing on targeting this process in order to better understand it and provide potential therapies. One potential target has been the EMT (epithelial- mesenchymal transition) molecule, a key molecule during embryogenesis that allows epithelial cells to break down cell-cell and cell-extracellular matrix connections and migrate to different locations in the body [16]. It has been found that this molecule provide cancer cells the ability to infiltrate surrounding tissues and ultimately metastasize [17].

Upon evasion from therapy and migration from the primary tumor, cancer stem cells remain in circulation or find a niche where they can remain dormant. Our current methods of detection and follow up for head and neck cancer lack the ability of tracking or detecting cancer stem cells since they have no markers to rely on. Recent studies have proposed three markers that when found in head and neck squamous cell carcinomas give the functional definition ability of a CSC to a subpopulation of cells in these tumors. These genetic markers, CD44, CD133 and ALDH have been implicated in head and neck CSC ability for self-renewal, tumor progression and aggressiveness, chemo resistance, increased migration and invasiveness, and poor cancer prognosis. Having specific markers that are unique to cancer stem cells would be a great tool in the fight against cancer and will enable us to identify and track cancer stem cells among tumor cells and to predict the likelihood of recurrence and metastases [18].

Despite recent advances in cancer stem cell biology, the understanding of cancer stem cells role in head and neck squamous cell carcinoma is still in its infancy. Several mechanisms may play a role in cancer stem cells ability to metastasize and to resist current therapies. However until a means of detecting and preventing occult distant metastases becomes available, the likelihood of translating loco regional control into free of cancer will remain difficult.

Our case highlights the need for a method to identify and track tumor cell lineage, the importance of thorough examination to be performed during routine oncologic follow-up visits and the need for better understanding of cancer stem cells role in head and neck squamous cell carcinoma in order to further develop cancer-stem-cell-based therapies that will help improve the survival of patients with head and neck cancer in the future and prevent recurrence or occurrence of delayed distant metastases. Testing isolated distal recurrences more than five years from the index case to identify possible stem cell metastases may provide insight into future treatment therapies.

References

1. Spector JG, Sessions DG, Haughey BH, Chao KS, Simpson J, et al. (2001) Delayed regional metastases, distant metastases, and second primary malignancies in squamous cell carcinomas of the larynx and hypopharynx. Laryngoscope 111: 1079-1087.
2. Okamoto M, Nishimine M, Kishi M, Kirita T, Sugimura M, et al. (2002) Prediction of delayed neck metastasis in patients with stage I/II squamous cell carcinoma of the tongue. J Oral Pathol Med 31: 227-233.
3. Brugère JM, Mosseri VF, Mamelle G, David JM, Buisset E, et al. (1996) Nodal failures in patients with NO N+ oral squamous cell carcinoma without capsular rupture. Head Neck 18: 133-137.
4. Carvalho AL, Kowalski LP, Borges JA, Aguiar S Jr, Magrin J (2000) Ipsilateral neck cancer recurrences after elective supraomohyoid neck dissection. Arch Otolaryngol Head Neck Surg 126: 410-412.
5. Hoch S, Fasunla J, Eivazi B, Werner JA, Teymoortash A (2012) Delayed lymph node metastases after elective neck dissection in patients with oral and oropharyngeal cancer and pN0 neck. Am J Otolaryngol 33: 505-509.
6. Shingaki S, Suzuki I, Kobayashi T, Nakajima T (1996) Predicting factors for distant metastases in head and neck carcinomas: an analysis of 103 patients with locoregional control. J Oral Maxillofac Surg 54: 853-857.
7. Papac RJ (1984) Distant metastases from head and neck cancer. Cancer 53: 342-345.
8. Schultz BM, Schwartz RA (1985) Hypopharyngeal squamous cell carcinoma metastatic to skin. J Am Acad Dermatol 12: 169-172.
9. Alvi A, Johnson JT (1997) Development of distant metastasis after treatment of advanced-stage head and neck cancer. Head Neck 19: 500-505.
10. Pitman KT, Johnson JT (1999) Skin metastases from head and neck squamous cell carcinoma: incidence and impact. Head Neck 21: 560-565.
11. León X, Quer M, Orús C, del Prado Venegas M, López M (2000) Distant metastases in head and neck cancer patients who achieved loco-regional control. Head Neck 22: 680-686.
12. Shiozawa Y, Nie B, Pienta KJ, Morgan TM, Taichman RS (2013) Cancer stem cells and their role in metastasis. Pharmacol Ther 138: 285-293.
13. Krivtsov AV, Twomey D, Feng Z, Stubbs MC, Wang Y, et al. (2006) Transformation from committed progenitor to leukaemia stem cell initiated by MLL-AF9. Nature 442: 818-822.
14. Prince ME, Sivanandan R, Kaczorowski A, Wolf GT, Kaplan MJ, et al. (2007) Identification of a subpopulation of cells with cancer stem cell properties in head and neck squamous cell carcinoma. Proc Natl Acad Sci U S A 104: 973-978.
15. Bonnet D, Dick JE (1997) Human acute myeloid leukemia is organized as a hierarchy that originates from a primitive hematopoietic cell. Nat Med 3: 730-737.
16. Radisky DC, LaBarge MA (2008) Epithelial-mesenchymal transition and the stem cell phenotype. Cell Stem Cell 2: 511-512.
17. Thiery JP (2002) Epithelial-mesenchymal transitions in tumour progression. Nat Rev Cancer 2: 442-454.
18. Horst D, Kriegl L, Engel J, Kirchner T, Jung A (2009) Prognostic significance of the cancer stem cell markers CD133, CD44, and CD166 in colorectal cancer. Cancer Invest 27: 844-850.

Documenting the Hypopharyngeal Environment of Patients Undergoing General Endotracheal Tube Anesthesia: A First Look at Intraoperative pH Characteristics

Elliot Regenbogen[1], Slawomir P. Oleszak[2], Thomas Corrado[3], A. Laurie W. Shroyer[4], Elizabeth Vanner[5], Jordan Goldstein[6] and Michael L. Pearl[7]

[1]*Division of Otolaryngology Head and Neck Surgery, Stony Brook University Medical Center, HSC T19-065, Stony Brook, NY 11794-8191, USA*
[2]*Division of Cardiothoracic Anesthesiology, Stony Brook University Medical Center, Stony Brook, NY 11794-8191, USA*
[3]*Division of Neuroanesthesia/ENT Anesthesia, Stony Brook University Medical Center, Stony Brook, NY 11794-8191, USA*
[4]*Department of Surgery, Stony Brook University, School of Medicine, Stony Brook, NY 11794-8191, USA*
[5]*Departments of Pathology and Bioinformatics, Stony Brook University School of Medicine, Stony Brook, NY 11794-8691, USA*
[6]*Stony Brook University School of Medicine, Stony Brook, NY 11794-8191.*
[7]*Division of Gynecologic Oncology, Stony Brook University Medical Center, Stony Brook, NY 11794-8191, USA*

Abstract

Objectives: While laryngeal injuries are important and not infrequent following both short and extended endotracheal tube exposure, little detailed information is available regarding the hypopharyngeal environment during intubation. The objective of this pilot study was to explore a simple method of accurately documenting hypopharyngeal pH values in surgical patients undergoing endotracheal tube anesthesia and to report the findings.

Methods: Twenty volunteers were continuously monitored intra-operatively using a commercially available hypopharyngeal pH monitoring system. Demographics, pre- and postoperative voice and reflux self reported survey data were also collected.

Results: No complications associated with the pH monitoring system occurred. Median pH was 6.5 (range 6.0-7.0); median recorded time in minutes was 183.9 (range 130.7 – 323.5). 13/20 patients had pH>5.0 ≤ 5.5 events, for up to 113 minutes of monitored time; 2/20 patients had pH>4.0 ≤ 5.0 events, for up to 8 minutes of monitored time; 2/20 patients had pH ≤ 4.0 events, for up to 61 minutes of monitored time.

Conclusions: The hypopharyngeal pH test was used successfully to intra-operatively record hypopharyngeal pH variations. Extended pharyngeal exposures to low pH environments were commonly documented. No associations were found with patient survey scores. Future research appears warranted to expand this study, identify "at-risk" populations and to rigorously evaluate an expanded set of voice-related and lower airway clinical outcomes measures.

Keywords: Anesthesia; Laryngopharyngeal reflux; Laryngeal diseases; Hoarseness; Voice disorders; Esophageal pH monitoring

Introduction

Common laryngopharyngeal complaints following general endotracheal tube anesthesia include hoarseness and sore throat. Post-extubation hoarseness has been reported in 12–25 % of patients, while post-extubation sore throat has been described in 6–90% [1]. A recent systematic review of the literature which looked at the occurrence and type of vocal cord injuries after short-term general anesthesia using an endotracheal tube (ET) or laryngeal mask in adults found hoarseness and vocal cord injuries to be common in most studies with several investigations reporting persistent hoarseness and injury for up to 6 months [2].

Several risk factors leading to ET-related laryngeal injury have been described. These include ET size, cuff design, cuff pressure, type of ET, use of an introducer, use of a gastric tube, use of a paralytic agent, use of Propofol, duration of the operation, intubation conditions, and movement of the ET. The pressure exerted on the adjacent laryngeal tissue can reach more than 200 mmHg and lead to ischemic necrosis of the posterolateral laryngeal mucosa since its capillary perfusion pressure is far below that [1]. Additional factors such as sex, weight, history of smoking, the type of operation and gastroesophageal reflux have also been cited [3].

Most studies that have focused on pH monitoring during surgical procedures have done so to answer questions related to aspiration risk. While the majority of such studies report the average pH as well as reflux episodes during surgery none have provided a more detailed evaluation of the exposure time at varied hypopharyngeal pH that might occur during the procedures and how this might relate to laryngeal morbidity.

Given the "gap" in knowledge as to the ET-related procedure-specific factors and patient-specific risk characteristics that may predispose to enhanced risk for laryngeal injury, our pilot study sought to describe the variations in hypopharyngeal pH observed intra-operatively during an ET surgical procedure. The possibility of a relationship between intraoperative prolonged pH environmental exposure with changes (from baseline to post-hospital discharge) of

***Corresponding author:** Elliot Regenbogen, Division of Otolaryngology Head and Neck Surgery, Stony Brook University Medical Center, HSC T19-065, Stony Brook, NY 11794-8191, USA; E-mail: elliot.regenbogen@stonybrookmedicine.edu

patient voice and reflux self-reported survey outcomes will also be reported. As a descriptive, exploratory pilot study, we sought to gather preliminary data regarding intraoperative pH measures that may be useful to guide future research to advance this important field forward.

Methods

Design, participants, and setting

As an observational cross-sectional study, twenty volunteers were recruited as a convenience sample between June and September 2013 from two surgical services, the Division of Otolaryngology Head and Neck Surgery and the Division of Gynecologic Surgery. Following study start-up, patients were recruited for the study based on the operating room schedule prepared by each service. All patients underwent surgery with general endotracheal (ET) anesthesia, at Stony Brook University Hospital, a tertiary care academic medical center located on Long Island, New York. Patients were excluded from study consideration if they were: < 18 years of age; considered unsafe to maintain the device trans-nasally (e.g. facial surgery); had a history of a deviated septum, frequent epistaxis, nasal polyps, fractured nose, or frequent hoarseness; received anesthesia for a head or neck procedure that might complicate the surgical process (bleeding into the pharynx); were pregnant; or were unwilling to provide informed consent.

Intervention

To obtain our intraoperative pH measures, the Restech® Dx-pH test (Respiratory Technology Corp., San Diego, CA, USA) was selected for this purpose as it was developed to measure reflux in patients suspected of having extraesophageal symptoms presumably related to GERD [4,5]. While traditional hypopharyngeal pH catheters are prone to drying-out effects, which may cause misleading results due to pseudoreflux, the Restech probe reportedly resists drying, and does not require contact with fluid or tissue for electrical continuity. This sensor detects aerosolized or liquid acid, records pH values twice every second (2 Hz) while other pH devices may detect pH values once every 4–6 seconds. The device utilizes a 1.5 mm diameter catheter that incorporates a flashing LED light at its tip to facilitate placement [6,7]. Data is sent from the probe to a wireless recording device and saved to an SD card for latter download and analysis.

Prior to the patient entering the operating room the pH probe was calibrated with the test kit's pH 7.0 and pH 4.0 calibration solutions. Just after intubation, an attending Otolaryngologist or Anesthesiologist performed trans-nasal placement of the calibrated pH probe. Probe placement was limited to two attempts to reduce potential trauma or irritation to the nose and/or throat. None of the patients were dropped from the study due to this. An intubating laryngoscope was used for direct visualization to confirm the position of the blinking LED probe tip at the level of the epiglottis. The probe was removed and recording terminated after extubation and prior to the patient leaving the operating room. The raw data was converted to pH values and analyzed as described below using Microsoft Excel.

Main outcomes and measures

The baseline pH for each patient was the initial value measured. The measured pH values at or below a defined threshold were recorded as a pH hypopharyngeal event; for example, pH ≤ 6.0 events are measured pH values that were recorded as initiating at a pH of ≤ 6.0 as a threshold value. To explore a wide diversity of pH environments (i.e., pH ≤ 5.5, pH ≤ 5.0, pH ≤ 4.5, and pH ≤ 4.0) we counted the number of events occurring as well as the duration of each event for this set of threshold values. We also attempted to divide the group at a 50th percentile, the pH value at which half the group had exposure and half did not.

All study participants were requested to complete two validated questionnaires, the Reflux Symptom Index (RSI) and a Voice Handicap Index-10 (VHI-10) questionnaires, preoperatively and two to four weeks postoperatively [8-10]. Additional data collected on other covariates included age, height, weight, sex, tobacco use, alcohol use, proton pump inhibitor (PPI) use, a patient given history of gastroesophageal reflux disease (GERD), type of surgical procedure, duration of surgery and any complications that may have been related to the pH monitoring device during surgery and in the immediate postoperative period.

An official GERD diagnosis based on the "gold standard" assessment using esophageal pH monitoring was not required for purposes of this pilot study. Each patient's past medical history of gastroesophageal reflux disease (GERD) was gathered as part of the pre-surgery assessment, as self-reported by study patients. With symptom relief described, moreover, the patient's use of reflux-related medications (PPI or H2 blockers) within the past month prior to their date of surgery was deemed to be an adequate verification of the presence of GERD. The use of antacids (or other over the counter medications) with symptom relief was not deemed sufficient, in and of itself, to document GERD history.

Statistical analysis

Due to our small, pilot studies sample size (n = 20), all comparisons for non-normally distributed variables were performed using non-parametric statistical tests. Comparisons of categorical data elements were made using a Fisher's exact test; comparisons of continuous variables were made using either a t-test or a Wilcoxon-Mann-Whitney test. Data analysis was done with Microsoft Excel 2010 (Redmond, WA, USA) and STATA 11.0 (College Station, Texas, USA). A p-value ≤ 0.05 was considered statistically significant. Due to the large number of statistical tests performed, some or all of the significant correlations may be false positives (type I errors). No multivariable adjustments were made due to small sample size. Moreover, no Bonferroni corrections were made due the exploratory nature of this pilot study.

Institutional review board approval

This pilot research project was approved by our Institutional Review Board (Committee on Research in Human Subjects [CORIHS]) at Stony Brook University (CORIHS # 2012-1914-R1).

Results

Twenty patients were voluntarily enrolled in this pilot study, as a convenience sample. Operative procedures performed included: microsuspension direct laryngoscopy (n = 1); thyroidectomies (n = 3); gynecologic oncology procedures (n = 16). The pH probe was successfully placed and tolerated throughout surgery without reported complication, including the immediate postoperative period. Six of the 20 study patients enrolled were lost to follow-up, and therefore did not complete the postoperative surveys.

Our enrolled patient characteristics are described in Table 1. In general, our study volunteers were 54.3 (mean age) years old, with only one male patient enrolled. Body mass index (BMI) classification was based upon WHO and NIH guidelines [11, 12]. The majority of

Variable	All Patients (n=20)
Age, mean (SD)	54.3 (14.1)
Height, mean (SD), cm	162.8 (8.9)
Weight, mean (SD), kg	85.2 (23.5)
BMI, mean (SD)	32.3 (9.5)
Monitored time, median (IQR), minutes	183.9 (126.7 - 324.5)
Median pH (IQR)	6.5 (6.0 - 7.0)
Baseline pH, median (IQR)	6.7 (6.2 - 7.2)
Female (yes)	19
Preop RSI > 10	8
Tobacco Use (n)	6
Alcohol Use (n)	5
PPI Use (n)	5
History of GERD (n)	9
BMI: Underweight (n)	2
BMI: Normal (n)	2
BMI: Overweight (n)	4
BMI: Class I obesity (n)	5
BMI: Class II obesity (n)	2
BMI: Class III obesity (n)	5

Table 1: Patient demographics.

patients (80%) were either overweight or obese. Of the study patients, 45% had a history of GERD, 25% had PPI use, and 30% were prior or current smokers. Median values for monitored time and baseline pH are also given.

Individual patient pH median values are shown in Figure 1. The median pH for five patients was > 7.0; nine patients were pH ≤ 7.0 > 6.0; six patients were pH ≤ 6.0. The percentage of recorded time at pH ≤ 7.0 and pH ≤ 6.0 is shown if Figure 2. The median percentage time at pH ≤ 6.0 was 14.4% (0.6 – 60.0).

The number of patients with recorded pH values within various pH ranges is shown in Figure 3. Looking at the range of pH < 7.0, 13/20 patients had pH>5.0 ≤ 5.5 events, for up to 113 minutes of monitored time; 2/20 patients had pH>4.0 ≤ 5.0 events, for up to 8 minutes of monitored time; 2/20 patients had pH ≤ 4.0 events, for up to 61 minutes of monitored time. Of the thirteen with pH ≤ 5.5 events, three patients events were of only 0.5 seconds each. It was therefore felt to be reasonable to place these three in the "without pH ≤ 5.5 events" group in order to create a better approximation of a 50th percentile of pH events for group analysis.

There was no difference in the incidence of pH ≤ 5.5 hypopharyngeal events and baseline patient characteristics, Table 2, with the exception that patients with pH ≤ 5.5 events had significantly lower mean weight and BMI. Comparisons of subgroups of patients with and without pH ≤ 5.5 events are summarized in Table 3. There were no significant differences between these sub-groups with regard to the incidence of pH ≤ 5.5 hypopharyngeal events with the exception of baseline pH that was significantly lower in those with pH ≤ 5.5 events.

The percentage of total monitored time at measured pH ≤ 5.5 for each of the ten patients is documented in Figure 4. Only two of the nine patients with a history of GERD had pH ≤ 5.5 events was higher in the sub-group without a history of gastroesophageal reflux disease. Two (2,18) of the five patients reporting PPI use had pH ≤ 5.5 events, one of which represented a third of the monitored time.

Patient self-reported survey findings are shown in Table 3. The average pre- and post-operative RSI values were 7.8 (6.6) and 4 (5.3) respectively; pre- and post-operative VHI-10 values were 1.5 (4.0) and 1.6 (3.6) respectively. Baseline and follow-up RSI and VHI-10 scores were not significantly different between patient sub-groups. The analysis of VHI-10 scores may have been affected by the consistently low scores reported pre- and postoperatively for both groups.

The number of pH ≤ 5.5 events categorized by duration of events

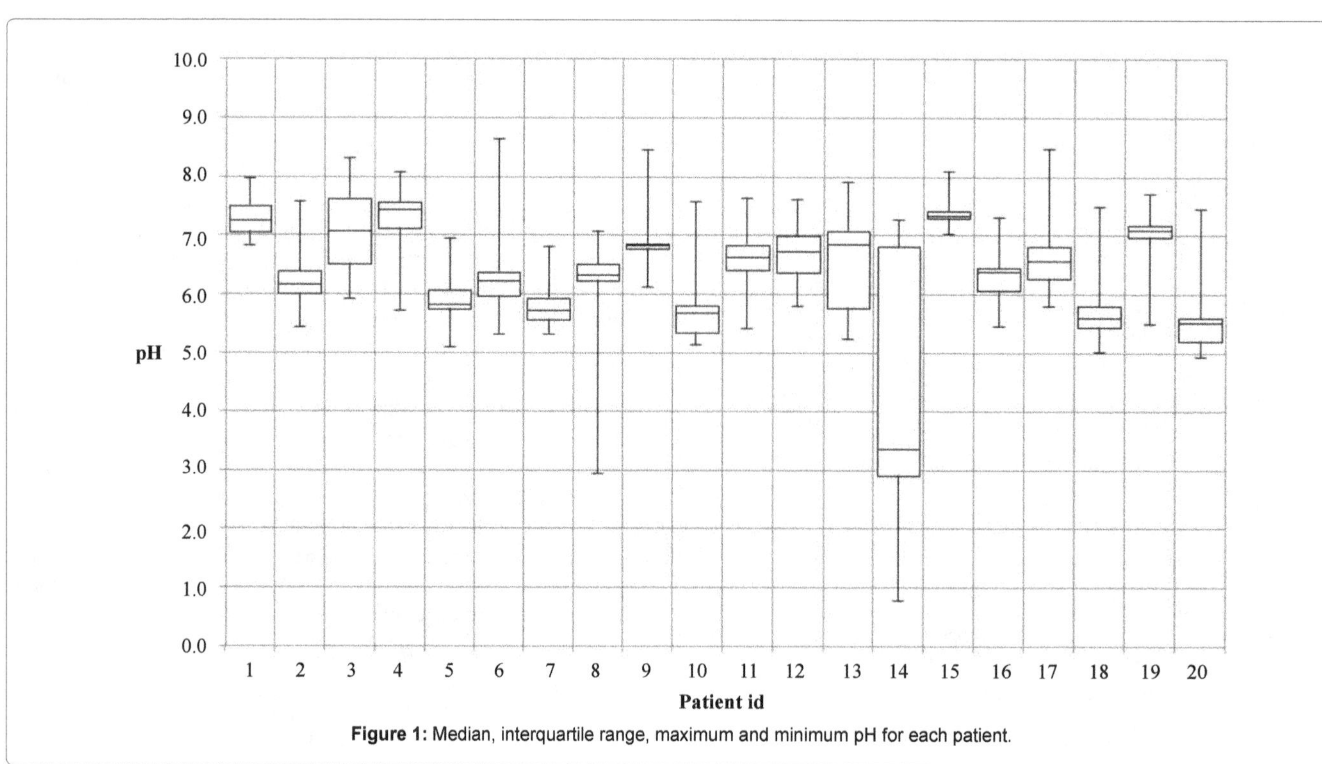

Figure 1: Median, interquartile range, maximum and minimum pH for each patient.

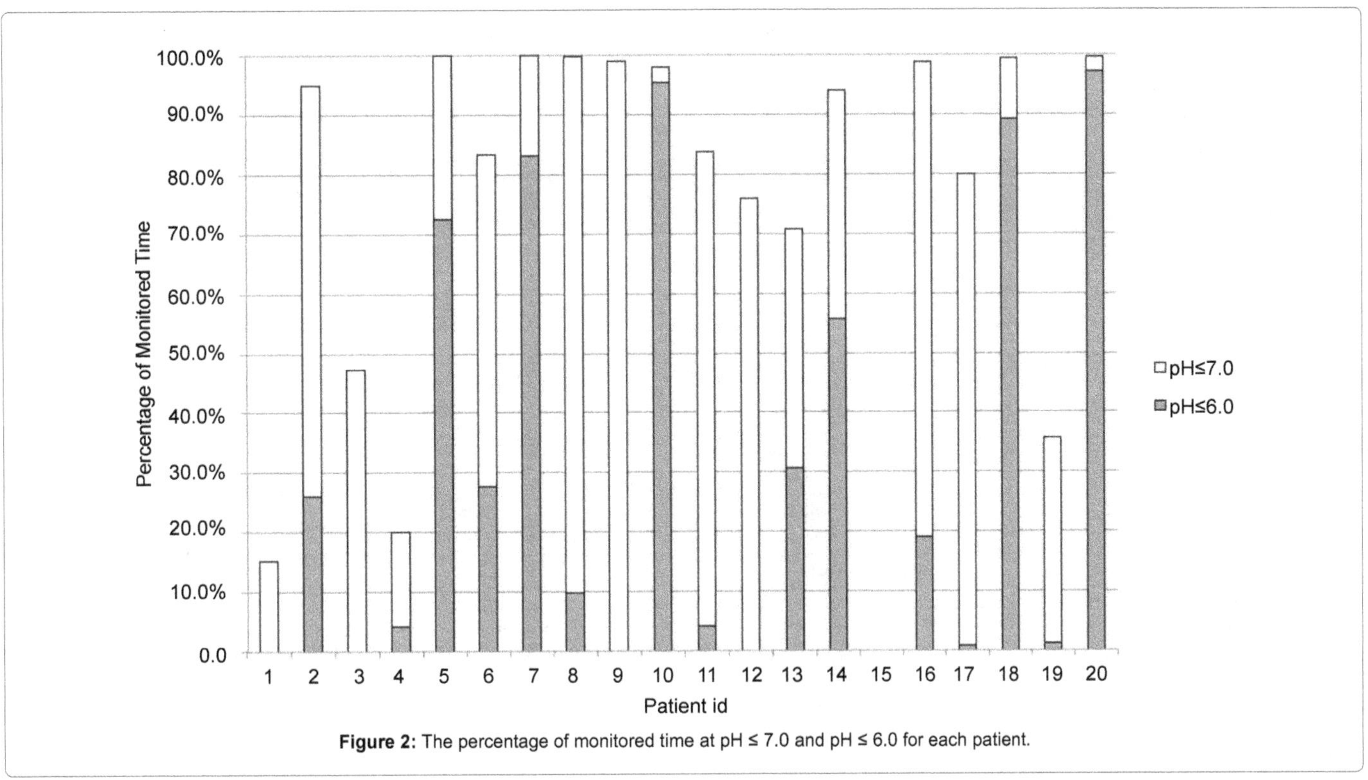

Figure 2: The percentage of monitored time at pH ≤ 7.0 and pH ≤ 6.0 for each patient.

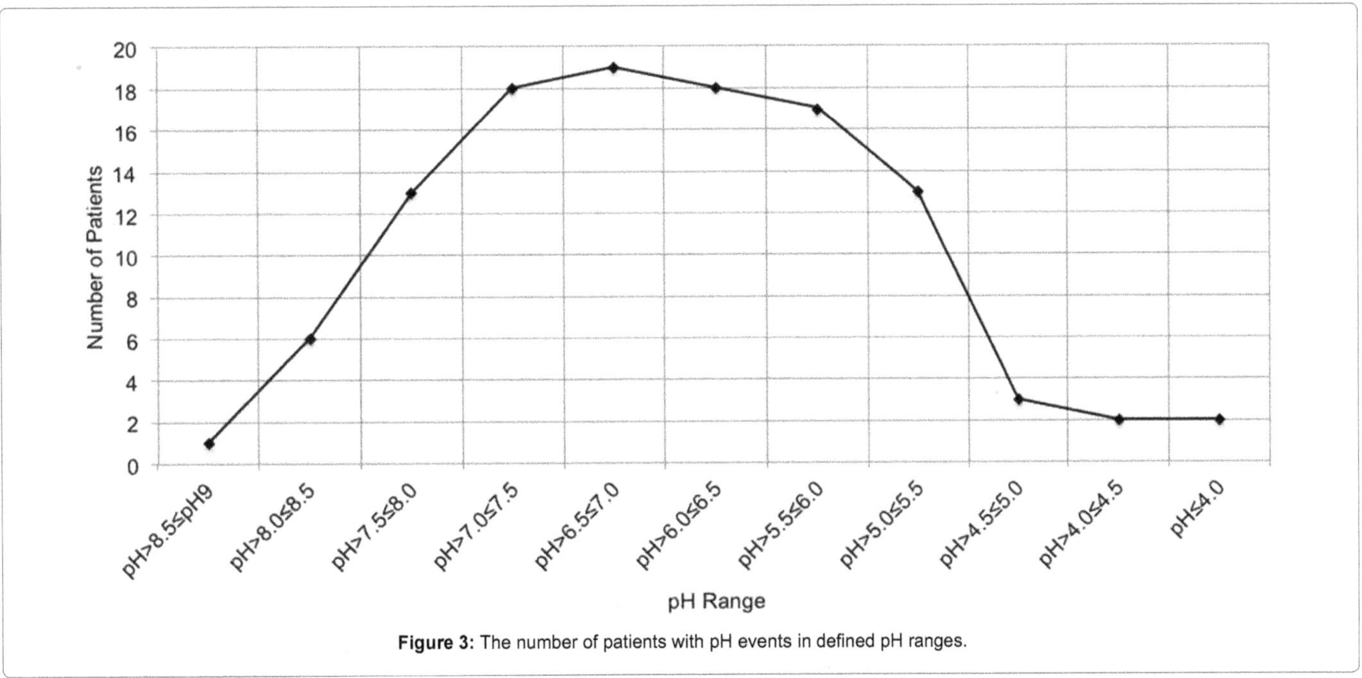

Figure 3: The number of patients with pH events in defined pH ranges.

is summarized in Table 4. The percentage of monitored time for the total number of events for each duration per patient is also shown. 81% of pH ≤ 5.5 events were less than one minute; 13% were 1-10 minute duration; 4% were 10 – 60 minute duration; 3% were over one hour duration.

Discussion

The risk of injury to the larynx and trachea from endotracheal tube anesthesia has been well known for many years. According to anesthesia-related claims in a closed claims database, 7% of all claims are related to airway injury [13]. The most frequent site of injury is the larynx. In addition to arytenoid subluxation and vocal fold paralysis, associated lesions have included inflammation, edema, hematoma, scarring and granuloma formation [14]. Regarding prolonged intubation, numerous studies have found various degrees of similar laryngeal injuries in nearly all patients intubated for more than 48 hours [15]. These injuries may result in severe, prolonged laryngeal dysfunction and the majority has been associated with extraesophageal

	without pH ≤ 5.5 events	with pH ≤ 5.5 events	P Value
n	10	10	
Age, mean (SD)	56 (14.5)	53.6 (14.1)	0.7[a]
Height, mean (SD), cm	163.4 (11.5)	162.3 (5.9)	0.8[a]
Weight, mean (SD), kg	96.8 (19.0)	73.7 (22.6)	0.02[a]
BMI, mean (SD)	36.6 (8.4)	28.2 (9.1)	0.04[a]
Preop RSI > 10 (n)	4	4	1[b]
Tobacco Use (n)	2	4	0.6[b]
Alcohol Use (n)	1	4	0.3[b]
PPI Use (n)	3	2	1[b]
History of GERD (n)	6	3	0.4[b]

[a]independent samples t-test assuming equal variance; [b]Fisher's exact test

Table 2: pH events.

	without pH ≤ 5.5 events	with pH ≤ 5.5 events	P Value[a]
n	10	10	
Monitored time, median (IQR), min	316.2 (136.5 - 365.5)	168.2 (122.8 - 205.2)	0.3
Baseline pH, median (IQR)	7.2 (6.8 - 7.2)	6.3 (5.9 - 6.5)	0.001
Baseline RSI, median (IQR)	6.5 (4.3 - 15.3)	3 (0.5 - 11.5)	0.2
Baseline VHI-10, median (IQR)	1.5 (0 - 2)	0 (0 - 0)	0.06
Follow-up RSI, median (IQR)	3 (1 - 9)	0 (0 - 3)	0.3
Follow-up VHI-10, median (IQR)	0 (0 - 3)	0 (0 - 0)	0.4

[a] Wilcoxon (Mann-Whitney)

Table 3: pH events.

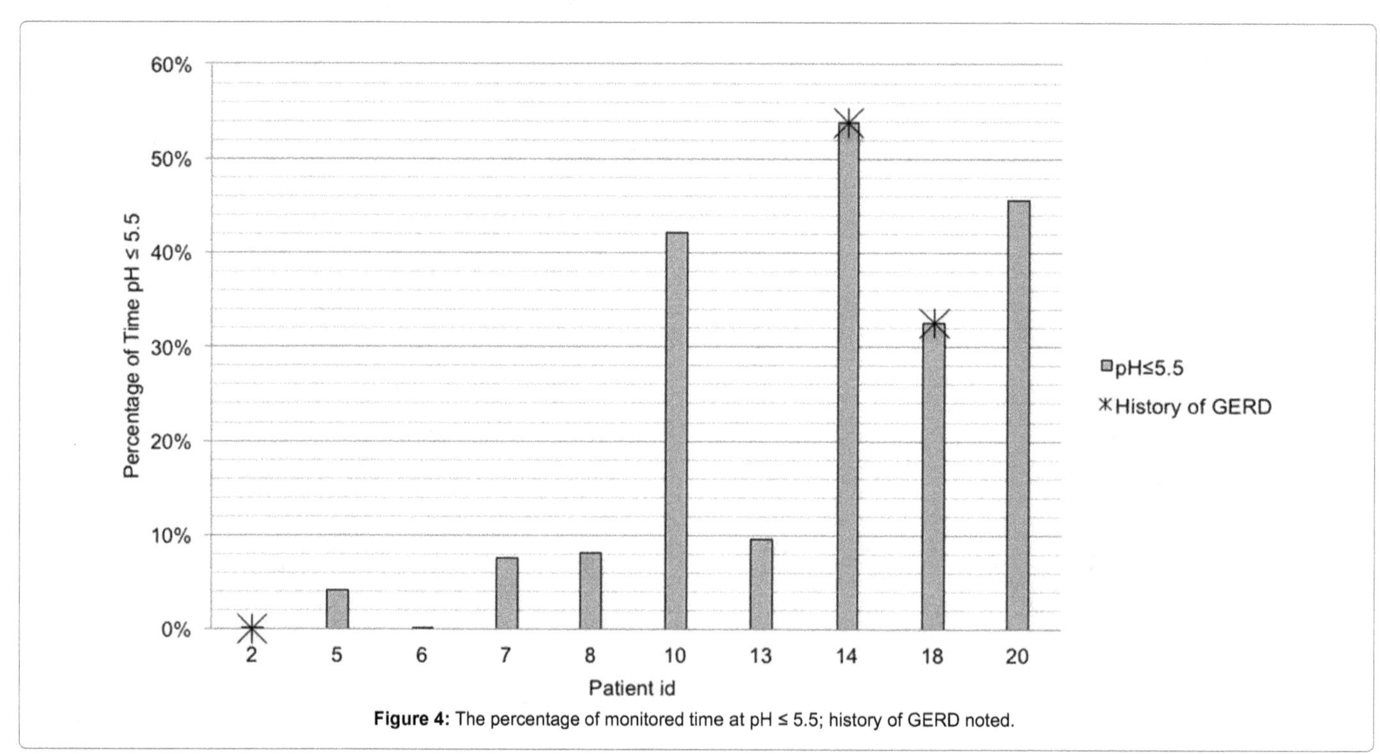

Figure 4: The percentage of monitored time at pH ≤ 5.5; history of GERD noted.

reflux [8]. Damage may occur due to a drop in pH and also due to exposure to noxious elements in the refluxate, including pepsin, bile salts and pancreatic enzymes [16].

Most studies that have included hypopharyngeal pH measures have done so in terms of understanding aspiration risk with various anesthesia devices. Turndorf et al and Blitt et al utilized dye instillation into the stomach to look for extraesophageal regurgitation in patients undergoing general anesthesia [17,18]. They found a regurgitation rate of 14.5% and 7.8% respectively. Carlsson and Islander used pH test paper at the end of surgery to assess hypopharyngeal pH, which was found to average pH 5.6 (1.0) [19]. Kofke et al. reported on hypopharyngeal pH during mask anesthesia. Patients were grouped by inhalation anesthetic [20]. They used a monocrystalline antimony electrode connected to a pH meter (Biosearch Medical Products, Somerville, NJ), recording readings at approximately five-minute intervals over one hour. The range of hypopharyngeal pH was

patient id	number of events (% monitored time)			
	<1 minute	1-10 minute	10-60 minute	>1hour
2	2 (<1%)	0	0	0
5	7 (<1%)	2 (3.3%)	0	0
6	3 (<1%)	0	0	0
7	13 (3.8%)	1 (3.7%)	0	0
8	4 (<1%)	0	1 (8%)	0
10	10 (<1%)	1 (<1%)	0	1 (40.8%)
13	5 (<1%)	1 (<1%)	1 (8.6%)	0
14	3 (1.2%)	1 (1.1%)	0	1 (51.6%)
18	23 (5.8%)	5 (4.9%)	0	1 (21.8%)
20	20 (4.5%)	3 (6.7%)	2 (34.5%)	0

Table 4: Duration of pH ≤ 5.5 events.

between 5.0 and 7.7. Joshi et al reported continuous hypopharyngeal monitoring comparing laryngeal mask to tracheal intubation [21]. A monocrystalline antimony electrode was used and measures stored in a portable pH data logger system (Reflux Monitoring System I; Sandhill, Littleton, CO). Four patients were eliminated from the study due to difficulty in retrieving pH data from the data logger. There were no episodes of hypopharyngeal regurgitation (pH < 4) detected during the course of measurement. At no time did the hypopharyngeal pH value decrease below 5.5.The hypopharyngeal pH values in both groups were similar, ranging between 5.5 and 7.5, with median values of 5.7 and 6.2. The pH in any given patient did not vary more than 1.0 unit from the initial value after placement of the airway device throughout the study period. Comparing six airway devices Khazin, et al focused on "regurgitation" episodes (pH<4), but reported minimal pH values ranging from approximately pH 1 - pH 8; twenty of 180 patients had episodes pH<4.0 [22]. They used nondisposable antimony catheters with an external reference electrode (Medtronic Functional Diagnostics,Inc, c/o Medtronic, Inc, Minneapolis, MN), measuring pH eight times per minute.

To our knowledge, this study is the first to report a more detailed analysis of intraoperative hypopharyngeal pH values from monitoring during surgery performed under general endotracheal tube anesthesia. The Restech® Dx-pH wireless system proved to be easy to setup, position and reliable in terms of data capture. No device-related complications were encountered.

While the results of our pilot study should not be generalized broadly, they are intriguing. Over 50% of monitored time for six patients studied had events of pH ≤ 6.0 and four of these were over 80% of monitored time. Looking in detail at pH ≤5.5 events, the majority of these events were of trivial duration of less than one minute; seven patients recorded short duration events of one to ten minutes; three patients experienced moderately long events of ten to sixty minutes and three experienced long events of over one hour. The long duration pH ≤ 5.5 events represented approximately 22% - 52% of the monitored time.

As a limitation of our current pilot study, we used a convenience sample of study volunteers, resulting in almost all female patients being recruited. Future studies should be designed to recruit both a larger and more diverse population, as well as to identify patient sub-populations (e.g., patients with a GERD history) that may be "at risk" for extended exposure to various pH hypopharyngeal environments. Our study was underpowered to detect a statistical difference across patient sub-groups.

The range of pH values recorded throughout the study was surprisingly broad. The stomach secretes acid at a pH of 1.5 to 2.0 and exhaled breath condensate has been found to have a pH range of 4-6 depending on disease state [23,24]. Correlative data utilizing multichannel intraluminal pH monitoring, impedance and other technologies will need to be performed to better understand the etiology of the pH fluctuations. Future studies will also need to include pre- and post-procedural laryngeal evaluations such as laryngoscopy, more extensive patient-reported outcome measures and objective measure of voice such acoustic analysis. Extending observations to intensive care settings, the role that various hypo pharyngeal pH environments may play in prolonged intubation (and re-intubation) clinical outcomes and resource utilization should also be explored.

Conclusion

Our pilot study documented a surprisingly wide range and dynamic pH environment during general endotracheal tube anesthesia. The Restech pH-Dx test appears to be a safe, simple to use tool that can be considered to support future investigations. The reasons for the unanticipated variability in the frequency and duration of low pH exposure during ET-related surgical procedures need to be elucidated. It is unclear what role various pH environments may play in the pathogenesis of laryngotracheal morbidity or voice-related performance challenges arising post-ET surgery. As this study has raised important questions regarding potential for laryngeal damage during routine surgical procedures, further research appears warranted to better understand the clinical significance of these preliminary findings.

References

1. Bottcher A, Mencke T, Zitzmann A, Knecht R, Jowett N, et al. (2014) Laryngeal injuries following endotracheal intubation in ENT surgery: predictive value of anatomical scores. Eur Arch Otorhinolaryngol 271: 345-352.

2. Mendels EJ, Brunings JW, Hamaekers AE, Stokroos RJ, Kremer B, et al. (2012) Adverse laryngeal effects following short-term general anesthesia: a systematic review. Arch Otolaryngol Head Neck Surg 138: 257-264.

3. Mencke T, Echternach M, Plinkert PK, Johann U, Afan N, et al. (2006) Does the timing of tracheal intubation based on neuromuscular monitoring decrease laryngeal injury? A randomized, prospective, controlled trial. Anesth Analg 102: 306-312.

4. Wiener GJ, Tsukashima R, Kelly C, Wolf E, Schmeltzer M, et al. (2009) Oropharyngeal pH monitoring for the detection of liquid and aerosolized supraesophageal gastric reflux. J Voice 23: 498-504.

5. Sun G, Muddana S, Slaughter JC, Casey S, Hill E, et al. (2009) A new pH catheter for laryngopharyngeal reflux: Normal values. Laryngoscope 119: 1639-1643.

6. Savarino E, Zentilin P, Savarino V, Tenca A, Penagini R, et al. (2013) Functional testing: pharyngeal pH monitoring and high-resolution manometry. Ann N Y Acad Sci 1300: 226-235.

7. Ayazi S, Lipham JC, Hagen JA, Tang AL, Zehetner J, et al. (2009) A new technique for measurement of pharyngeal pH: normal values and discriminating pH threshold. J Gastrointest Surg 13: 1422-1429.

8. Belafsky PC, Postma GN, Koufman JA (2002) Validity and reliability of the reflux symptom index (RSI). J Voice 16: 274-277.

9. Arffa RE, Krishna P, Gartner-Schmidt J, Rosen CA (2012) Normative values for the Voice Handicap Index-10. J Voice 26: 462-465.

10. Rosen CA, Lee AS, Osborne J, Zullo T, Murry T (2004) Development and validation of the voice handicap index-10. Laryngoscope 114: 1549-1556.

11. http://apps.who.int/bmi/index.jsp?introPage=intro_3.html

12. http://www.nhlbi.nih.gov/health/public/heart/obesity/lose_wt/bmi_dis.htm

13. Metzner J, Posner KL, Lam MS, Domino KB (2011) Closed claims' analysis. Best Pract Res Clin Anaesthesiol 25: 263-276.

14. Domino KB, Posner KL, Caplan RA, Cheney FW (1999) Airway injury during anesthesia: a closed claims analysis. Anesthesiology 91: 1703-1711.

15. Colton House J, Noordzij JP, Murgia B, Langmore S (2011) Laryngeal injury from prolonged intubation: a prospective analysis of contributing factors. Laryngoscope 121: 596-600.

16. Ylitalo R, Baugh A, Li W, Thibeault S (2004) Effect of acid and pepsin on gene expression in laryngeal fibroblasts. Ann Otol Rhinol Laryngol 113: 866-871.

17. Turndorf H, Rodis ID, Clark TS (1974) "Silent" regurgitation during general anesthesia. Anesth Analg 53: 700-703.

18. Blitt CD, Gutman HL, Cohen DD, Weisman H, Dillon JB (1970) "Silent" regurgitation and aspiration during general anesthesia. Anesth Analg 49: 707-713.

19. Carlsson C, Islander G (1981) Silent gastropharyngeal regurgitation during anesthesia. Anesth Analg 60: 655-657.

20. Kofke WA, Fasano M, Keamy MF 3rd, Derr JA (1987) Continuous hypopharyngeal pH during anesthesia via mask. Anesthesiology 67: 434-436.

21. Joshi GP, Morrison SG, Okonkwo NA White PF (1996) Continuous hypopharyngeal pH measurements in spontaneously breathing anesthetized outpatients: laryngeal mask airway versus tracheal intubation. Anesth Analg 82: 254-257.

22. Khazin V, Ezri T, Yishai R, Sessler DI, Serour F, et al. (2008) Gastroesophageal regurgitation during anesthesia and controlled ventilation with six airway devices. J Clin Anesth 20: 508-513.

23. Wood JM, Hussey DJ, Woods CM, Watson DI, Carney AS (2011) Biomarkers and laryngopharyngeal reflux. J Laryngol Otol 125: 1218-1224.

24. Paget-Brown AO, Ngamtrakulpanit L, Smith A, Bunyan D, Hom S, et al. (2006) Normative data for pH of exhaled breath condensate. Chest 129: 426-430.

10

Dynamics of Swallowing Tablets during the Recovery Period following Surgery for Tongue Cancer

Yu Yoshizumi[1], Shinya Mikushi[2*], Ayako Nakane[1], Haruka Tohara[1] and Shunsuke Minakuchi[1]

[1]Gerodontology and Oral Rehabilitation, Department of Gerontology and Gerodontology, Graduate School of Medical and Dental Sciences, Tokyo Medical and Dental University, Japan
[2]Department of Special Care Dentistry, Clinic for Oral Health Care and Dysphagia Rehabilitation, Nagasaki University Hospital, Japan

Abstract

Objective: Medicinal tablets are sometimes difficult to swallow, even for healthy individuals. Accordingly, it is likely more difficult for patients to swallow tablets after oral surgery for tongue tumors. In this study, we aimed to investigate the dynamics of swallowing tablets in the recovery period following surgery for tongue tumors.

Methods: Two experiments were conducted (Experiment 1 and Experiment 2). In Experiment 1, 20 tongue cancer patients swallowed simulated tablets and underwent videofluoroscopic (VF) examination of swallowing before and after surgery. The ability or inability to pass the tablet to the esophagus and the number of swallowing attempts required to ingest the tablet were evaluated. In Experiment 2, 48 similar subjects swallowed thickened barium and simulated tablets and underwent VF examination of swallowing after surgery. The ability or inability to pass the tablet to the esophagus, the number of swallows required to ingest the tablet, the tablet position after the initial and the final swallowing reflexes, and the oral transit time and pharyngeal transit time for swallowing the thickened barium solution and simulated tablets were evaluated.

Results: After subtotal glossectomy, more subjects were unable to pass the tablet to the esophagus after surgery rather than before surgery. However, after surgery, patients needed more numbers of swallowing reflex attempts in order to successfully swallow tablets. Also, the tablets remained not only in the mouth, but also in the epiglottic vallecula and pyriform sinus. In the patients who could pass the tablet, the oral transit time of the thickened barium solution was shorter than in the patients who could not.

Conclusion: In cases of subtotal glossectomy, tablet intake should be avoided, particularly in the recovery phase, and VF or endoscopic evaluation of swallowing should be performed when tablets are prescribed. After tongue cancer surgery, patients should be recommended to make multiple swallowing attempts when swallowing tablets.

Keywords: Deglutition; Deglutition disorders; Medical tablets; Tongue cancer; Videofluoroscopic examination of swallowing; Glossectomy; Mandibulectomy; Neck dissection

Introduction

Compared to foods, medicinal tablets are difficult to swallow: even 10-20% of healthy subjects have trouble swallowing tablets [1,2]. Compared to healthy subjects, patients with dysphagia reportedly experience more difficulty swallowing tablets and require an increased volume of water for tablet ingestion, a longer ingestion time, and an increase in the number of swallowing attempts [2-4]. In order to improve compliance with taking medication, investigations into the dosage forms and physical properties of tablets that can be easy to ingest have been conducted in the past [5,6]. The larger the tablets, the harder they are to ingest; conversely, if they are too small, they can be difficult to handle. A tablet size of 7-8 mm in diameter is considered the easiest for Japanese people to swallow [4,7,8].

Immediately after surgery for tongue tumors, dysphagia occurs. The mobility of the tongue is reduced due to glossectomy, and mastication and passage of food from the oral cavity to the pharynx become difficult. Furthermore, since the range of movement of the root of the tongue is restricted, pharyngeal constriction becomes dysfunctional. When neck dissection is performed to prevent metastasis of the tumor to the lymph nodes, dysfunctions of raising and closing the larynx and opening the entry to the esophagus occur. When the range of the tumor excision is enlarged, dysphagia can be severe [9-14]. In particular, when the root of the tongue is excised, dysphagia is more likely to occur [15-17]. For patients in an advanced tumor stage, and especially for those who need subtotal glossectomy, an increase in the food bolus passage time occurs preoperatively [18,19]. Therefore, in patients who have undergone tongue cancer surgery, retention of tablets in the oral cavity or pharynx may occur due to dysphagia, and so the decision to prescribe tablets can be difficult. Moreover, retention of tablets can cause ulcers in the esophageal mucosa, and similar caution is relevant for the mucous membranes of the oral cavity and pharynx [20].

To date, reports on the dynamics of swallowing tablets are limited, and in particular, investigations in patients after tongue cancer surgery have not been conducted. In this study, the aim was to investigate the dynamics of swallowing tablets during the recovery period after surgery, a period in which dysphagia can readily occur.

Materials and Methods

Tongue cancer patients who underwent tumor excision followed by immediate reconstruction and neck dissection at the Tokyo Medical

***Corresponding author:** Shinya Mikushi, Department of Special Care Dentistry, Clinic for Oral Health Care and Dysphagia Rehabilitation, Nagasaki University Hospital, 1-7-1 Sakamoto, Nagasaki 852-8501, Japan; E-mail: sirokori5@yahoo.co.jp

and Dental University Hospital Faculty of Dentistry between May 2010 and October 2012 were enrolled in the present study.

Patient images were collected from the VF image database and analyzed and investigated using a personal computer (FMVA53CW, Fujitsu, Tokyo, Japan). For VF examinations, an X-ray fluoroscopic table (Medix-900DR, Hitachi Medical Corporation, Tokyo, Japan; 30 frames/sec) was used. For image recording and time measurement, a digital video recorder (GV-D1000, Sony, Tokyo, Japan) and video timer (VTG-33, FOR-A, Tokyo, Japan) were used. The simulated tablet was manufactured using barium (baritogensol, baritogen HD, Fushimi Pharmaceutical, Kagawa, Japan), and had a cylindrical shape with a diameter of 8 mm and a length of 4 mm. The swallowing of the simulated pill was performed in a sitting position in the following manner: the patients put the tablet on the dorsum of the tongue by themselves; then, after instruction from the investigator, swallowed the tablet while drinking a cup of water thickened with a thickening agent and prepared as a purée, containing no barium. The viscosity was adjusted using a thickening agent (Toromi Up Perfect, Nisshin Oillio, Tokyo, Japan). Cases where the tablet did not pass the entry point to the esophagus 30 seconds after the instruction to swallow were deemed 'unable to ingest'. Subjects who had problems with arousal or dementia, and thus had difficulties with communication, were excluded from the study.

Experiment 1: Pre- and postoperative comparison

A total of 20 patients who underwent swallowing assessment pre and postoperatively by VF using a simulated tablet were investigated in this study arm.

VF was performed an average of 2.6 ± 1.5 (range, 1-19) days before surgery and an average of 17.3 ± 5.7 (9-29) days after surgery. The patients were 15 men and 5 women with a mean age of 56 ± 15 (36-77) years. The assessment criteria were the ability or inability to ingest the tablet, and the number of swallowing attempts required to ingest the tablet.

Experiment 2: Assessment of postoperative swallowing dynamics

Simultaneously with Experiment 1, for postoperative VF investigation of tongue cancer patients who underwent tumor excision/immediate reconstruction and neck dissection, 48 patients were enrolled and underwent assessment of both the swallowing of 4 mL of a thick barium solution and a simulated tablet.

VF was performed 20.3 ± 7.1 (9-29) days postoperatively. The patients were 38 men and 10 women, and the mean age was 58 ± 14 (20-82) years.

Regarding the barium solution with a thickener added, a thickening agent was added to a 50% barium solution and then prepared into a purée form. The barium solution with thickener was applied to the dorsum of the tongue of the subjects by the investigator using a syringe. The solution was swallowed after instruction from the investigator.

The assessment criteria were as follows: ability or inability to pass the tablet to the esophagus; the number of swallows required to ingest the tablet; the tablet position after the initial and the final swallowing reflex (after initial swallowing reflex, after final swallowing reflex); and the oral transit time (OTT) and pharyngeal transit time (PTT) for swallowing the barium solution with thickener and the simulated tablet. The time measurements were performed based on the following standards: OTT was measured from the initiation of tongue movement for passing the test food to when the tail end of the test food passed the inferior border of the mandible, and the PTT was defined as the time from when the leading end of the test food passed the inferior border of the mandible until the tail end of the test food passed the upper esophageal sphincter (UES).

Statistical analyses were performed using SPSS 11.0J for Windows (IBM, New York, NY). The Mann-Whitney test was used for comparisons of OTT and PTT, and the chi-square and Fisher's exact tests were used for the comparison of the ability or inability to pass the tablet. Significance levels were set at <5%.

This study was performed with the approval of the Tokyo Medical and Dental University Faculty of Dentistry ethics committee (receipt number 962).

Results

Experiment 1: Pre- and postoperative comparison

Experiment 1 data of patients is shown in Table 1. Based on the VF performed before surgery, all subjects were able to pass the tablet to the esophagus. In cases of subtotal glossectomy, many subjects were unable to pass the tablet to the esophagus after surgery (Fisher's exact test, p=0.02) (Table 2). In cases of hemiglossectomy, many patients were able to pass the tablet after surgery, and no significant differences were observed between pre- and postoperative states (Table 3).

In the 12 cases where the tablet could be passed to the esophagus, the number of swallowing reflex actions required for passage was investigated. The number of swallows required to pass the tablet to the esophagus was 1 for all cases preoperatively, and an average of 2.8 ± 1.6 (1-6) swallows postoperatively. Even in the cases where passage was possible, the number of swallowing times was significantly increased postoperatively (Mann-Whitney test, p<0.01) (Figure 1).

Case #	Sex	Age	Primary site	TNM stage	Glossectomy	Mandibulectomy	Reconstruction	Neck dissection
1	F	37	Left	4	SG	SM	FRAF and Plate	Both
2	M	43	Right	4	SG	SM	FRAF and Plate	Left
3	F	77	Right	4	SG	SM	FRAF and Plate	Both
4	F	42	Left	4	SG	MM	FRAF	Left
5	M	74	Right	3	SG		FRAF	Right
6	F	39	Right	3	SG		FFF	Both
7	M	50	Right	2	SG		FFF	Right
8	M	58	Left	4	HG		FFF	Left
9	M	69	Right	4	HG		FFF	Right
10	M	76	Left	3	HG		FFF	Left
11	F	55	Left	3	HG		FFF	Left
12	M	36	Left	3	HG		ALTF	Left
13	M	40	Left	2	HG		FFF	Left
14	M	39	Left	2	HG		FFF	Left
15	M	61	Right	2	HG		FFF	Right
16	M	68	Right	2	HG		FFF	Right
17	M	45	Left	2	HG		FFF	Right
18	M	73	Right	2	HG		FFF	Right
19	M	62	Right	2	HG		FFF	Right
20	M	76	Right	1	HG		FFF	Right

SG: subtotal glossectomy; HG: hemiglossectomy; SM: segmental mandibulectomy; MM: marginal mandibulectomy;FRAF: free rectus abdominis flap; Plate: mandibular plate reconstruction; FFF: free forearm flap; ALTF: anterolateral thigh flap.

Table 1: Experiment1 data of patients.

	Able to pass	Unable to pass
Preoperative	7	0
Postoperative	2	5
* p = 0.02 Fisher's exact test		

Table 2: Tablet passage ability or inability in subtotal glossectomy cases (n =7).

	Able to pass	Unable to pass
Preoperative	13	0
Postoperative	10	3
p = 0.59 Fisher's exact test		

Table 3: Tablet passage ability or inability in hemimglossectomy cases (n = 13).

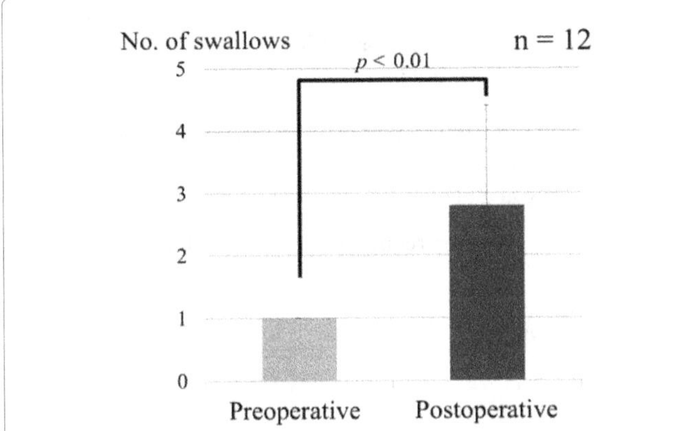

Figure 1: The number of swallows required for tablet passage.
The number of swallows required for passage is significantly is increased postoperatively (Mann-Whitney test, p<0.01).

Experiment 2: Assessment of postoperative swallowing dynamics

Experiment 2 data of patients is shown in Table 4. Based on postoperative VF, 22 of 48 (45.8%) cases could not pass the tablet to the esophagus. According to TNM stage classifications, the cases where the tablet could not be passed to the esophagus were: 2 cases in Stage I (66.7%); 5 cases in Stage II (31.3%); 7 cases in Stage III (58.3%); and 8 cases in Stage IV (47.1%). A significant difference was not observed in the ability or inability to pass the tablet (chi-square test, p=0.26) based on the TNM stage classification.

For the extent of glossectomy, the numbers of subjects who could not pass the tablet to the esophagus were: 3 cases for partial glossectomy (42.9%); 9 cases for hemiglossectomy (36.0%); and 10 cases for subtotal glossectomy (62.5%). A significant difference was not observed in the ability or inability to pass the tablet (chi-square test, p=0.16) based on the extent of glossectomy.

Regarding mandibulectomy, the numbers of subjects who could not pass the tablet to the esophagus were: 6 cases for segmental mandibulectomy (75.0%); 2 cases for marginal mandibulectomy (33.3%); and 14 cases for no excision of the mandible (41.2%). A significant difference was not observed in the ability or inability to pass the tablet (chi-square test, p=0.15) according to the extent of mandibulectomy.

From the method of reconstruction, the numbers of subjects who could not pass the tablet to the esophagus were: 12 cases for free forearm flap (38.7%); 4 cases for free rectus abdominis flap (50.0%); 5 cases

Case #	Sex	Age	Primary site	TNM stage	Glossectomy	Mandibulectomy	Reconstruction	Neck dissection
1	F	77	Right	4	SG	SM	FRAF and Plate	Both
2	M	46	Right	4	SG	SM	FRAF and Plate	Both
3	F	37	Left	4	SG	SM	FRAF and Plate	Both
4	M	49	Right	4	SG	SM	FRAF and Plate	Both
5	M	49	Right	4	SG	SM	FRAF and Plate	Both
6	M	43	Right	4	SG	SM	FRAF and Plate	Left
7	M	82	Left	4	SG		FRAF	Both
8	M	55	Right	4	SG		FRAF	Both
9	F	42	Left	4	SG	MM	FRAF	Left
10	M	66	Right	4	SG		FRAF	Right
11	M	65	Left	3	SG	MM	FRAF	Left
12	M	57	Left	3	SG	MM	FRAF	Left
13	M	74	Right	3	SG		FRAF	Right
14	F	39	Right	3	SG		FFF	Both
15	M	41	Right	2	SG		FRAF	Right
16	M	50	Right	2	SG		FFF	Right
17	M	68	Left	4	HG	SM	VOSF	Left
18	M	59	Left	4	HG		FFF	Left
19	M	58	Left	4	HG		FFF	Left
20	M	69	Right	4	HG		FFF	Right
21	F	76	Right	3	HG		FFF	Both
22	M	76	Left	3	HG		FFF	Left
23	F	55	Left	3	HG		FFF	Left
24	M	62	Left	3	HG		FFF	Left
25	M	20	Right	3	HG		FFF	Left
26	M	64	Left	3	HG		FFF	Left
27	M	75	Right	3	HG		FFF	Right
28	M	36	Left	3	HG		ALTF	Left
29	F	48	Left	2	HG	MM	FFF	Left
30	M	40	Left	2	HG		FFF	Left
31	M	58	Left	2	HG		FFF	Left
32	M	39	Left	2	HG		FFF	Left
33	F	55	Right	2	HG		FFF	Right
34	M	61	Right	2	HG		FFF	Right
35	M	61	Right	2	HG		FFF	Right
36	M	68	Right	2	HG		FFF	Right
37	M	45	Left	2	HG		FFF	Right
38	M	65	Right	2	HG		FFF	Right
39	M	73	Right	2	HG		FFF	Right
40	M	62	Right	2	HG		FFF	Right
41	M	76	Right	1	HG		FFF	Right
42	F	62	Left	4	PG		FFF	Both
43	M	63	Left	4	PG	MM	FFF	Both
44	F	67	Left	4	PG		FFF	Both
45	M	53	Right	2	PG		FFF	Right
46	M	65	Right	2	PG		FFF	Right
47	M	52	Right	1	PG	SM	VOSF	Both
48	M	63	Left	1	PG	MM	FFF	Left

HG: hemiglossectomy; PG: partial glossectomy; MM: marginal mandibulectomy; SM: segmental mandibulectomy; FFF: free forearm flap; ALTF: anterolateral thigh flap; VOSF: vascularized osteocutaneous scapular flap; SG: subtotal glossectomy; HG: hemiglossectomy; SM: segmental mandibulectomy; MM: marginal mandibulectomy; FRAF: free rectus abdominis flap; Plate: mandibular plate reconstruction; FFF: free forearm flap; VOSF: vascularized osteocutaneous scapular flap.

Table 4: Experiment 2 data of patients.

for free rectus abdominis flap and mandibular plate reconstruction (83.3%); 1 case for vascularized osteocutaneous scapular flap (50.0%); and no cases for anterolateral thigh flap. A significant difference was not observed in the ability or inability to pass the tablet (chi-square test, p=0.23) regarding the reconstruction.

The number of swallows required to pass the tablet from the oral cavity to the esophagus was 2.8 ± 1.7 (1-6) times in the 26 cases (of the 48 investigated) where passage was possible.

Of the 48 subjects, the tablet location after the initial swallowing reflex was in the: oral cavity in 29 cases; epiglottic vallecula in 7 cases; pyriform sinus in 5 cases; and esophagus in 7 cases. The tablet location after the final swallowing attempt was in the: oral cavity in 16 cases; epiglottic vallecula in 4 cases; pyriform sinus in 2 cases; and esophagus in 26 cases (Figure 2 and Table 5).

Of the 26 cases where tablet passage was possible, the OTT and PTT were measured for the thickened barium solution and the tablets. For the thickened barium solution, the OTT was 2.6 ± 1.6 seconds, and the PTT was 1.5 ± 0.7 seconds. For the tablets, the OTT was 3.2 ± 2.8 seconds, and the PTT was 3.9 ± 5.0 seconds. For both the OTT and PTT, there were no significant differences in food bolus passage time between the thickened barium solution and the tablets (Mann-Whitney test, p>0.05) (Figure 3).

Comparison of the OTT and PTT of the thickened barium solution between cases that could pass the tablet (able to pass group) and that could not pass the tablet (unable to pass group) revealed that, in the unable to pass group, the OTT of the thickened barium solution was 3.4 ± 1.7 seconds, and the PTT was 2.2 ± 1.8 seconds. The OTT of the thickened barium solution was significantly longer in the unable to pass group (Mann-Whitney test, p=0.02), but no significant difference was observed in the PTT (Mann-Whitney test, p=0.28) (Figure 4).

Discussion

When comparing the passage of tablets based on the extent of glossectomy, there was no significant difference. However, a high proportion of patients were unable to pass the tablets after subtotal glossectomy, and when comparing the pre- and postoperative findings, a significant increase was observed in the proportion of those who could not pass the tablets after surgery. When the extent of glossectomy increases, swallowing function is known to decrease [9,11,15] and subtotal glossectomy in particular results in difficulties with passing a food bolus and an increase in mealtime duration [19,21]. Moreover, when compared with subtotal glossectomy, partial glossectomy and hemiglossectomy result in a more mild form of dysphagia, which is known to improve within a few months to 1 year postoperatively [19,22-24]. Therefore, in patients who undergo subtotal glossectomy, it is considered that tablet intake should be avoided, particularly in the recovery phase. Over time, resolution of dysphagia can be expected; however, assessments of the ability to ingest tablets should be performed using VF or endoscopy while confirming food intake status. With surgical procedures, no significant differences were observed in the pass ability. However, patients undergoing segmental mandibulectomy and accompanying rectus abdominis flap/plate reconstruction had an increased tendency to be unable to pass.

Moreover, there was no significant difference in the proportion of individuals able or unable to pass according to the TNM classification. Further investigation based not on the stage of the tumor but on the site of excision, occurrence of neck dissection, and the extent of dissection is required. Regarding retention in the oral cavity, the entry of the tablet into the dead space was the cause; therefore, avoiding the creation of dead space with the use of a flap and of dentures may be important [25].

Preoperatively, all cases required only one swallow to ingest the

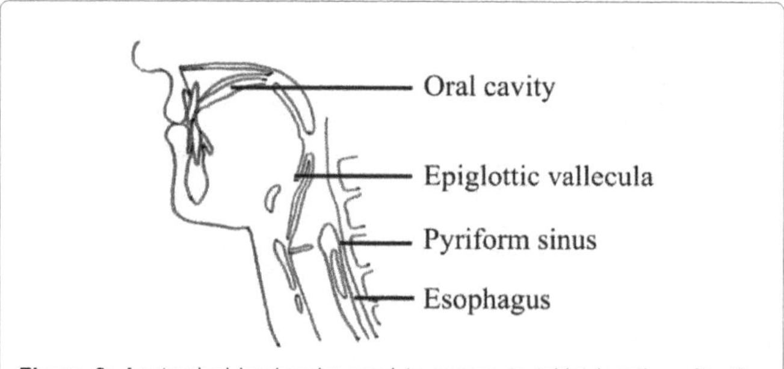

Figure 2: Anatomical landmarks used to assess to tablet location after the swallowing reflex.

	Initial	Final
Oral cavity	29	16
Epiglottic vallecula	7	4
Pyriform sinus	5	2
Esophagus	7	26

Table 5: Tablet location after swallowing reflex (n= 48).

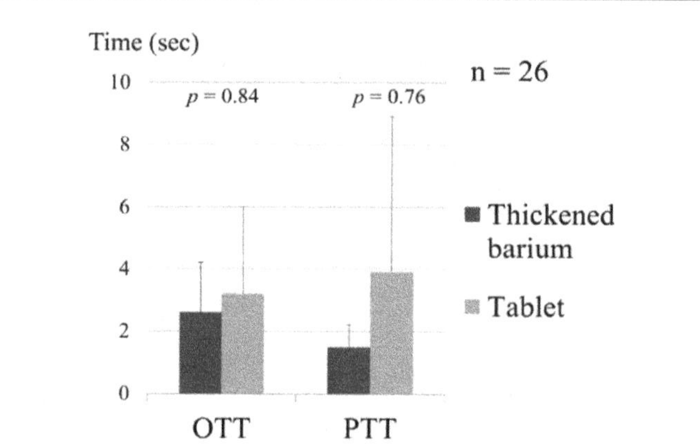

Figure 3: Oral transit time and pharyngeal transit time.
For both OTT and PTT, there are no significant differences in food bolus passage time after placing thickened barium solution into the mouth compared to the tablet (Mann-Whitney test, p>0.05).

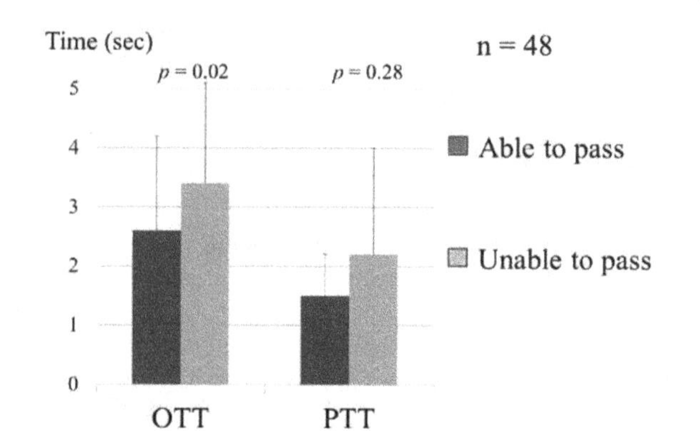

Figure 4: Oral transit time and pharyngeal transit time.
The OTT of the thickened barium solution is significantly longer in the unable to pass group (Mann-Whitney test, p=0.02). No significant difference in PTT is observed (Mann-Whitney test, p=0.28).

tablet. However, when only considering postoperative cases where passage was possible, an average of 2.8 (median 2) swallows were required. Mann et al. reported that outpatients with dysphagia require a median of 3 swallows to ingest a tablet [3]. Furthermore, the location of tablet retention was predominantly in the oral cavity due to the effect of glossectomy; however, there were also retentions in the epiglottic vallecula and pyriform sinus. Therefore, even in cases where there is no tablet retention in the oral cavity after ingestion, the possibility of retention in the pharynx must be considered, and a confirmation of the sensation of retention within the pharynx and additional swallowing should be performed.

The normal OTT and PTT values for liquids in healthy individuals are 1-1.5 and 0.38-0.48 seconds, respectively [26-31]. In the current study, a thickened barium solution resulted in an OTT of 2.6 ± 1.6 seconds. A lengthening of the OTT is known to occur in tongue tumor patients [32,33]. Pauloski et al. reported that the OTT of thick solutions 1 month post-surgery is 2.33 seconds, which is similar to the present findings [34]. Regarding PTT, a lengthening compared to normal healthy individuals was seen for both the thickened solution and tablets, and the tablets in particular showed an increase in the transit time through the pharynx. However, a longer transit time through the pharynx occurred in cases of tablet retention in the pharynx, and there was large variability in the values. In cases where the tablet passage was not possible, the OTT of the thickened solution was longer than in cases where passage was possible. Therefore, in patients where the passage of a thickened solution is difficult, the passage of tablets is also likely to be difficult. In institutions where assessments using simulated tablets are not performed, an extrapolation of the ability or inability to pass may be made from the passage of thickened solutions.

Conclusion

After subtotal glossectomy, many patients are unable to swallow tablets, and confirmation using VF or endoscopic evaluation of swallowing should be performed when prescribing tablets. For the swallowing of tablets after tongue cancer surgery, patients should be instructed to attempt multiple swallows. Even in cases where tablet retention in the pharynx is not seen in the oral cavity, investigation of the sensation of retention should be performed.

Acknowledgements

Funding: This research was carried out with a research grant from the Japanese Society of Dysphagia Rehabilitation, Japan (2010) from August 1st, 2010 to July 31st, 2011.

References

1. Kottke MK, Stetsko G, Rosenbaum SE, Rhodes CT (1990) Problems encountered by the elderly in the use of conventional dosage forms. J Geriatr Drug Ther 5: 77-92.
2. Roy N, Stemple J, Merrill RM, Thomas L (2007) Dysphagia in the elderly: preliminary evidence of prevalence, risk factors, and socioemotional effects. Ann Otol Rhinol Laryngol 116: 858-865.
3. Carnaby-Mann G, Crary M (2005) Pill swallowing by adults with dysphagia. Arch Otolaryngol Head Neck Surg 131: 970-975.
4. Miura H, Kariyasu M (2007) Effect of size of tablets on easiness of swallowing and handling among the frail elderly. Nihon Ronen Igakkai Zasshi 44: 627-633.
5. Overgaard AB, Højsted J, Hansen R, Møller-Sonnergaard J, Christrup LL (2001) Patients' evaluation of shape, size and colour of solid dosage forms. Pharm World Sci 23: 185-188.
6. Hey H, Jørgensen F, Sørensen K, Hasselbalch H, Wamberg T (1982) Oesophageal transit of six commonly used tablets and capsules. Br Med J (Clin Res Ed) 285(6356): 1717-1719.
7. Oshima T, Hori S, Maida C, Miyamoto E (2006) Effect of size and shape of tablets and capsules on ease of grasping and swallowing (1): Comparison between elderly and students. Jpn J Pharm Health Care Sci 32: 842-848.
8. Sugihara M, Hidaka M, Saito A (1986) Discriminatory features of dosage form and package. Jpn J Hosp Pharm 12: 322-328.
9. Hosoda M, Koshima I, Rata T, Deguchi H, Katayama Y (1998) Assessment of swallowing function following reconstruction of base of tongue and/or lateral pharyngeal wall with microvascular tissue transfer. Jpn J Head Neck Cancer 24: 352-357.
10. Hirano M, Kuroiwa Y, Tanaka S, Matsuoka H, Sato K, et al. (1992) Dysphagia following various degrees of surgical resection for oral cancer. Ann Otol Rhinol Laryngol 101: 138-141.
11. Fujimoto Y, Matsuura H, Kawabata K, Takahashi K, Tayama N (1997) [Assessment of Swallowing Ability Scale for oral and oropharyngeal cancer patients]. Nihon Jibiinkoka Gakkai Kaiho 100: 1401-1407.
12. Schliephake H, Jamil MU (2002) Prospective evaluation of quality of life after oncologic surgery for oral cancer. Int J Oral Maxillofac Surg 31: 427-433.
13. Diz Dios P, Fernández Feijoo J, Castro Ferreiro M, Alvarez Alvarez J (1994) Functional consequences of partial glossectomy. J Oral Maxillofac Surg 52: 12-14.
14. Nicoletti G, Soutar DS, Jackson MS, Wrench AA, Robertson G (2004) Chewing and swallowing after surgical treatment for oral cancer: functional evaluation in 196 selected cases. Plast Reconstr Surg 114: 329-338.
15. Kuroiwa Y (1992) Dysphagia following various degrees of surgical resection for oral and oropharyngeal cancer. Jibi To Rinsho 38: 812-824.
16. Sato K, Kuroiwa Y, Matsuoka H, Yoshida T, Hirano M (1993) [Dysphagia following extensive oral cancer surgery.] Jibi To Rinsho 39: 326-328.
17. Joo YH, Hwang SH, Park JO, Cho KJ, Kim MS (2013) Functional outcome after partial glossectomy with reconstruction using radial forearm free flap. Auris Nasus Larynx 40: 303-307.
18. Pauloski BR, Rademaker AW, Logemann JA, Stein D, Beery Q, et al. (2000) Pretreatment swallowing function in patients with head and neck cancer. Head Neck 22: 474-482.
19. Matsunaga K, Oobu K, Ohishi M (2002) [The clinical study on pre and postoperative swallowing function in tongue cancer patients.] Jpn J Dysphagia Rehab 6: 53-64.
20. Bailey RT Jr, Bonavina L, McChesney L, Spires KJ, Muilenburg MI, et al. (1987) Factors influencing the transit of a gelatin capsule in the esophagus. Drug Intell Clin Pharm 21: 282-285.
21. Yanai C, Kikutani T, Adachi M, Thoren H, Suzuki M (2008) Functional outcome after total and subtotal glossectomy with free flap reconstruction. Head Neck 30(7): 909-918.
22. Hsiao HT, Leu YS, Chang SH, Lee JT (2003) Swallowing function in patients who underwent hemiglossectomy: comparison of primary closure and free radial forearm flap reconstruction with videofluoroscopy. Ann Plast Surg 50: 450-455.
23. Uwiera T, Seikaly H, Rieger J, Chau J, Harris JR (2004) Functional outcomes after hemiglossectomy and reconstruction with a bilobed radial forearm free flap. J Otolaryngol 33: 356-359.
24. Panchal J, Potterton AJ, Scanlon E, McLean NR (1996) An objective assessment of speech and swallowing following free flap reconstruction for oral cavity cancers. Br J Plast Surg 49: 363-369.
25. Okuno K, Nohara K, Tanaka N, Sasao Y, Sakai T (2014) The efficacy of a lingual augmentation prosthesis for swallowing after a glossectomy: a clinical report. J Prosthet Dent 111: 342-345.
26. Mandelstam P, Lieber A (1970) Cineradiographic evaluation of the esophagus in normal adults. A study of 146 subjects ranging in age from 21 to 90 years. Gastroenterology 58: 32-39.
27. Blonsky ER, Logemann JA, Boshes B, Fisher HB (1975) Comparison of speech and swallowing function in patients with tremor disorders and in normal geriatric patients: a cinefluorographic study. J Gerontol 30: 299-303.
28. Tracy JF, Logemann JA, Kahrilas PJ, Jacob P, Kobara M, et al. (1989) Preliminary observations on the effects of age on oropharyngeal deglutition. Dysphagia 4: 90-94.

29. Lof GL, Robbins J (1990) Test-retest variability in normal swallowing. Dysphagia 4: 236-242.

30. Robbins J, Hamilton JW, Lof GL, Kempster GB (1992) Oropharyngeal swallowing in normal adults of different ages. Gastroenterology 103: 823-829.

31. Rademaker AW, Pauloski BR, Logemann JA, Shanahan TK (1994) Oropharyngeal swallow efficiency as a representative measure of swallowing function. J Speech Hear Res 37: 314-325.

32. Logemann JA, Bytell DE (1979) Swallowing disorders in three types of head and neck surgical patients. Cancer 44: 1095-1105.

33. Zu Y, Narayanan SS, Kim YC, Nayak K, Bronson-Lowe C, et al. (2013) Evaluation of swallow function after tongue cancer treatment using real-time magnetic resonance imaging: a pilot study. JAMA Otolaryngol Head Neck Surg 139: 1312-1319.

34. Pauloski BR, Logemann JA, Rademaker AW, McConnel FM, Heiser MA, et al. (1993) Speech and swallowing function after anterior tongue and floor of mouth resection with distal flap reconstruction. Speech Hear Res 36: 267-276.

Endoscopic Repair of Carotid Artery Injury

Irit Duek[1,2], Gill E Sviri[3], Moran Amit[1,2] and Ziv Gil[1,2*]

[1]*Department of Otolaryngology Head and Neck Surgery, Rambam Health Care Campus, Haifa, Israel*

[2]*The Laboratory for Applied Cancer Research, the Clinical Research Institute, Rambam Health Care Campus, The Technion, Haifa, Israel*

[3]*Department of Neurosurgery, Rambam Health Care Campus, Haifa, Israel*

***Corresponding author:** Ziv Gil, Department of Otolaryngology Head and Neck Surgery, Rambam Medical Center, the Technion, Israel Institute of Technology, 6 Ha'Aliya Street, POB 9602, Haifa 31096, Israel, E-mail: ziv@baseofskull.org

Abstract

Background: Injury to the cavernous portion of the Internal Carotid Artery (ICA) during endoscopic skull base surgery is a well-recognized rare complication, which can be associated with high rates of morbidity and mortality. Many techniques have been suggested to manage ICA injury with varying degrees of success. A detailed technical description of an operative technique for endoscopic management of carotid artery injury is provided.

Methods: A case of ICA injury during endoscopic skull base surgery is presented. The immediate treatment measurements include: 1) early recognition of ICA injury; 2) briefing of the team and preparations; 3) packing; 4) harvesting of temporalis muscle patch; 5) placement of the muscle patch over the defect; 6) gentle compression for 10 minutes.

Results: The technique presented facilitates quick repair, restoring normal blood flow through the damaged artery and thereby preventing exsanguination or the symptoms of stroke that may occur from prolonged occlusion of the ICA.

Conclusions: This protocol has been useful for the management of this life-threatening complication.

Keywords: Carotid artery injury; Endoscopic endonasal skull base surgery

Abbreviations: CN: Cranial Nerve; CT: Computed Tomography; ESS: Tomography; EES: Endoscopic Endonasal Surgery; FESS: Functional Endoscopic Sinus Surgery; ICA: Internal Carotid Artery; MRI: Magnetic Resonance Imaging

Introduction

Intraoperative injury to the Internal Carotid Artery (ICA) during Endoscopic Endonasal Surgery (EES) of the skull base is a rare and well recognized complication which can potentially be associated with high rates of morbidity and mortality [1-3]. In the event of a traumatic injury to the ICA during EES, hemorrhage might be massive, difficult to control as the access to the sphenoid sinus is limited and the visual field becomes quickly obscured. Bleeding from this vital artery can become lethal within minutes and even when the bleeding is controlled, permanent neurological deficits frequently persist [4-6]. According to the literature, the risk for injury to the ICA following endoscopic tumor resection is around 1% [7-11]. Many techniques have been developed to manage ICA injury including controlled hypotension, ipsilateral and contralateral neck pressure, proximal control through neck dissection and distal control, with varying degrees of success. The size of the arterial damage, its nature (small perforator avulsion vs. large, direct injury) and its site would determine its treatment and the ability to control the injury while preserving the vessel. The ability to repair the ICA using endoscopic techniques is limited by the narrow surgical field and inability of suturing. Pressure application or bipolar cautery were suggested when the defect in the vessel wall was small. However, in cases of significant bleeding during EES, endovascular treatment was suggested as definitive treatment.

In this paper, we provide a detailed description of an endoscopic repair after carotid artery injury with a temporalis muscle patch.

Surgical Anatomy

The bony separation between the sphenoid sinus and the cavernous portion of the ICA is very thin [12], and injury to the ICA can occur via penetration to the lateral sphenoid wall. According to Fujii et al. 88% of 50 carotid arteries in cadavers had a bony thickness less than 0.5 mm [13], and in 8% of cases, the bone overlying the internal carotid artery was dehiscent. Vincentelli et al. noted that 4% of 116 cadavers had minimal bone [14] while Kennedy et al. found that 20% of postmortem specimens had a dehiscent intrasphenoid carotid artery [15]. Similarly, in a review of 500 consecutive axial CT scans Johnson et al. observed that 14.4% radiographs had minimal to no bone between the two structures [16].

Case Report

A 57 years old otherwise healthy woman was referred to our institution due to complaints of intense headaches, speech difficulties and dysphagia for 2 weeks. At physical examination the patient demonstrated slurred speech with tongue deviation towards the left. Neck examination and endoscopic flexible fiber optic were normal, and no other neurological deficits were observed.

Magnetic Resonance Imaging (MRI) scan demonstrated an enhanced clival mass, 48×36×55 mm, invading the right sphenoid sinus, the occipital condyles, the dense and the anterior arch of C1 (Figure 1). The mass was pushing the pituitary gland upward, invading the parapharyngeal space, upper middle and lower parts of the clivus with intradural extension through the midclivial region pushing the pons and the basilary trunk. Inferiorly the mass invaded the occipital condyl at both sides, the anterior ring of C1 and the upper dens. Radiological features were consistent with chordoma, and the patient was scheduled for an extended trans sphenoidal endonasal resection.

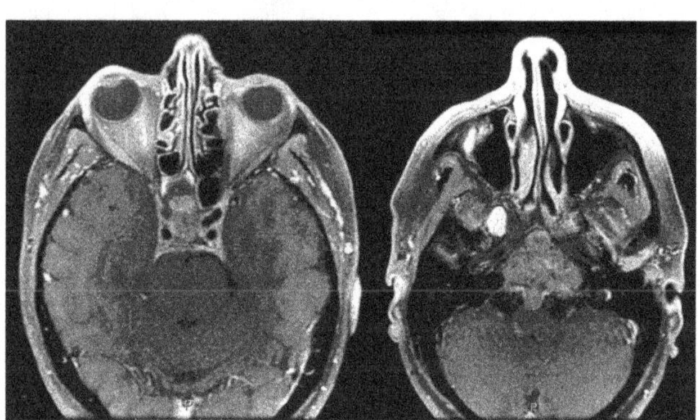

Figure 1: Pre-operative gadolinium-enhanced T1-weighted axial magnetic resonance imaging (MRI) sections. An enhanced clival mass, 48X36x55 mm, is demonstrated, invading the right sphenoid sinus, the occipital condyles, the dense and the anterior arch of C1. Radiological features were consistent with chordoma.

Surgical Technique

The operation was performed under general anesthesia using an intraoperative frameless navigation. The surgery was conducted under electrophysiological monitoring. After inferior turbinate lateralization, middle turbinectomy, middle antrostomy, anterior and posterior ethmoidectomy, posterior septectomy and elevation of a nasoseptal flap, the tumor was exposed in the sphenoid sinus. Using a high speed coarse drill, the rostrum and clival tumor extensions were drilled out. The anterior wall of the sphenoid sinus was removed in order to provide a better access. The tumor was of rubbery consistency and non-suckable and therefore tumor removal was performed with a Kerrison rongeur forceps and a drill. When the tumor was extirpated from the left sphenoid wall, bleeding was identified from the left ICA at the cavernous part. The exact location, size and configuration of the defect at the vessel's wall was not identified. The operating team and the anesthesiologist were immediately notified. Packed cells and fresh frozen plasma were ordered to the operating room and a second anesthesiologist joined the team. Vital signs were monitored carefully; arterial blood was drawn to monitor blood gases and hematocrit levels. No hemodynamic compromise nor deviation from normal ranges of any of the monitored parameters were noted.

Using two-surgeon four-hand technique, two attempts to correct the injury with Surgicel (Ethicon, West Somerville, NJ, USA) were unsuccessful. Then, a decision to repair the injury with a temporalis muscle patch was made. A 4×4 cm warm saline soaked gauze was inserted under vision into the nasal cavity, with its tip placed directly on the injured part of the left ICA applying packing using local pressure. Full control of the bleeding was achieved. Next, a 2×2 cm muscle patch flap, not including the fascia, was harvested from the left temporalis muscle through a small scalp incision at the superior temporal line in a coronal plane. After harvesting, the gauze was removed, and the muscle flap was inserted and positioned directly over the injured ICA. Gentle pressure was applied with overlying cotton patties for exactly 10 minutes. During that time, the blood pressure was kept above 100/60 mmHg. After 10 minutes the cotton patties were removed without evidence of residual bleeding. The total blood loss was <250 cc, and that there was no hemodynamic compromise (vital signs, including blood pressure were at normal ranges, so as lab results including arterial blood gases, hemoglobin and hematocrit levels). The patient received 1 unit of packed red blood cells (300 mL/unit) and 2 units of fresh frozen plasma, and tumor resection was completed. The right CN XII was monitored during the surgery and preserved while the left nerve was non-functional prior to surgery.

Postoperative Management

After the operation, the patient was extubated uneventfully and transferred to the postsurgery care unit for observation. No postoperative complications were encountered. Postoperative CT scan with contrast material demonstrated no pneumocephalus, pseudoaneurysm or intracranial bleeding. On 1 month follow-up the patient was asymptomatic, maintained good outpatient oral intake, with great relief of her pre-operative complaints. There have been no neurological deficits except for the known preoperative left CN XII palsy, which was improved following surgery. The surgical wounds were intact, without evidence of infection or inflammation, without local pain. The specimen's pathology analysis demonstrated clival chordoma. The patient was referred for adjuvant radiotherapy.

Discussion

Dissection around the cavernous, paraclival, and petrous segments of the ICA with a drill or microdissection may be associated with vascular injury [7-11,17,18].

Gardner et al. [18] described their experience of seven ICA injuries in 2,015 endoscopic endonasal skull base cases over a 13-year period, giving an incidence of 0.3%. Most injuries (5 of 7) involved the left ICA, and the most common diagnosis was chondroid neoplasm (chordoma, chondrosarcoma; 3 of 7 [2% of 142 cases]). Two injuries occurred during 660 pituitary adenoma resections (0.3%). The paraclival ICA segment was the most commonly injured site (5 of 7). Four of 7 injured ICAs were sacrificed either intraoperatively or postoperatively. No patient suffered a stroke or neurological deficit. There were no intraoperative mortalities; 1 patient died postoperatively of cardiac ischemia. One of the 3 preserved ICAs developed a pseudoaneurysm over a mean follow-up period of 5 months that was treated endovascularly [18]. Injury of the ICA might be associated with long-term neurological deficits [1,4,6]. Therefore, when such a life-threatening complication occurs, prompt identification and intervention is crucial. Identification of the ICA is essential when operating in the cavernous region. The posterior wall of the sphenoid sinus, which has the optic and carotid prominences, should not be considered sufficient protection of the carotid and optic nerve and avoiding injury is the best management. Valentine and Wormald [19] developed a sheep model to recreate and train surgeons in the management of ICA injury.

A number of hemostatic techniques were tested, including muscle patch treatment (harvested sternocleidomastoid), Floseal (Baxter International, Deerfield, IL, USA), oxidized regenerated cellulose (Surgicel Nu-Knit, Ethicon, West Somerville, NJ, USA), MicroFrance Wormald vascular clamps (Medtronic, Jacksonville, FL, USA), and U-Clip anastomotic sutures (Medtronic) to suture the vascular defect. Muscle patch treatment was effective at achieving vascular control, as was use of the MicroFrance Wormald vascular clamp and U-Clips [19]. Packing and placing adequate pressure has the potential to stop the bleeding, however, applying enough pressure to stop the bleeding can lead to complete occlusion of the artery [1,4,6]. Thus, despite controlling the bleeding, the same complications of exsanguination may occur as a result of reduced blood flow to the brain. Applying pressure can lead to pseudoaneurysm formation, especially following endovascular recanalization [20,21]. As Liskey et al. reported in their literature review, abrupt ICA occlusion is associated with a stroke rate of up to 26% and a mortality rate of 12% [22]. Roski et al. had a 16.6% incidence of strokes in their long-term follow-up (average 12.5 years) after ligation of the ICA for an ICA aneurysm [23].

Endovascular techniques remain valid option if endonasal repair is not achived [24]. In such cases, following packing, the patient is delivered intubated to the endovascular suite. Two commonly used endovascular techniques include balloon occlusion and coil embolization, by endovascular stent graft placement [25].

Conclusion

The mortality and morbidity of an ICA injury during EES can be decreased if the team is properly trained for this event. The following steps are the basis of successful control of ICA bleeding: 1) Early recognition of the ICA injury 2) briefing of the team and preparations; 3) packing; 4) harvesting of temporalis muscle patch; 5) placement of the muscle patch over the defect; 6) Gentle compression for 10 minutes. Using this technique the continuity of the vessel is maintained and neurological complications can be avoided.

References

1. Laws ER Jr (1999) Vascular complications of transsphenoidal surgery. Pituitary 2: 163-170.
2. Isenberg SF, Scott JA (1994) Management of massive hemorrhage during endoscopic sinus surgery. Otolaryngol Head Neck Surg 111: 134-136.
3. Hudgins PA, Browning DG, Gallups J, Gussack GS, Peterman SB, et al. (1992) Endoscopic paranasal sinus surgery: radiographic evaluation of severe complications. AJNR Am J Neuroradiol 13: 1161-1167.
4. Cavallo LM, Briganti F, Cappabianca P, Maiuri F, Valente V, et al. (2004) Hemorrhagic vascular complications of endoscopic transsphenoidal surgery. Minim Invasive Neurosurg 47: 145-150.
5. Berker M, Aghayev K, Saatci I, Palaoglu S, Onerci M (2010) Overview of vascular complications of pituitary surgery with special emphasis on unexpected abnormality. Pituitary 13: 160-167.
6. Fukushima T, Maroon JC (1998) Repair of carotid artery perforations during transsphenoidal surgery. Surg Neurol 50: 174-177.
7. Dessi P, Castro F, Triglia JM, Zanaret M, Cannoni M (1994) Major complications of sinus surgery: a review of 1192 procedures. J Laryngol Otol 108: 212-215.
8. Freedman HM, Kern EB (1979) Complications of intranasal ethmoidectomy: a review of 1,000 consecutive operations. Laryngoscope 89: 421-434.
9. Stevens HE, Blair NJ (1988) Intranasal sphenoethmoidectomy: 10-year experience and literature review. J Otolaryngol 17: 254-259.
10. May M, Levine HL, Mester SJ, Schaitkin B (1994) Complications of endoscopic sinus surgery: analysis of 2108 patients--incidence and prevention. Laryngoscope 104: 1080-1083.
11. Stankiewicz JA (1989) Complications in endoscopic intranasal ethmoidectomy: an update. Laryngoscope 99: 686-690.
12. Wigand ME, Hosemann WG (1991) Results of endoscopic surgery of the paranasal sinuses and anterior skull base. J Otolaryngol 20: 385-390.
13. Fujii K, Chambers SM, Rhoton AL Jr (1979) Neurovascular relationships of the sphenoid sinus. A microsurgical study. J Neurosurg 50: 31-39.
14. Vincentelli F, Grisoli F, Bartoli JF, Leclerc T, de Smedt E, et al. (1982) Anatomico-radiological basis of sellar surgery and its nasoseptal approach. J Neuroradiol 9: 284-303.
15. Kennedy DW, Zinreich SJ, Hassab, MH (1990) The internal carotid artery as it relates to endonasal sphenoethmoidectomy. Am J Rhino I4: 7-12.
16. Johnson DM, Hopkins RJ, Hanafee WN, Fisk JD (1985) The unprotected parasphenoidal carotid artery studied by high-resolution computed tomography. Radiology 155: 137-141.
17. Renn WH, Rhoton AL Jr (1975) Microsurgical anatomy of the sellar region. J Neurosurg 43: 288-298.
18. Gardner PA, Tormenti MJ, Pant H, Fernandez-Miranda JC, Snyderman CH, et al. (2013) Carotid artery injury during endoscopic endonasal skull base surgery: incidence and outcomes. Neurosurgery 73: ons261-269.
19. Valentine R, Wormald PJ (2011) Controlling the surgical field during a large endoscopic vascular injury. Laryngoscope 121: 562-566.
20. Raymond J, Hardy J, Czepko R, Roy D (1997) Arterial injuries in transsphenoidal surgery for pituitary adenoma; the role of angiography and endovascular treatment. AJNR Am J Neuroradiol 18: 655-665.
21. Casler JD, Doolittle AM, Mair EA (2005) Endoscopic surgery of the anterior skull base. Laryngoscope 115: 16-24.
22. Linskey ME, Jungreis CA, Yonas H, Hirsch WL Jr, Sekhar LN, et al. (1994) Stroke risk after abrupt internal carotid artery sacrifice: accuracy of preoperative assessment with balloon test occlusion and stable xenon-enhanced CT. AJNR Am J Neuroradiol 15: 829-843.
23. Roski RA, Spetzler RF, Nulsen FE (1981) Late complications of carotid ligation in the treatment of intracranial aneurysms. J Neurosurg 54: 583-587.
24. Kocer N, Kizilkilic O, Albayram S, Adaletli I, Kantarci F, et al. (2002) Treatment of iatrogenic internal carotid artery laceration and carotid cavernous fistula with endovascular stent-graft placement. AJNR Am J Neuroradiol 23: 442-446.
25. Park YS, Jung JY, Ahn JY, Kim DJ, Kim SH (2009) Emergency endovascular stent graft and coil placement for internal carotid artery injury during transsphenoidal surgery. Surg Neurol 72: 741-746.

12

Factors Affecting Recurrence of T1 and T2 Tongue Cancer Undergoing Intraoral Resection

Takeshi Mohri[1,2], Yasuhiko Tomita[3]*, Takashi Fujii[2], Miki Tomoeda[3], Shota Kotani[3], Tomonori Terada[1], Nobuo Saeki[1], Nobuhiro Uwa[1], Kousuke Sagawa[1] and Masafumi Sakagami[1]

[1]*The Department of Otolaryngology, Hyogo Medical University, Japan*
[2]*The Departments of Otolaryngology, Osaka Medical Center for Cancer and Cardiovascular Diseases, Japan*
[3]*The Departments of Pathology, Osaka Medical Center for Cancer and Cardiovascular Diseases, Japan*

Abstract

Background: Intraoral resection of early tongue cancer minimally affects the quality of life (QOL) of patients; however, local recurrence of the tumor requires radical resection and negatively affects QOL as well as patient prognosis. The present study was performed to clarify factors affecting recurrence of tongue cancers undergoing intraoral resection.

Methods: In total, 174 patients (T1: 105 patients and T2: 69 patients) with squamous cell carcinoma of the tongue receiving intraoral resection were enrolled in the study, including 106 male patients and 68 female patients (aged 27-88 years, mean 58 years). Tumor recurrence was observed in 10 of 105 patients with T1 stage cancer (9.5%) and in 6 of 69 patients with T2 stage cancer (8.7%). The clinicopathological factors, including immunohistochemistry for p53, Ki67, and vimentin, were analyzed.

Results: An infiltration pattern and vimentin expression were associated with tongue cancer recurrence. Specifically, tumors with positive vimentin expression exhibited a higher ratio of endophytic growth, and multivariate analysis revealed that the Ki67 labeling index and vimentin expression were independent factors affecting tumor recurrence.

Conclusion: The mode of tumor invasion and the epithelial-to-mesenchymal transition, as evidenced by vimentin immunohistochemistry, assisted the identification of high-risk patients with tongue cancer undergoing intraoral resection. Intense follow-up with the aid of multimodal therapies after surgery is necessary in this group of high-risk patients.

Keywords: Tongue cancer; Recurrent; Infiltration gamma; Vimentin expression

Background

Oral cancer represents 2.1% of the total cancer incidence, and more than 200,000 new cases are estimated to occur annually worldwide [1]. More than 80% of oral cancers are histologically squamous cell carcinomas, among which tongue cancer is most predominant. Several prognostic factors have been proposed for tongue cancer, including tumor depth and lymph node metastasis, which are the main factors affecting prognosis [2,3]. Furthermore, the Tumor-Node-Metastasis (TNM) classification has been widely employed for the staging of tongue cancer [4]. Intraoral resection performed in patients with early (pT1 and T2) tongue cancer minimally affects the swallowing ability and cosmetics of the patient and is thus superior to radical resection with respect to patient quality of life (QOL). Nevertheless, local recurrence of the tumor requires radical resection and negatively impacts patient QOL and prognosis. Postoperative chemo- and/or radiotherapy may prevent tumor recurrence. However, the negative effects of adjuvant therapy on tongue function and the body suggest that adjuvant therapy is a poor choice when applied indiscriminately to all patients with early tongue cancer. Therefore, the identification of patients at high risk for tumor recurrence is necessary to establish appropriate treatment modalities for patients with early tongue cancer.

During tumor development, the communication between tumor cells and the surrounding microenvironment is important. In particular, epithelial tumor cells (carcinomas) often change their morphology to undergo local invasion and metastatic dissemination, which is termed the epithelial-to-mesenchymal transition (EMT) [5,6]. Lines of evidence have revealed the correlation between EMT and cancer invasion [7-9]. With the developmental of cancer EMT, the cell intermediate filament status changes from a keratin-rich network connected to adherens junctions and hemidesmosomes to a vimentin-rich network connected to focal adhesions [9]. In the present study, clinicopathological factors were analyzed to clarify factors affecting the recurrence of tongue cancers subjected to intraoral resection. Additionally, to study the EMT status of cancer cells, vimentin expression was examined using immunohistochemistry.

Methods

This study comprised 174 patients (T1: 105 patients and T2: 69 patients) with squamous cell carcinoma of the tongue who underwent intraoral resection between January 1990 and January 2008 at the Osaka Medical Center for Cancer and Cardiovascular Diseases. The study included 106 male patients and 68 female patients (aged 27–88 years, mean 58 years). The observation period ranged from 4 months to 24 years (median 6 years and 1 month). Tumor recurrence was observed in 10 of 105 patients with T1 stage cancer (9.5%) and 6 of 69 patients with T2 stage cancer (8.7%). Resected specimens were cut into slices at a thickness of 5 mm, fixed in 10% formalin and routinely processed for paraffin embedding. Histological sections cut at 4 μm

***Corresponding author:** Yasuhiko Tomita, MD, PhD, Department of Pathology, Osaka Medical Center for Cancer and Cardiovascular Diseases, 1-3-3 Nakamichi, Higashinari-ku, Osaka 537-8511, Japan; E-mail:yasuhiko-tomita@umin.ac.jp

were stained with hematoxylin and eosin (H and E) and subjected to immunoperoxidase procedures (avidin-biotin complex (ABC) method). Tumor stages were defined based on the pTNM classification [4]. The following characteristics were compared between patients with and without tumor recurrence: age, sex, macroscopic tumor growth pattern, histologic classification, tumor size, depth of tumor, lymphatic invasion, venous invasion, and mode of tumor invasion.

Macroscopic growth patterns were classified as follows with the use of visual examination and palpation: superficial type, lesions with no protrusion from the surrounding mucous membrane or with some ulceration and white spots in the event of protrusion but no palpable induration; exophytic type, growth defined as a main lesion that protrudes externally; and endophytic type, growth defined as a deep induration in the main lesion (Figure 1). The mode of tumor invasion was defined as follows: infiltration (INF)-alpha invasion, lesions with extensible growth that were clearly distinguishable from the surrounding tissue; INF-gamma invasion, lesions with invasion and proliferation that was indistinct from the surrounding tissue; and INF-beta, lesions in which the state of invasion and proliferation were intermediate between INF-alpha- and INF-gamma-positive regions (Figure 2). If the tumor contained various patterns of infiltration at the edge, the most infiltrative pattern was chosen. To further clarify influential factors affecting local recurrence of tongue cancer, immunohistochemistry using antibodies against p53, Ki67, and vimentin (all from Dako, Glostrup, Denmark) was performed using samples from 15 patients who experienced local tumor recurrence and 14 patients without local recurrence. All the procedures of the present study were approved by the internal revenue service of Osaka Medical Center for Cancer and Cardiovascular Diseases. Written informed consent was obtained from all patients.

a) superficaial pattern

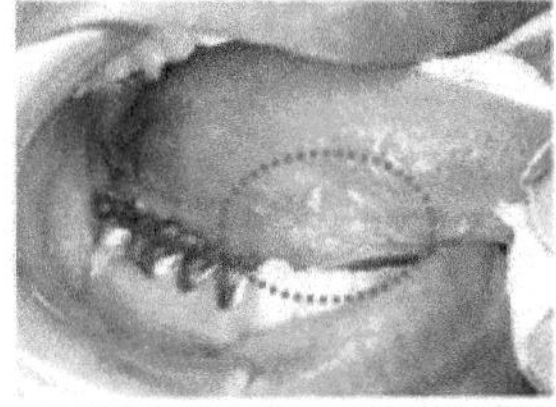

b) exophytic pattern

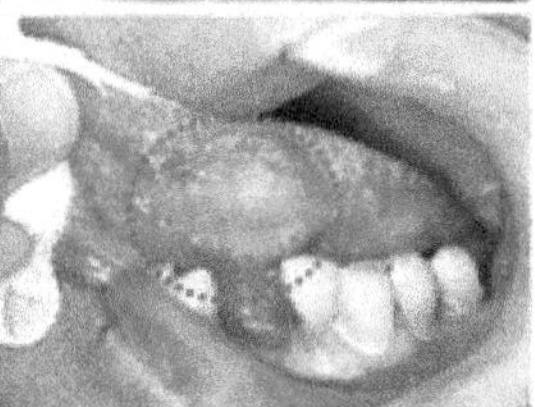

c) endophytic pattern

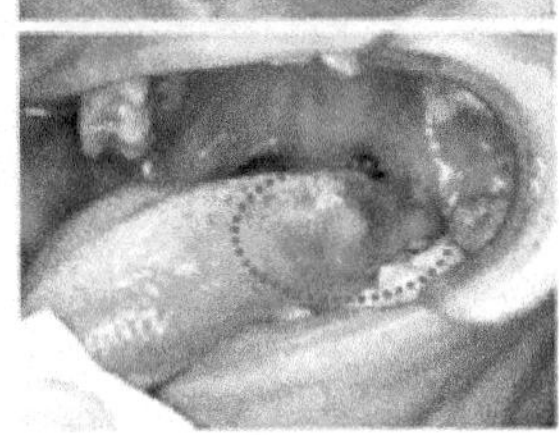

Figure 1: Typical tongue cancer cases showing a) Superficial, b) Exophytic, and c) Endophytic growth patterns.

a) Tumors with superficial growth patterns exhibit no elevation from the surrounding mucosa or a palpable tumor but may exhibit occasional erosion or white spots.

b) Tumors with exophytic growth patterns expand outward from the tongue. Induration inside the tongue is smaller than the main tumor outside of the original tongue.

c) Tumors with endophytic growth patterns exhibit the tumor mainly as an induration inside the tongue.

Statistical analysis

SAS software (Statistical Analysis System Institute, Cary, NC) was used for all statistical analyses. The significance of differences was tested using the log-rank test, Wilcoxon signed-rank sum test, and the chi-squared test. Multivariate analysis of factors related to tumor recurrence was performed using logistic regression analysis. Statistical significance was set at $p<0.05$.

Results

The correlation between tumor recurrence and clinicopathological factors is presented in Table 1. Patients with primary tumors with INF-gamma invasion exhibited a higher ratio of tumor recurrence compared with those with INF-alpha and INF-beta invasion ($p<0.0001$). Other factors did not affect tumor recurrence. Vimentin expression was examined in 15 cases with recurrence and 14 without recurrence. Eleven recurrent tumors and two without recurrence exhibited various percentages of vimentin expression in cancer cells (3-100%, median 30%, Figure 3). The remaining 18 cancers were completely negative for vimentin expression. The correlation between vimentin expression and the incidence of local recurrence was statistically significant ($p=0.01$). The correlation between vimentin expression and other factors is presented in Table 2. Tumors with positive vimentin expression were more likely to exhibit the endophytic growth pattern. Other factors did not correlate with vimentin expression. Multivariate analysis was performed using samples with full information (Table 3). The Ki67 labeling index and vimentin expression were identified as independent factors affecting tumor recurrence.

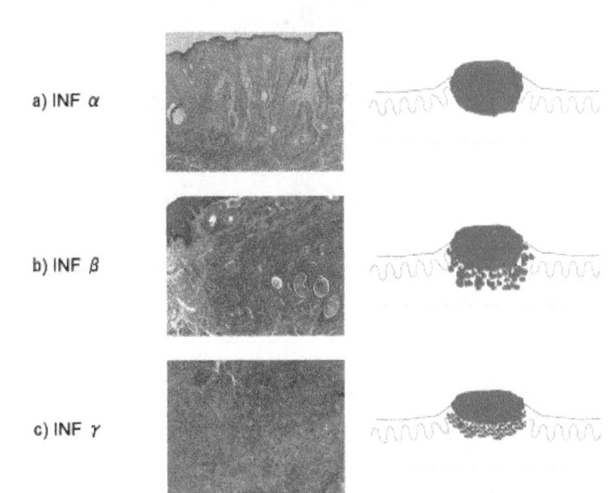

Figure 2: Types of infiltration.

a) Tumors with infiltration (INF)-alpha invasion grow expansively, and the border between the tumor and the surrounding tissue is clearly marginated.b) Tumors with INF-beta invasion exhibit the coexistence of clusters of tumor cells and surrounding tissue at the edge, but the two components are distinct from each other.

c) Tumors with INF-gamma invasion exhibit small clustered tumor cells at the edge, and the distinction of tumor cells from surrounding tissue is obscured.

Original magnification: X20

		With local recurrence	Without local recurrence	p-value
Age		57.2 ± 3.4	57.5 ± 1.1	0.9
Sex	Male	7	102	0.1
	Female	9	56	
Tumor size		17.9 ± 2.1	18.4 ± 0.6	0.8
Tumor depth	pT1	10	95	0.7
	pT2	6	63	
Growth pattern	Superficial	6	70	0.1
	Exophytic	1	32	
	Endophytic	9	56	
Tumor differentiation	Well differentiated	12	111	0.8
	Moderately differentiated	4	42	
	Poorly differentiated	1	4	
Mode of tumor invasion	Infiltration α	3	16	<0.0001
	Infiltration β	6	103	(Infiltration γ vs. others)
	Infiltration γ	7	7	
Lymphatic invasion	Absent	14	107	0.5
	Present	2	27	
Venous invasion	Absent	15	129	0.5
	Present	1	4	
p53 expression	Absent	11	9	0.6
	Present	4	5	
Ki67 labeling index	<10%	12	8	0.2
	>10%	3	6	
Vimentin expression	Absent	6	12	0.01
	Present	9	2	

Table 1: Correlation of clinicopathological factors with tumor recurrence.

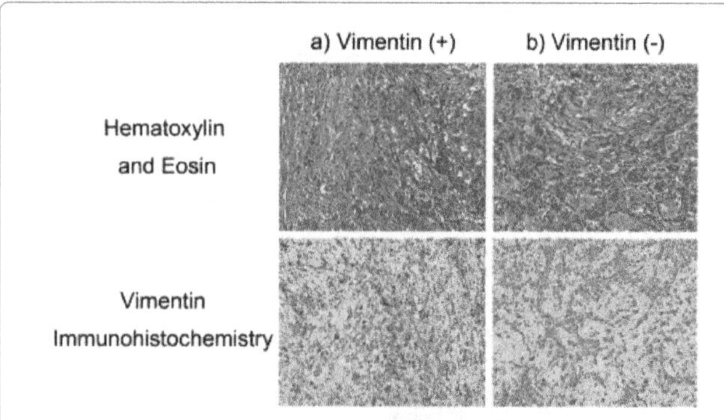

Figure 3: Immunohistochemistry of vimentin.

a) Case showing positive vimentin expression. Vimentin is widely expressed in tumor cells.

b) Case showing negative vimentin expression. Vimentin is expressed in the surrounding tissue but not in tumor cells.

Original magnification: X100

Discussion

The choice of treatment modalities for T1 and T2 tongue cancer remains controversial among physicians; some recommend simple resection, whereas others suggest intensive treatment such as surgery combined with chemoradiotherapy accompanied by neck lymph node dissection. To establish an appropriate treatment strategy for each patient, it is necessary to clarify the risk of local recurrence in each cancer. The present analysis revealed that the mode of tumor invasion and vimentin expression were predictive of local recurrence in patients undergoing intraoral resection. Tumors with a Ki67 labeling index less than 10% exhibited a higher ratio of local recurrence compared to those with indices greater than 10%, although this difference was not significant. Nevertheless, the Ki67 labeling index was identified as an independent factor affecting local recurrence in the multivariate analysis. The mode of tumor invasion exhibited a close correlation with tumor recurrence. Among 14 tumors with the INF-gamma pattern, seven experienced tumor recurrence. However, 9 out of 119 showing INF-alpha or INF-beta invasion developed recurrent tumors. Previous reports indicate that the most severe pattern of invasion is a strong risk factor for local recurrence and mortality [10]. In the present study, the most infiltrative pattern was selected in tumors with mixed patterns of infiltration at the tumor edge, and INF classification proved to be a useful marker to predict local recurrence.

Originally observed in morphogenesis during embryonic development, EMT has subsequently been observed in various pathological conditions in adults, including cancer and fibrosis [7]. During EMT, the disruption of tight junctions, loss of cell polarity, cytoskeletal changes, and formation of actin stress fibers are observed. Moreover, EMT causes cells to acquire mesenchymal features, including a spindle-shaped morphology, and express mesenchymal proteins, including vimentin [9,11]. TGFβ signaling activates many transcriptional factors involved in EMT, such as Snail, Slug, ZEB1/deltaEF1, and ZEB2/SIP1, and is considered a master regulator of EMT [8]. The present study clearly demonstrated that EMT, as evidenced by vimentin immunohistochemistry, represents a risk factor for tongue cancer recurrence. Recently, Jensen et al. reported the expression of factors involved in EMT, including TGFβ activation, in tumor budding of oral squamous cell carcinoma [12]. Tumor budding was identified

		Vimentin (-)	Vimentin (+)	p value
Age		57.5 ± 3.2	59.4 ± 4.1	0.7
Sex	Male	11	4	0.2
	Female	7	7	
Tumor size		19.2 ± 1.7	18.5 ± 2.2	0.8
Tumor depth	pT1	10	5	0.6
	pT2	8	6	
Growth pattern	Superficial	9	2	0.016
	Exophytic	4	1	(endophytic type vs. others)
	Endophytic	5	8	
Tumor differentiation	Well differentiated	15	7	0.3
	Moderately differentiated	3	3	
	Poorly differentiated	0	1	
Mode of tumor invasion	Infiltration α	2	2	0.14
	Infiltration β	12	5	
	Infiltration γ	2	4	
Lymphatic invasion	Absent	15	9	0.6
	Present	2	2	
Venous invasion	Absent	17	0	0.2
	Present	0	1	
p53 expression	Absent	12	8	0.7
	Present	6	3	
Ki67 labeling index	< 10%	13	7	0.5
	> 10%	5	4	

Table 2: Correlation of clinicopathological factors with vimentin expression in tumors.

		chi-square value	p-value
Age	1: <58	1.48	0.22
	0: >58		
Sex	1: Male	0.87	0.35
	0: Female		
Tumor size	1: <18 mm	0.09	0.75
	0: >18 mm		
Tumor depth	1: pT1	0.01	0.93
	0: pT2		
Growth pattern	1: Superficial and exophytic types	0.03	0.86
	0: Endophytic type		
Tumor differentiation	1: Well differentiated	1.35	0.24
	0: Moderately and poorly differentiated		
Mode of tumor invasion	1: Infiltration α and β	3.18	0.07
	0: Infiltration γ		
Lymphatic invasion	1: Absent	0.01	0.97
	0: Present		
Venous invasion	1: Absent	2.18	0.13
	0: Present		
p53 expression	1: Absent	0.41	0.52
	0: Present		
Ki67 labeling index	1: <10%	5.33	0.02
	0: >10%		
Vimentin expression	1: Absent	4.54	0.03
	0: Present		

Table 3: Multivariate analysis of clinicopathological factors affecting tumor recurrence.

as a risk factor for tongue cancer recurrence [10], although further investigation is necessary to clarify the correlation between EMT and the budding grade of tumors.

The clinical growth pattern has also been recognized as an important factor affecting local recurrence; in this study, the growth pattern was classified as superficial, endophytic, or exophytic. In the present study, tumors with exophytic growth exhibited the lowest rate of recurrence, whereas those with endophytic growth exhibited the highest recurrence rate, although this difference was not significant. Similarly, previous studies reported high risks of recurrence in tongue cancers exhibiting endophytic growth [13,14]. Thus, circumspect estimation of the surgical procedure prior to operation is needed for tongue cancers with endophytic growth patterns. Positive surgical margins are also associated with local recurrence. For instance, recurrence is twice as likely when tumor cells are found within 5 mm of the resection stump compared to when no tumor cells are observed [15]. In the present study, a margin of more than 10 mm was observed in all of the primary tumor specimens from patients who developed recurrent tumors (data not shown); thus, recurrence was unlikely to be due to tumor cells remaining in the resection stump. In the present study, previously reported factors affecting recurrence, such as size, depth, differentiation, and lymphatic and vascular invasion of the tumor, showed no influence on tumor recurrence. The present study included patients receiving intraoral resection but not radical operation; therefore, the factors affecting recurrence might differ from previous reports. Increased tumor size has been linked to cervical nodal involvement, high recurrence rate and poor prognosis [16].

Conclusion

In conclusion, the mode of tumor invasion and EMT, as evidenced by vimentin immunohistochemistry, represent useful markers for the identification of high-risk patients with tongue cancer receiving intraoral resection. Intense follow-up after surgery with the aid of multimodal therapies is necessary for patients in this high-risk category.

Acknowledgement

There were no conflicts of interest in the study. This work was supported by grants from the Japan Society for the Promotion of Science (15K08391).

References

1. Curado MP, Edwards B, Shin HR, Ferlay J, Heanue M et al (2009) Cancer Incidence in Five Continents, Volume IX. IARC Scientific Publication, Lyon.

2. Thiagarajan S, Nair S, Nair D, Chaturvedi P, Kane SV, et al. (2014) Predictors of prognosis for squamous cell carcinoma of oral tongue. J Surg Oncol 109: 639-644.

3. Rodrigues PC, Miguel MC, Bagordakis E, Fonseca FP, de Aquino SN, et al. (2014) Clinicopathological prognostic factors of oral tongue squamous cell carcinoma: A retrospective study of 202 cases. Int J Oral Maxillofac Surg 43: 795-801.

4. Sobin LH, Gospodarowicz MK, Wittekind CE (2009) TNM Classification of Malignant Tumours, 7th Edition. Wiley-Blackwell, Oxford.

5. Li L, Li W (2015) Epithelial-mesenchymal transition in human cancer: comprehensive reprogramming of metabolism, epigenetics, and differentiation. Pharmacol Ther 150: 33-46.

6. Thompson EW, Torri J, Sabol M, Sommers CL, Byers S, et al. (1994) Oncogene-induced basement membrane invasiveness in human mammary epithelial cells. Clin Exp Metastasis 12: 181-194.

7. Thiery JP (2002) Epithelial-mesenchymal transitions in tumour progression. Nat Rev Cancer 2: 442-454.

8. Ombrato L, Malanchi I (2014) The EMT universe: space between cancer cell dissemination and metastasis initiation. Crit Rev Oncog 19: 349-361.

9. Thiery JP, Sleeman JP (2006) Complex networks orchestrate epithelial-mesenchymal transitions. See comment in PubMed Commons below Nat Rev Mol Cell Biol 7: 131-142.

10. Almangush A, Bello IO, Keski-Säntti H, Mäkinen LK, Kauppila JH, et al. (2014) Depth of invasion, tumor budding, and worst pattern of invasion: prognostic indicators in early-stage oral tongue cancer. Head Neck 36: 811-818.

11. Xu J, Lamouille S, Derynck R (2009) TGF-beta-induced epithelial to mesenchymal transition. Cell Res 19: 156-172.

12. Jensen DH, Dabelsteen E, Specht L, Fiehn AM, Therkildsen MH, et al. (2015) Molecular profiling of tumour budding implicates TGFÎ²-mediated epithelial-mesenchymal transition as a therapeutic target in oral squamous cell carcinoma. J Pathol 236: 505-516.

13. Spiro RH, Guillamondegui O Jr, Paulino AF, Huvos AG (1999) Pattern of invasion and margin assessment in patients with oral tongue cancer. Head Neck 21: 408-413.

14. Sharma P, Shah SV, Taneja C, Patel AM, Patel MD (2013) A prospective study of prognostic factors for recurrence in early oral tongue cancer. J Clin Diagn Res 7: 2559-2562.

15. Loree TR, Strong EW (1990) Significance of positive margins in oral cavity squamous carcinoma. Am J Surg 160: 410-414.

16. Woolgar JA (2006) Histopathological prognosticators in oral and oropharyngeal squamous cell carcinoma. Oral Oncol 42: 229-239.

13

Functional Appliances in the Treatment of Sleep Apnea in Children

Rosa Carrieri Rossi[1*], Nelson Jose Rossi[2], Nelson Carrieri Rossi[2], Reginaldo Raimundo Fujiya[3] and Shirley Nagata Pignatari[3]

[1]*Division of Paediatric Otolaryngology, Federal University of Sao Paulo- UNIFESP SP, Brazil*

[2]*Professor of Postgraduate of Orthodontics, North of Minas Foundation- FUNORTE, Brazil*

[3]*Associate Professor, Division of Paediatric Otolaryngology, Department of Otolaryngology and Head and Neck Surgery, Federal University of Sao Paulo- UNIFESP, Brazil*

***Corresponding author:** Rosa Carrieri Rossi, Division of Paediatric Otolaryngology, Federal University of Sao Paulo- UNIFESP SP, Brazil; E-mail: rosacrossi@gmail.com

Abstract

Obstructive Sleep Apnea in children (OSA) is a Sleep-Disordered Breathing (SDR) characterized by partial or complete obstruction of the Upper Airways (UA) during sleep and interfere with sleep patterns and growth and development in children. The gold standard treatment in children is the removal of lymphoid tissue surgery. Disease recurrence can happen and is believed to be due to craniofacial concomitant problems, among others. The objective of this systematic review was demonstrate the effect of the use of functional appliances in the treatment of OSA in children. The search was in the databases included "pubmed, scholar, Medline, scielo" with the filters, "human, children, in all languages, with the key words "obstructive sleep apnea and children and orthodontic appliance" between the years 1988-2015. Initially were obtained 49 studies, but only 8 studies were eligible by level of evidence. The researches presented clinical positive results but not statistical results. This systematic literature review showed that orthopaedic devices seem to be a good treatment option for children with OSA. Although the level of evidence of the effectiveness of these devices is weak to moderate.

Keywords: Functional appliances; OSA; Children; Treatment

Abbreviations

AHI: Apnea/Hypopnea Index; OSA: Obstructive Sleep Apnea; REM: Rapid Eye Movement; SDB: Sleep Disordered Breathing; UA: Upper Airways; PS: Primary Snoring; OB: Oral Breathing; PSG: Polysomnography Exam; CPAP or BPAP: Air Pressure Devices; FA: Functional Appliances

Introduction

Obstructive Sleep Apnea (OSA) is a breathing disorder sleep characterized by partial or complete obstruction of the Upper Airways (UA) interfering with the normal sleep pattern. The prevalence of this disease in children is 0.2 to 3% [1-4]. Children with OSA usually present insidious signs and symptoms such as Primary Snoring (PS), Oral Breathing (OB), behavioural disorders, hyperactivity daytime, which cannot be recognized as part of that disease [5-11].

The Polysomnography Exam (PSG) is considered the gold standard for diagnosis, expressed by the apnea and hypopnea index (AIH), classified according to the number of occurrences per hour of sleep: the diagnosis is confirmed when the AHI is higher than [1,12,13]. The criteria diagnostic for children are different from adults and have not been completely established yet [4]. Many studies suggest more diagnostic tools and options should be considered, such as parents reports, clinical examination, questionnaires addressing behavioral and cognitive information and 3D imaging studies [14-23]. The multi displinary and multi professional nature of the disease, recommending an interactive diagnostic approach [24-28]. Adenotonsillar hypertrophy is known to be the main risk factor for the disease [1-11] followed by obesity, neuromuscular disorders and craniofacial anomalies [29-34]. The gold standard treatment for children is removal of the oropharyngeal lymphoid tissue [9,11,30-34]. Treatment during childhood is believed to be crucial; the delay in its recognition may play a negative influence on the quality in their adult life [35-38].

The most common non-surgical types of treatment include devices of air pressure (CPAP or BPAP), however, they are expensive and little accepted by children [39,40]. Recurrence of the clinical condition can happen after adenotonsillectomy, and it is believed to be due to concomitant craniofacial problems, among others [41-43]. These alterations can be easily recognized and treated by the orthodontist [23-26]. The persistence of OB and PS during the growing and developmental period may lead or exacerbate dental skeletal changes [39,42,43]. The incurred changes coupled with genetic predisposition make the OSA even more severe, allowing the development of a vicious circle. Orthodontic appliances can be used before or after surgery as preventive or curative [5,6,34,39,42-49]. The FA is widely used in children to promote mandibular growth and to improve craniofacial changes [50-56]. The mandibular advancement devices protrude the mandible and the tongue, increasing the passage diameter of the UA, improving the tonicity of the muscles in the region, particularly the genioglossus muscle, and consequently preventing the collapse of the soft tissue [57-63].

FA offer no risks, they are well tolerated by the patients, they minimize the overall costs of the treatment and are an alternative for the children treatment with OSA who persist with the disease after surgery [42,44]. The best results are obtained when the child enters in the pubertal growth spurt [51-57]. The restriction of this treatment is the lack of children´s cooperation by not using the device properly. Good results depend on the appropriate device use, at least for 12 months, all day long [59-65]. The objective of this research was to demonstrate through a systematic review, the effectiveness of a FA in the treatment of OSA in children.

Search of Databases

The search was in the databases included "pubmed, scholar, Medline, scielo" with the filters, "human, children, in all languages, with the key words "obstructive sleep apnea and children and orthodontic appliance" between the years 1988-2015. Initially were obtained 49 studies and 14 studies were excluded from the first selection by checking their overall goals as Osa and enuresis, OSA and syndromes. This pre-selection was made by three researchers individually. The selected 35 studies were requested by subjects in a comprehensive manner, including etiology of the disease, related to other sicknesses such as OB, PS, size of UA, diagnostic and treatment. The results of research we could see in Table 1.

Year	Author	Subject	Evidence	N	Conclusion
2011	Van Holsbeke et al.	OSA x 3D x FAx x resistence AU	Clinical cross	143	Women respond better to treatment
2011	Matter et al.	OB x NB x cephal skeletal pattern	Clinical longitudinal	33	Surgery restored normal growth in children pattern
2007	Vos et al.	OSA x 3D x PSG	Clinical observational	20	All tests should be used for effective diagnosis of OSA
2006	Ramos et al.	OSA PSG x x INDEX	Clinical observational	93	RA and adenoid and tonsil hypertrophy are large alerts in OSA
2008	Gregório et al.	OSA x most frequent symptoms	Clinical observational	38	PS, bruxism, early age appeared in children with severe OSA
2011	Godt et al.	OSA x UA x FA x Class II x HG x Rx	Clinical observational		There was no significant change in the UA after treatments
2002	Villa et al.	OSA x FA x tolerance x results	Clinical rand controlled	32	FA treated group had reduced OSA and well toletou the device
2013	Gullerminoult et al.	OSA surgery x relapse	Clinical retrospective	29	RecidiUA in adolescents were confirmed, I need to study better
2011	Kizinger et al.	OSA x UAX Cefalom x FA	Clinical retrospective	43	Ap fixed not improve OSA and cephalometric does not evaluate UA
1988	Cheng et al.	OB x mallocclusion	ClinicalControlled obser	71	OB should be recognized early to avoid malformations
2011	Moraes ME	CBCT x 2D in dry skulls	Experimental Study	10	3D survey looks better than 2D on dry skulls
2005	Nixon et al.	OSA diagnostic x	Literature review		Importance of early diagnosis of the disease to prevent greater evils
2009	Capua, Ahmadi, Shapiro	OSA and growth	Literature review		OSA has cognitive and functional negative impact
2011	Shott	OSA Persistent x risk factors	Literature review		Risk factors for persistent OSA
2006	Gozzal and Gozzal	OSA diagnostic	Literature review		Because of the multifactorial nature of the disease there is no rule to day
2013	Chen e Lowe	OSA x FA	Literature review		Are effective but lack methods for real evidence
2012	Villa, Miano e Rizzoli	OSA x FA x tonsillectomy	Literature review		Both methods are effective but the FA seems to be more efficient
2012	Pliska e Almeida	OSA x x FA treatment	Literature review		FA are the first choice for mild to moderate OSA for effectiveness
2013	Tapia e Marcus	OSA x Obesity and risk	Literature review		Obese child remains with OSA, and new hair salon should be applied
2001	Guilleminault e Quo	OSA x FA	Literature review		Importance of dentists and orthodontists for treatment options

1990	Guilleminault e Stoohs	OSA HS x x B x PSG	Literature review		Importance of recognizing and treating these diseases
2015	Huynh et al.	OSA x FA x ERM	Systematc review		Without consistens results
2007	Carvalho et al.	OSA x FA	Systematic review		No enough evidence in the treatment of OSA with FA

Table 1: First selection.

A second selection was made, only including studies which are related to OSA with FA and Orthodontics. Articles dealing with OSA and other diseases as OSA and weight, OSA and rapid maxillary expansion, Osa and surgical treatments, OSA and diagnosis, were excluded, so were obtained 13 specific studies on this subject but, only 8 of them were eligible by level of evidence [66]. Some review and clinical studies that dealt with OSA and other variants which were excluded from the systematic review but some helped to explain the matter. These articles were citaded in the introduction of the study. The search methodology, is illustrated in the Figure 1.

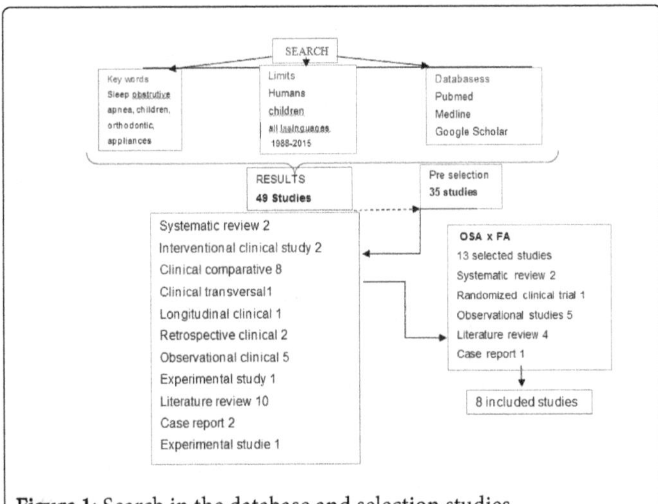

Figure 1: Search in the database and selection studies.

Results

Eight studies addressed to FA impact in the treatment of OSA, but the results, could not answer yet the question whether the use of the device type can improve OSA. These studies were listed below by chronological order and methodologically summarized in Table 2.

Selected Studies- Chronological order

Villa et al. [47], evaluated the clinical use and tolerance of FA for OSA treatment in 32 children at an average age of 7.1 ± 2.6 years, 20 boys and 12 girls who had OSA symptoms an AHI>1 event per hour and malocclusion. Randomly were selected 19 patients (SG) with AHI=6, which used the FA and the remaining patients formed the CG. After the treatment, the polysomnography exam showed the SG achieved a significant decrease in the AHI compared to the same index at the treatment beginning, and the CG showed no change. Clinical symptoms examination before and after the appliance use showed that 7 of the 14 subjects, had reduced 2 points in the score of respiratory symptoms, and 7 had solved the main complaints of respiratory symptoms compared to the CG which continued with baseline symptoms. Therefore, they concluded the treatment of OSA with FA is effective and well tolerated.

Cozza et al. [51], in a comparative clinical study evaluated 20 children (10 boys and 10 girls) aged between 4 and 8 years with OSA and 20 control children (10 boys and 10 girls) aged 5 and 7 years without OSA to determine the differences between groups and check the FA effects with PSG and cephalometric. Anatomic differences statistically significant were detected among CG and SG. Polysomnography was repeated after six months in the group with OSA, having noticed that the use of FA, promoted a statistically significant reduction in AHI (P=0.0003). The use of the device reduced daytime sleepiness and subjectively improved sleep quality. Parents and patients reported good cooperation in dealing with intra-oral appliance.

Year	Author	Subject	Evidence	N	Conclusion
2007	Carvalho et al [48]	OSA x FA	Systematic review		There are insufficient evidence in the OSA treatment with FA
2015	Huynh et al. [65]	OSA x FA x ERM	Systematic review, metan		Only 6 studied for meta-analysis and no definitive results
2002	Villa MP et al. [47]	OSA x FA X tolerance X results	Clinical Controlled rdz	32	FA SG had reduction of OSA and well toletou the device
2011	Godt et al. [44]	OSA x FA x cephalog x HG	Clinical observational	209	There was no significant change in UA in the 3 SG
2011	Kizinger et al. [42]	OSA x FA x UA x Cephalom	Clinical retrospective c	43	Ortodontic appliances not improve OSA and cephalometric does not evaluate UA

2011	Van Holsbeke et al. [64]	OSAx FA x 3D x resistenc UA	Clinical comparative	143	Women respond better to the OSA treatment
2004	Cozza et al. [51]	OSA x FA x GC	Clinical comparative	20	dDfferences between groups were big and FA improved disease
2014	Iwasaki et al. [60]	OSA x Fax fixed x Herbst	Clinical comparative	24	Herbst increased UA in patients with OSA
Excluded					
2006	Rose e Schessl	OSA x FA x Frankel II	Case report	2	Success of FA in OSA treatment
2001	Guilleminault e Quo	OSA e FA	Literature review		Importance of dentists and orthodontists for treatment options
2013	Chen e Lowe	OSA e FA	Literature review		Are effective but lack methods for real evidence
2012	Pliska e Almeida	OSA x FA x treat	Literature review		FA are the first choice for mild to moderate OSA
2012	Villa et al.	OSA x FA x surgery	Literature review		Both methods are effective but FA seems to be more efficient

Table 2: Evidence vased included studies (OSA e FA).

Carvalho et al. [48], through a systematic review investigated the effectiveness of treatment of OSA in children with FA. Randomized studies were selected and do not have randomized trials comparing all types of orthopedic devices with placebos or not, in children at 15 years old. They demonstrated through the results the improvement in the AHI, in the dento skeletal relations, sleep parameters, cognitive and speech, behavioral problems, quality of life, side effects, and economic and social aspects. Therefore, the authors concluded that there is no evidence enough to confirm the effectiveness of the devices for sleep disorders. The devices improve the craniofacial characteristics of children who have risk factors for OSA but there is no way to prove these.

Godt et al. [44] investigated the width of the upper airway in different facial patterns and changes during the various treatments including FA for Class II. They used cephalograms before and after the three treatment modalities (headgear, FA and bite jumping). Little increase in UA was observed around the vertical level during the treatment, and they concluded that no significant changes occurred in those segments during treatment. In addition, with headgear, the UA size decreased.

Van Holsbeke et al. [64] conducted a study with 143 patients with OSA, who used FA. CT scans were performed with minimal radiation dose before and after placement of the apparatus and the changes were verified using a bite simulator able to show resistance change in the UA. They demonstrated that ideal patients for the success were women with small UA and high early strength.

Kizinger et al. [42] in a retrospective cephalometric study found that the two forms of fixed functional appliances to correct Class II (Herbst and FA) influenced the morphology of the UA. The sample consisted of 43 patients, 18 patients used the FA and 25 used the conventional Herbst (fix FA). Measures of cephalometric analyzes were verified and compared in two times. Both devices had similar effects. They concluded that treatment with FA cannot prevent the risk of OSA although studies cephalogram are not able to measure the depth of the upper airways.

Iwasaki et al. [60], in a clinical study, observed a sample of 24 patients of Angle class II, who opted for Edwise fixed therapy compared to a group that used Herbst Fixed FA. The three dimensions of the oropharynx through CT scans, were verified in 11 children at mean age of 11.6 years old, who had already taken 3D Cone Beam before and after Herbst´s therapy. The CG was obtained in a sample of 20 patients Angle Class I, who opted for treatment with fixed orthodontic and had the same tests. The group opted for the Herbst´s appliance (SG) found a significant increase in the volume of the upper UA compared to CG.

Huynh, et al. [65] conducted a systematic review and meta-analysis to check the effectiveness of orthodontic appliances in the treatment of OSA in children and adolescents. Eligible studies were investigated in Pubmed, Medline, Embase, and Internet published until April 2014 were identified, in a total of 58 studies. Only eight studies were included in the review. Among these, six were included in the meta-analysis. The search yielded only a small number of studies. Consequently, any findings of diagnostic parameters grouped and their interpretation should be treated carefully (Table 2). The researches in which patients used FA, presented clinical positive results but not statistical results. The results showed decreasing or disappearance of the OSA symptoms and also an improvement of the clinical outcome regarding craniofacial deformities caused by the sleep respiratory disorder [6,48,49,62,63,65].

Discussion

OSA has a negative impact on child growth, affecting their quality of life. If the condition persists, it may affects the quality of life in their adulthood [1-1,15,35-38]. Tonsil hypertrophy is considered the leading cause of OSA [1-11,13,23,27,30]and tonsillar removal is the optional treatment [3,5,6,9,10,27- 29,31-34]. Common diseases such as oral breathing and primary snoring are related to OSA and if there is an association with craniofacial abnormalities, this may lead to the recurrence of the OSA after adenotonsillectomy [23,24,32-34,39,44,45,63]. The literature showed the most frequent complaints of patients with OSA were PS and troubled sleep. Allergic rhinitis RA was the most frequent comorbidity accompanying OSA, followed by hypertrophy of the tonsils [1,2,4,8,11,20,26,29]. The most severe apnea indexes were found in younger children, and African descendants had a higher prevalence of the disease [9]. One study [33] reported that the tonsillectomy surgery was effective for the treatment of OSA in a group of children aged between 3 to 6 years old, who returned to a normal growth pattern. On the other hand, other studies reported that adolescents aged between 11 and 14 years old, continued with OB after the removal of the tonsils, presented the worst AHI and reduction of UA lumen [5,6,9,10,29,34]. The causal effect between tonsil hypertrophy and OSA has not been established yet [40,45].

Treatments for persistent apnea are not completely known yet. Treatment approaches must be better evaluated [10,11]. Anti-inflammatory therapies, masks for ventilation and oral appliances are offered to the treatment of recurrent OSA but the disease remains a challenge due to its multifactorial nature [1-3,11,39,48,63,65]. Some authors consider as the best form of clinical treatment of OSA the use of CPAP or BPAP but such treatment does not get a good patients cooperation and the discontinuance is large [26,27,39,40,41].

Two reports of clinical case studies demonstrated OSA improvement with the use of FA [49,50]. In both studies, high AHI were reported, but the patients did not have tonsillar hypertrophy and craniofacial deformities were treated with FA. The treatment improved the OSA and normalized the craniofacial deformities. Reports of clinical cases do not represent a high level of evidence and do not show statistical significance, but can be considered a warning about the clinical need of new approaches. Isolated cases, out of average, should be considered for further investigation. Early intervention of the orthodontist with FA in patients with disorders of the craniofacial structures in cooperation with other specialists should be considered [26,27]. The FA promotes an increase in mandibular growth and permanently changes in the craniofacial structure, facilitating the breathing mode and preventing obstructions of the UA. [42]Orthodontists are professionals trained to recognize and treat OSA with FA in patients with craniofacial anomalies [5,6,15,25,28] promoting a harmonious facial growth and avoid aggressive surgery in adulthood and cardiovascular comorbidities resulting from sleep disorders [16,41,42,62].

The FA are simple, silent, well tolerated and effective, but some challenges still remain, as the need for monthly monitoring by the professional for more than twelve months, which may discourage the patient[43-66]. Studies have shown that the use of FA can eliminate or reduce the symptoms of the OSA, promoting a better long-term quality of life [35-38]. The PSG tests have been considered the gold standard in OSA diagnosis. Perhaps due to the difficulty in performing these exams, by of the lack of specialized centers and the high cost, making most of the clinical researches outcomes were not investigated with this exam. Some of the studies were not able to include enough patients for an statistical result maybe because of the difficulty of suitable sample allocation in the inclusion criteria [5,6,14,42-50,52,59-65].

Some researchers used 2D image parameters to check UA [42,44,51] and did not obtain reliable results. Few studies included patients monitored with polysomnography [42,44,47] and were not able to report improvement of OSA based on AHI parameters.

The difficulty in assessing the results of the studies was due to the differences in the used methodologies. The different investigated devices and patient maturity were not homogeneous, creating difficulties in the methodological comparisons. Many of them, showed positive results in the improve of OSA with FA but the parameters used to measure the effectiveness were not similar and acceptable [42,44,47,51,60,64]. A recent study of systematic review [65] evaluated several types of orthodontic therapy, and did not answer the purpose of our research. Due to the difficulty of conducting well-designed studies with samples and suitable tests for good results, there is no strong evidence that FA is indeed effective in the treatment of obstructive sleep apnea in children.

Conclusion

This systematic literature review showed that orthopedic devices seem to be a good treatment option for children with OSA. Although the level of evidence of the effectiveness of these devices is weak to moderate, as there are no randomized controlled clinical studies that support this hypothesis (H0), but either do not reject it. There is still need for more well designed controlled research, with large enough case series in order to accurately obtain the answer.

References

1. Pignatari SSN, Pereira FC, Avelino MAG, Fujita RR (2002) Noções gerais sobre a síndrome da apnéia e da hipopnéia obstrutiva do sono em crianças e o papel da polissonografia.Tratado de Otorrinolaringologia. (1stedn), São Paulo, Brazil, South America.
2. Ramos RTT, Daltro, CHDC, Gregório (2006) em crianças: perfil clínico e respiratório polissonográfico. Rev Bras Otorrinolaringol 72.
3. Rosen CL (2004) Obstructive sleep apnea syndrome in children: controversies in diagnosis and treatment. Pediatr Clin North Am 51: 153-167, vii.
4. Powell S, Kubba H, O'Brien C, Tremlett M (2010) Paediatric obstructive sleep apnoea. BMJ 340: c1918.
5. Guilleminault C, Stoohs R (1990) Chronic snoring and obstructive sleep apnea syndrome in children. Lung 168 Suppl: 912-919.
6. Guilleminault C, Quo SD (2001) Sleep-disordered breathing. A view at the beginning of the new Millennium. Dent Clin North Am 45: 643-656.
7. Marcus CL (2001) Sleep-disordered breathing in children. Am J Respir Crit Care Med 164: 16-30.
8. Gregório PB, Athanazio RA, Bitencourt AG, Neves FB, Terse R, et al. (2008) [Symptoms of obstructive sleep apnea-hypopnea syndrome in children]. J Bras Pneumol 34: 356-361.
9. American Academy of Pediatrics (AAP). (2002) Subcommittee on Obstructive Sleep Apnea Syndrome. Clinical practice guideline: diagnosis and management of childhood obstructive sleep apnea syndrome. Pediatrics 109: 704-712.
10. Nixon GM, Brouillette RT (2005) Sleep . 8: paediatric obstructive sleep apnoea. Thorax 60: 511-516.
11. Gozal D, Kheirandish-Gozal L (2006) Sleep apnea in children--treatment considerations. J Orofac Orthop. 67: 58-67.
12. Wise MS, Nichols CD, Grigg-Damberger MM, Marcus CL, Witmans MB, et al. (2011) Executive summary of respiratory indications for polysomnography in children: an evidence-based review. Sleep 34: 389-398AW.
13. Avelino MA, Pereira FC, Carlini D, Moreira GA, Fujita R, et al. (2002) Avaliação polissonográfica da síndrome da apnéia obstrutiva do sono em crianças, antes e após adenoamigdatomia. Rev Bras Otorrinolaringol 68: 308-311.
14. Iwasaki T, Saitoh I, Takemoto Y, Inada E, Kanomi R, et al. (2011) Evaluation of upper airway obstruction in Class II children with fluid-mechanical simulation. Am J Orthod Dentofacial Orthop 139: e135-145.
15. Weber SA, Montovani JC, Matsubara B, Fioretto JR (2007) Echocardiographic abnormalities in children with obstructive breathing disorders during sleep. J Pediatr (Rio J) 83: 518-522.
16. Mello Junior CF, Guimarães Filho HA, de Brito Gomes CA, de Amorim Paiva CC (2013) Achados radiológicos em pacientes portadores de apneia obstrutiva do sono. Jornal Brasileiro de Pneumologia 39(1).
17. Vos W, De Backer J, Devolder A, Vanderveken O, Verhulst S, et al. (2007) Correlation between severity of sleep apnea and upper airway morphology based on advanced anatomical and functional imaging. J Biomech 40: 2207-2213.

18. Aboudara C, Nielsen IB, Huang J C, Maki K, Miller AJ, et al. (2009) Comparison of airway space with conventional lateral headfilms and 3-dimensional reconstruction from cone-beam computed tomography. American Journal of Orthodontics and Dentofacial Orthopedics 135: 468-479.

19. Moraes de MEL, Hollender LG, Chen (2011) Evaluating craniofacial asymmetry with digital cephalometric images and cone-beam computed tomography. American Journal of Orthodontics and Dentofacial Orthopedics 139: 523-531.

20. Schendel SA, Hatcher D (2010) Automated 3-dimensional airway analysis from cone-beam computed tomography data. J Oral Maxillofac Surg 68: 696-701.

21. Zinsly SDR, Moraes LCD, Moura PD, Ursi W (2015) Assessment of pharyngeal airway space using Cone-Beam Computed Tomography. Dental Press Journal of Orthodontics 15: 150-158.

22. El H, Palomo JM (2010) Measuring the airway in 3 dimensions: a reliability and accuracy study. Am J Orthod Dentofacial Orthop 137: S50.

23. Abramson Z, Susarla S, August M, Troulis M, Kaban L (2010) Three-dimensional computed tomographic analysis of airway anatomy in patients with obstructive sleep apnea. J Oral 68: 354-362.

24. Kapila S, Conley RS, Harrell Jr WE (2011) The current status of cone beam computed tomography imaging in orthodontics. DentomaxillofaciaRadiology 40: 24-34.

25. Ianni DF, Bertolini MM, Lopes ML (2006) Contribuição multidisciplinar no diagnóstico e no tratamento das obstruções da nasofaringe e da respiração bucal R Clin Ortodon Dental Press 4: 90-102.

26. Capua M, Ahmadi N, Shapiro C (2009) Overview of obstructive sleep apnea in children: exploring the role of dentists in diagnosis and treatment. J Can Dent Assoc 75: 285-289.

27. Tapia IE, Marcus CL (2013) Newer treatment modalities for pediatric obstructive sleep apnea. Paediatr Respir Rev 14: 199-203.

28. Mora R, Salami A, Passali FM, Mora F, Cordone MP, et al. (2003) OSAS in children. Int J Pediatr Otorhinolaryngol 67 Suppl 1: S229-231.

29. Ferguson KA, Cartwright R, Rogers R, Schmidt-Nowara W (2006) Oral appliances for snoring and obstructive sleep apnea: a review. Sleep 29: 244-262.

30. Vieira FMJ, Diniz F (2003) Hemorragia na adenoidectomia e/ou amigdalectomia: estudo de 359 casos. Rev bras Otorrinolaringol 69: 338-341.

31. Samuel C Leong Sujata De (2010) Changing trends of adeno-tonsillectomy for paediatric obstructive sleep apnoea. BMJ.

32. Morton S, Rosen C, Larkin E, Tishler P, Aylor J, et al. (2001) Predictors of sleep-disordered breathing in children with a history of tonsillectomy and/or adenoidectomy. Sleep 24: 823-829.

33. Mattar SE, Valera FC, Faria G, Matsumoto MA, Anselmo-Lima WT (2011) Changes in facial morphology after adenotonsillectomy in mouth-breathing children. International Journal of Paediatric Dentistry 21: 389-396.

34. Shott SR (2011) Evaluation and management of pediatric obstructive sleep apnea beyond tonsillectomy and adenoidectomy. Curr Opin Otolaryngol Head Neck Surg 19: 449-454.

35. Goldstein NA, Fatima M, Campbell TF, Rosenfeld RM (2002) Child behavior and quality of life before and after tonsillectomy and adenoidectomy. Arch Otolaryngol Head Neck Surg 128: 770-775.

36. Eckenhoff JE (1953) Relationship of anesthesia to postoperative personality changes in children. AMA Am J Dis Child 86: 587-591.

37. Silva VC, Leite AJ (2006) Quality of life in children with sleep-disordered breathing: evaluation by OSA-18. Braz J Otorhinolaryngol 72: 747-756.

38. Gomes Ade M, Santos OM, Pimentel K, Marambaia PP, Gomes LM, et al. (2012) Quality of life in children with sleep-disordered breathing. Braz J Otorhinolaryngol 78: 12-21.

39. Marcus CL, Rosen G, Ward SL, Halbower AC, Sterni L, et al. (2006) Adherence to and effectiveness of positive airway pressure therapy in children with obstructive sleep apnea. Pediatrics 117: e442-451.

40. Balbani AP, Weber SA, Montovani JC (2005) Update in obstructive sleep apnea syndrome in children. Braz J Otorhinolaryngol 71: 74-80.

41. Cheng MC, Enlow DH, Papsidero M, Broadbent BH Jr, Oyen O, et al. (1988) Developmental effects of impaired breathing in the face of the growing child. Angle Orthod 58: 309-320.

42. Kinzinger G, Czapka K, Ludwig B, Glasl B, Gross U, et al. (2011) Effects of fixed appliances in correcting Angle Class II on the depth of the posterior airway space: FMA vs. Herbst appliance: a retrospective cephalometric study. J Orofac Orthop.72: 301-320.

43. Guilleminault C, Huang YS, Quo S, Monteyrol PJ, Lin CH (2013) Teenage sleep-disordered breathing: recurrence of syndrome. Sleep Med 14: 37-44.

44. Godt A, Koos B, Hagen H, Göz G (2011) Changes in upper airway width associated with Class II treatments (headgear vs activator) and different growth patterns. Angle Orthod 81: 440-446.

45. Rossi RC, Rossi NJ, Rossi NJ, Yamashita HK, Pignatari SS (2015) Dentofacial characteristics of oral breathers in different ages: a retrospective case-control study. Prog Orthod 16: 23.

46. Schütz TC, Dominguez GC, Hallinan MP, Cunha TC, Tufik S (2011) Class II correction improves nocturnal breathing in adolescents. Angle Orthod 81: 222-228.

47. Villa MP, Bernkopf E, Pagani J, Broia V, Montesano M, et al. (2002) Randomized controlled study of an oral jaw-positioning appliance for the treatment of obstructive sleep apnea in children with malocclusion. Am J Respir Crit Care Med 165: 123-127.

48. Carvalho FR, Lentini-Oliveira D, Machado MA, Prado GF, Prado LB, et al. (2007) Oral appliances and functional orthopaedic appliances for obstructive sleep apnoea in children. Cochrane Database Syst Rev : CD005520.

49. Rose E, Schessl J (2007) Orthodontic procedures in the treatment of obstructive sleep apnea in children. Paediatr Respir Rev 7: S58-61.

50. Horihata A, Ueda H, Koh M, Watanabe G, Tanne K (2013) Enhanced increase in pharyngeal airway size in Japanese class II children following a 1-year treatment with an activator appliance. Int J Orthod Milwaukee 24: 35-40.

51. Cozza P, Polimeni A, Ballanti F (2004) A modified monobloc for the treatment of obstructive sleep apnoea in paediatric patients. Eur J Orthod 26: 523-530.

52. Cozza P, Baccetti T, Franchi L, De Toffol L, McNamara JA Jr (2006) Mandibular changes produced by functional appliances in Class II malocclusion: a systematic review. Am J Orthod Dentofacial Orthop 129: 599.

53. Baccetti T, Franchi L (2001) The Fourth Dimension in Dentofacial Orthopedics: Treatment Timing for Class II and Class III Malocclusions. World Journal of Orthodontics 2: 159-167

54. Rossi RC, Rossi NJ, Rossi NCJ, Pignatari SSN (2015) Effects of the Rossi activator over Class II treatment of pre-adolescent patients – randomized controlled trial Ortho Scienc 30: 173-179.

55. Rossi NJ (1993) The Rossi orthopedic appliance: model preparation and appliance construction. Funct Orthod 10: 22-24, 26-9.

56. Rossi NJ, Rossi RC (1996) Indication of the Rossi orthopedic appliance: a case study. Funct Orthod 13: 36-40.

57. Rossi NJ, Rossi RC (1988) Ortopedia funcional integrada à ortodontia corretiva. São Paulo:Editora Pancast.

58. Fox NA (2007) Insufficient evidence to confirm effectiveness of oral appliances in treatment of obstructive sleep apnoea syndrome in children. Evid Based Dent 8: 84.

59. Ghodke S, Utreja AK, Singh SP, Jena AK (2014) Effects of twin-block appliance on the anatomy of pharyngeal airway passage (PAP) in class II malocclusion subjects. Prog Orthod 15: 68.

60. Iwasaki T, Takemoto Y, Inada E, Sato H, Saitoh I, et al. (2014) Three-dimensional cone-beam computed tomography analysis of enlargement of the pharyngeal airway by the Herbst appliance. Am J Orthod Dentofacial Orthop 146: 776-785.

61. Hänggi MP, Teuscher UM, Roos M, Peltomäki TA (2008) Long-term changes in pharyngeal airway dimensions following activator-headgear and fixed appliance treatment. Eur J Orthod 30: 598-605.

62. Pliska BT, Almeida F (2012) Effectiveness and outcome of oral appliance therapy. Dent Clin North Am 56: 433-444.

63. Villa MP, Milano S, Rizzoli A (2012) Mandibular advancement devices are an alternative and valid treatment for pediatric obstructive sleep apnea syndrome. Sleep Breath. 16: 971-976.

64. Van Holsbeke C, De Backer J, Vos W, Verdonck P, Van Ransbeeck P, et al. (2011) Anatomical and functional changes in the upper airways of sleep apnea patients due to mandibular repositioning: a large scale study. J Biomech 44: 442-449.

65. Huynh NT, Desplats E, Almeida FR (2015) Orthodontics treatments for managing obstructive sleep apnea syndrome in children: A systematic review and meta-analysis. Sleep Med Rev.

66. Sackett DL (2000) Evidence-based medicine. John Wiley & Sons, Ltd., USA.

Giant Cystic Parathyroid Adenoma Masquerading as a Retropharyngeal Abscess

Diom ES[1]*, Fagan JJ[2] and Dhirendra Govender[3]

[1]*Otolaryngologist, Dakar, Senegal*
[2]*Professor and Chairman, Division of Otolaryngology, University of Cape Town, Cape Town, South Africa*
[3]*Professor and Chairman, Division of Anatomical Pathology University of Cape Town, Cape Town, South Africa*

Abstract

Objective: A case report of a retropharyngeal cystic parathyroid adenoma and a review of its embryology, differential diagnosis and management are presented.

Material and Method: A 34-year-old woman presented with a 2-year history of a right-sided discrete, cystic, submucosal cervical mass displacing the oropharynx anteriorly. MRI showed a large, cystic hyperdense mass occupying the parapharyngeal and retropharyngeal spaces. Surgical resection revealed a right-sided multinodular neck mass originating from the thyroid gland and extending along the prevertebral space and towards the contralateral neck, displacing the pharynx and larynx. Histology was consistent with a cystic parathyroidadenoma.

Discussion: Cystic parathyroid adenoma has rarely been reported and may mimic a retropharyngeal abscess. The unusual location of parathyroid tissue can be explained by its origin from ectopic superior parathyroid glands or tumor extension from parathyroid glands intothe retropharyngeal space.

Conclusion: The differential diagnosis of a retropharyngeal mass should include parathyroid tumours.

Keywords: Parathyroid adenoma; Ectopic parathyroid; Retropharyngeal space; Retropharyngeal abscess

Introduction

Cysts of the parathyroid glands are uncommon and account for <0.001% of neck masses [1]; less than 200 cases of cystic parathyroid adenomas have been reported [2,3]. The diagnosis is therefore unlikely to be consideredand islikely to be confused with a retropharyngeal abscess. We report a case of a giant retropharyngeal cystic parathyroid adenoma and review the pathophysiology and management of this unusual condition.

Clinical Case

A 34-year-old female presented with a 2-year history of discomfort and a foreign body-like sensation in the throat. There was no history of dysphagia or dyspnoea. Palpation revealed a non-tender right-sided neck mass which was discrete, moved with swallowing, and had normal overlying skin. A diffuse, fluctuant retropharyngeal masscovered by a healthy, non-ulcerated mucosa displaced the posterior wall of the oropharynx anteriorly. Aspiration yielded 120 ml of thick, sticky, chocolate-brown fluid following which there was partial resolution of the mass. Bacteriological and cytologic examinations of the fluid were unremarkable.

Six weeks later the patient represented with discomfortand partial obstruction of the oropharynx due to recurrence of the retropharyngeal mass. MRI revealed a large; hyperdense cystic mass occupying the right parapharyngeal and retropharyngeal spaces with significant mass effect whichdisplaced the larynx and pharynx anteriorly (Figures 1a and b).

Transcervical surgical exploration yielded a slightly vascular, thinly encapsulated,nodular mass. It measured10cm in length and was situated behind the visceral compartment of the neck i.e. behind the trachea and esophagus. It involved the right lobe of the thyroid, and extended superiorly along the prevertebral space. A right thyroid lobectomy was done without difficulty, with delivery of the superior pole of the tumor by finger dissection. Histological examination of the surgical specimen was consistent with a cysticparathyroid adenoma. Macroscopic examination of the surgical specimen showed an encapsulated multiloculated cystic lesion with focal solid areas and adjacent thyroid tissue. Histological examination confirmed an encapsulated lesion composed predominantly of a cystic component with peripheral solid areas.The solid areas consisted of sheets, nests, and cords of regular cells with pale granular cytoplasm and regular round nuclei (Figure 2a). In addition, focal microscopic nodules of larger cells with water clear cytoplasm were present. Mitotic figures and necrosis was not seen. Some of the solid sheets and islands showed central cystic degeneration (Figure 2b). The large cyst was lined by similar regular small cells (Figure 2c). There was evidence of recent and old haemorrhage. Adjacent thyroid tissue was present. The histopathological features were those of a cystic parathyroid adenoma.

Discussion

Astriking feature of this parathyroid mass was its extension to the retropharynx. The retropharyngeal space is a virtual space comprising fat and lymphoid elements. It is more commonly the seat of infections such as retropharyngeal abscesses, including cervical Pott's disease (tuberculosis), or tumors lymphoma, or lymph node metastases from papillary and anaplastic cancers of the thyroid [4]. Causes of retropharyngeal cysts are listed in Table 1 [5,6].

Non-functioning parathyroid adenomassuch as was found in our

***Corresponding author:** Evelyne SigaDiom, Otolaryngologist, Dakar, Senegal; E-mail: evelynediom@yahoo.com

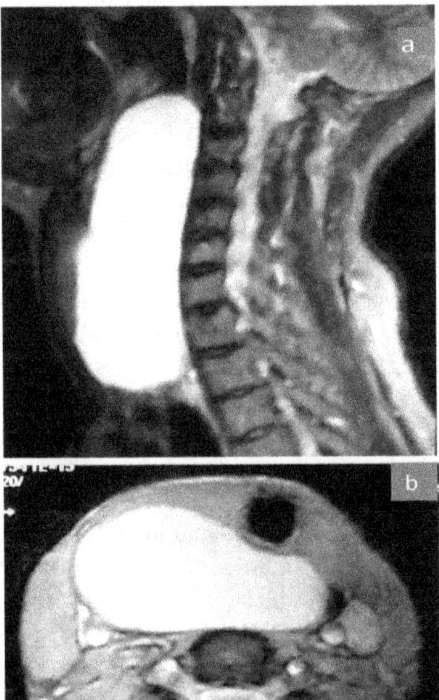

Figure 1a,b: Sagittal and axial (T1) MRI scans demonstrating a hyperdense neck mass located in the retropharyngeal space and having a mass effect on the trachea which is deviated to the left.

case are very rare; hypotheses found in the literature include:

- Tissue necrosis secondary to cystic degeneration
- "Autoparathyroidectomy" or "parathyroid apoplexy" caused by haemorrhage and infarction; this has to be supported by histopathological evidence of necrosis and degeneration of the adenoma. Generally the haemorrhage is spontaneous [7,8], but may be provoked by multiple needle punctures
- Pressure from ahaematoma causing ischaemia [9,10]
- Rapid growth leading to vascular insufficiency and infarction [11]
- Parathyroid Hormone (PTH) secreted into the lumen of the cyst instead of into the blood stream

The parathyroid cyst in our case is likely to have originated from an ectopic parathyroid gland located either within the retropharynx or intrathyroidally, or may have represented an extension of a large tumour of a normally situated parathyroid gland. Ectopic superior parathyroids are uncommon (1%) and may be found in the posterior neck, retropharyngeal and retroesophageal spaces and intrathyroidally [4,12]. The superior parathyroid glands originate from the 4th pharyngeal pouch. They adhere to the posterior surface of the caudally migrating thyroid. As the larger thymus and thyroid gland migrate from the upper neck into the lower neck and upper chest, they carry the "small passenger" parathyroids with them. The superior parathyroid glands have a much shorter distance to migrate than the inferior parathyroids; this might account for their more predictable location. The superior parathyroids are usually found posteriorly at the level of the upper two thirds of the thyroid gland, about 1 cm above the point where the Recurrent Laryngeal Nerve (RLN) crosses the inferior

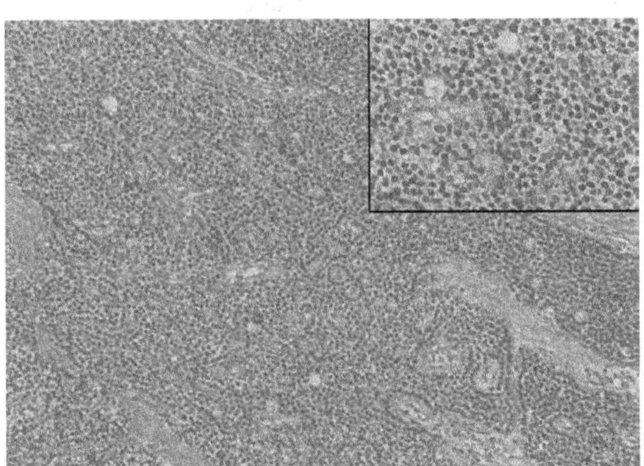

Figure 2a: Sheets of regular small cells with pseudorosettes, inset shows uniform small cells with minimal pale granular cytoplasm.

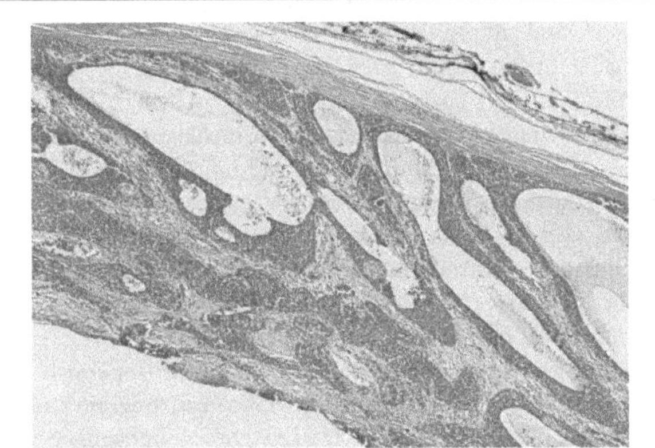

Figure 2b: Nests and islands of neoplastic cells with central cystic degeneration.

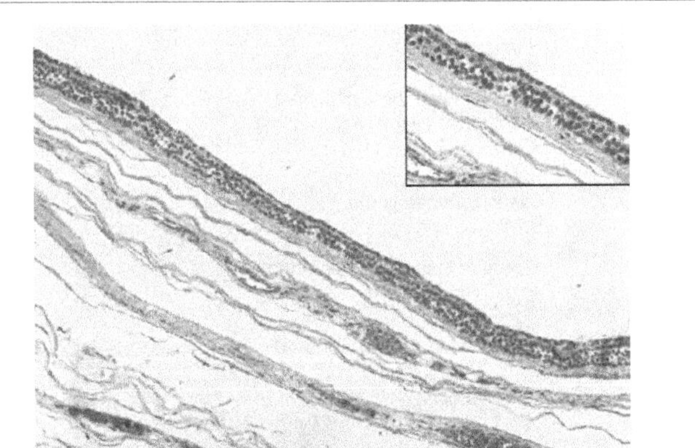

Figure 2c: The large multilocular cyst was lined by 2 to 5 layers of uniform small cells, inset confirms the uniformity of the cells and their similarity to the solid sheets.

thyroid artery and are embryologically and anatomically closely related to the Tubercle of Zuckerkandl. The superior parathyroid gland may be trapped within the thyroid parenchyma; this would explain why intrathyroid ectopic superior parathyroids account for 5% of ectopic parathyroids [4,13,14]. In our case, a nodular enlargement of the right thyroid lobe was discovered during surgical exploration and was the reason for doing a right hemithyroidectomy (Figure 2). The pathologists did not indicate the presence or absence of a parathyroid capsule; hence it is not possible to state unequivocally whether it was indeed an intrathyroidal parathyroid adenoma. Other pathological locations of ectopic parathyroid tissue have been reported i.e. posterior mediastinum [15], retrosternally in the anterior mediastinum within the thymus, in the carotid sheath, in the vagus nerve, the pericardium and also in the retrotracheal space [10,15]. Miller et al. [9] also described ectopic parathyroid glands located submucosallyinthe piriform sinus. He reported that in 1200 cervical explorations of parathyroid glands done over 58 years, 0.08%was situated in retropharyngeal space. An embryological explanation is the failure of the superior parathyroid gland to separate from the piriform sinus during its transcervical migration. According to Foroulis and Somparaoesophageal or retro-oesophageal parathyroid tumours originating from the superior parathyroid gland should embryologically have a normal blood supply from a branch of inferior thyroid artery [15,16].

Knowledge of the anatomical spaces of the neck is needed to understand the pathophysiology of retropharyngeal extension of parathyroidand thyroid tumours [16,17]. The pretracheal, retro-oesophageal and retropharyngeal spaces are a continuum [1,3]; this explains the extension of a large retropharyngeal thyroid or parathyroid into these spaces. Tahim [18] reported a case of a cystic parathyroid adenoma that extended into the mediastinum. The thyroid compartment is located in the anterior and inferior parts of the neck and overlies the tracheal rings; the thyroidcapsule is formed by the deep layer of the deep cervical fascia or visceral layer of the pretracheal fascia and is limited posteriorly and laterally by the visceral and vascular axes of the neck respectfully. Anteriorly it is covered by strap muscles, which in turn arecovered by the middle layer of deep cervical fascia. The muscular layer of the pretracheal fascia is limited superiorly by the inferior edge of the hyoid bone.This visceral compartmentincludes the thyroid gland, parathyroid gland, trachea and oesophagus. Superior and anterior extension is hindered by the attachment of the pretracheal fascia to the hyoid bone. The retrovisceral space is a single virtual space that extends laterally around the larynx and trachea and joins pretracheal space. Itstretches from the base of the skull to the posterior mediastinum at the tracheal bifurcation. Behind the pharynx it is called the retropharyngeal space; behind the oesophagus it is called the retro-oesophageal space.

Inflammatory	Retropharyngeal abscess (bacterial) Pott's disease (tuberculosis) Hydatid cyst
Miscellaneous	Hemangioma Thyroid cyst Papillary carcinoma of thyroid Parathyroid cyst 3rdBranchial cyst [5] Ectopic thymus [6] Cystic lymphangioma Bronchogenic cysts

Table 1: Causes of retropharyngeal cysts.

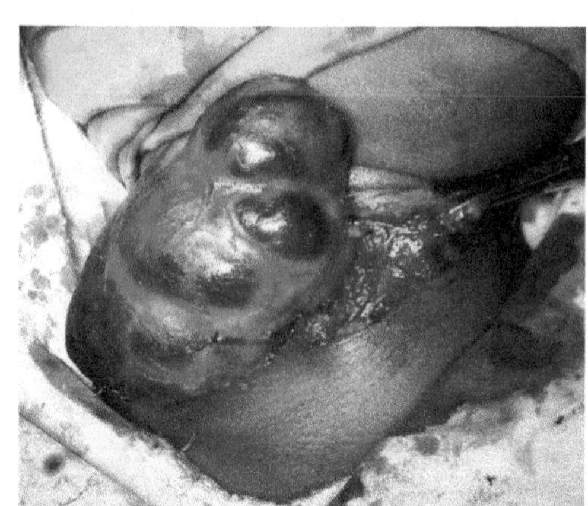

Figure 2: Intraoperative view of hemithyroidectomy. Note the multinodulargoitre. The upper pole of the thyroid was situated in the retropharyngeal space.

The clinical diagnosis of a cystic parathyroid adenoma is often missed especially when the parathyroid adenoma is non-functional as in our case [19]. Our patient presented with symptoms of dyspnoea following haemorrhage into a cervical cystic parathyroid adenoma, as has been previously described [8]. Other clinical signs associated with a cervical cystic parathyroid adenoma may include primary hyperparathyroidism [1,15], manifesting as hypercalcemia and even multiple organ failure; parathyroid crisis complicating hyperparathyroidism, also called acute hyperparathyroidism or parathyroid intoxication or parathyrotoxicosis are also reported in the literature [18]. Although it may be negative, Sestamibiscan is the gold standard for making a diagnosis of a parathyroidadenoma;CT and MRI are not 1st line investigations as their accuracy is too poor [9,20].

Conclusions

The diagnosis of a non-functional cystic parathyroid adenoma can be confusing especially when in a retropharyngeal position. Delimitations and connections between the neck spaces explain why such cases may be confused with other causesof retropharyngeal masses.PTH and calcium levels should be included in the diagnostic workup of cervical masses whenthe diagnosis is unclearin order to exclude parathyroid aetiology.

- Retropharyngeal cystic parathyroid adenomas can mimic a retropharyngeal abscess
- Cystic non-functional parathyroid adenomas are rare and may result for haemorrhage in a parathyroid gland and rapid growth of an adenoma
- Diagnostic workup of cervical masses of uncertain aetiology should include serum PTH and calcium levels to exclude parathyroid aetiology

Tc-sestamibiscintigraphy is the gold standard for diagnosing ectopic parathyroid adenomas

References

1. Asghar A, Ikram M, Islam N (2012) A case report: Giant cystic parathyroid adenoma presenting with parathyroid crisis after Vitamin D replacement. BMC Endocr Disord 12: 14.
2. Jha BC, Nagarkar NM, Kochhar S, Mohan H, Dass A (1999) Parathyroid cyst: a rare cause of an anterior neck mass. J Laryngol Otol 113: 73-75.
3. Davies ML, Middleton SB, Mellor SG (2002) Mistaken Identity: Cystic parathyroid adenoma masquerading as goitre. The Internet Journal of Surgery 3.
4. Lezrek M, Kabiri H, Al Bouzidi A, Sair K, Rachid K, et al. (1997) Glandeparathyroide intra-thyroidienne. Médecine Du Maghreb 62:61.
5. Huang RY, Damrose EJ, Alavi S, Maceri DR, Shapiro NL (2000) Third branchial cleft anomaly presenting as a retropharyngeal abscess. Int J Pediatr Otorhinolaryngol 54: 167-172.
6. Meyer E, Mulwafu W, Fagan JJ, Brown RA, Taylor K (2010) Ectopic thymic tissue presenting as a neck mass in children: a report of 3 cases. Ear Nose Throat J 89: 228-231.
7. Taniguchi I, Maeda T, Morimoto K, Miyasaka S, Suda T, et al. (2003)

Spontaneous retropharyngeal hematoma of a parathyroid cyst: report of a case. Surg Today 33: 354-357.

8. Shim WS, Kim IK, Yoo SD, Kim DH (2008) Non-functional parathyroid adenoma presenting as a massive cervical hematoma: a case report. Clin Exp Otorhinolaryngol 1: 46-48.

9. Miller DL, Craig W, Haine GA (1997) Retropharyngeal parathyroid adenoma: Precise preoperative localization with CT and arterial infusion of contrast material. Am J Roentgenol 169: 695-696.

10. Wang CA (1977) Parathyroid re-exploration. A clinical and pathological study of 112 cases. Ann Surg 186: 140-145.

11. Efremidou EI, Papageorgiou MS, Pavlidou E, Manolas KJ, Liratzopoulos N (2009) Parathyroid apoplexy, the explanation of spontaneous remission of primary hyperparathyroidism: a case report. Cases J 2: 6399.

12. Panieri E, Fagan JJ (2012) Parathyroidectomy: The Open Access Atlas of Otolaryngology, Head and Neck Operative Surgery.

13. Korukluoglu B, Kiyak G, Celik A et al. (2008) Our surgical approach to parathyroid adenoma and the role of localization studies. Turk Clin J Med Sci 28: 24-29.

14. Korukluoglu B, Ergul E, Yalcin S (2008) Giant intrathyroidal parathyroid cystic adenoma. J Pak Med Assoc 58: 592.

15. Foroulis CN, Rousogiannis S, Lioupis C, Koutarelos D, Kassi G, et al. (2004) Ectopic paraesophageal mediastinal parathyroid adenoma, a rare cause of acute pancreatitis. World J Surg Oncol 2: 41.

16. Som PM, Shugar JM (1991) Retropharyngeal mass as a rare presentation of a goiter: CT findings. J Comput Assist Tomogr 15: 823-825.

17. Shamim M (1978) Retropharyngeal goitre. J R Coll Surg Edinb 23: 367-368.

18. Tahim AS, Saunders J, Sinha P (2010) A parathyroid adenoma: benign disease presenting with hyper parathyroid crisis. Case Rep Med 2010: 596185.

19. Sekine O, Hozumi Y, Takemoto N, Kiyozaki H, Yamada S, et al. (2004) Parathyroid adenoma without hyperparathyroidism. Jpn J Clin Oncol 34: 155-158.

20. Wieneke JA, Smith A (2008) Parathyroid adenoma. Head Neck Pathol 2: 305-308.

Is Marriage a Risk Factor for Allergic Rhinitis?

Sara Safar AlShehri and Kamal-Eldin Ahmed Abou-Elhamd*

Department of ENT Surgery, College of Medicine, King Faisal University, Al-Ahsa, Saudi Arabia

***Corresponding author:** Kamal-Eldin Ahmed Abou-Elhamd, Doctorate Degree of ENT, Professor, Department of ENT Surgery, College of Medicine, King Faisal University, Al-Ahsa 31982, Box 400, Saudi Arabia; E-mail: kamal375@yahoo.com

Abstract

Objective: Our study aimed to determine the effect of marriage and sexual activity as risk factors for allergic rhinitis and to figure out degree of impact of consanguinity in the Saudi population on allergic rhinitis.

Study design: A cross sectional study.

Methods: The study was conducted at the outpatient ENT clinic of King Faisal University polyclinic centre at the period from October 2015 to February 2016. A random of 60 patients of age group 20-55 years old including both sex. The inclusive criteria were patients experienced symptoms related to out- door, indoor allergic rhinitis in the past 12 months. All of them were married and subjected to a questionnaire. It included 21 questions assessing symptoms of allergic rhinitis to verify the diagnosis, and its frequency and severity. It also included the marital details and patterns of consanguinity.

Results: Seven female patients (out of 24=29%) and 4 male ones (out of 25=16%) admitted experience of post coital exacerbation of allergic rhinitis attacks.

Conclusion: Marriage and sexual activity are risk factors for allergic rhinitis as 18% of our study experienced post coital exacerbation of allergic rhinitis attacks. However, vasomotor rhinitis might be a possible diagnosis if the patient age is above 35 with no family history of allergies.

Keywords: Allergic rhinitis; Allergy; Vasomotor rhinitis; Marriage; Sexual activity, Coital; Saudi arabia

Introduction

Allergic rhinitis is a chronic inflammatory disease characterized by recurrent attacks of nasal obstruction, nasal discharge and sneezing. It is hypersensitivity reaction type 1 with release of chemical mediators and cytokines on exposure to an allergen and is mediated by antibody IgE [1]. Several known link factors of allergic rhinitis have been documented. There is clear evidence to support the concept that allergic diseases are influenced by genetic predisposition and environmental exposure [2].

Vasomotor rhinitis is non-allergic rhinitis with symptoms and signs which are closely resemble those of allergic rhinitis and are difficult to differentiate from those resulting from allergy [3]. Its pathophysiology is unknown, and it is often classified as idiopathic rhinitis [4]. However, patients with symptoms onset later in life above age of 35 years, no family history of allergies and no seasonality have about 95% likelihood of having a physician diagnosis of non-allergic rhinitis and vasomotor if happens with exposure to a certain factor such as sexual activity [5].

The effect of marriage as an environmental stressor on exposure and exacerbation of AR is not well understood nor it is comprehensively studied, and thus, it needs more detailed research to study such correlation. Emotional stress and exercise were reported as stimuli for allergic rhinitis. Shah and Sircar in 1991 reported that sexual intercourse is a stimulus for AR too [6]. Post coital rhinitis can easily be overlooked due to patient embarrassment and unawareness of physicians. Sexual activity can trigger off asthma in more than one way.in some asthmatic subjects. Sexual excitement associated with anxiety can cause asthma as well as AR.

This has been recognized as post coital asthma and rhinitis and can occur in both males and females [6]. Falliers in 1976 described Sexercise-induced asthma as asthmatic episodes that cannot ascribed to any cause other than sexual excitement [7]. Intense emotional stimuli during sexual intercourse can lead to autonomic imbalance with parasympathetic over reactivity, thereby causing release of mast cell mediators that can provoke post coital rhinitis in these patients [8].

Earlier studies in psychosomatic medicine have linked type I on immunoglobulin E (IgE) mediated allergic disease as allergic rhinitis with psychological disturbance, particularly negative affecting states including depression and unhappy marriage [9]. An immune diversity of reactions may be encountered in female patients with hypersensitivity to seminal fluid (Human Seminal Plasma Allergy; HSPA). Bernstein et al. in 1981 reported disruption of maternal immune response during pregnancy, especially IgE specific suppresses T-cell [10].

1-Name written as a number: 2-Age .... 3-Sex: ☐ Male ☐ Female

4-Occupation.................................. 5-Residency: ☐ Urban ☐ Rural

6-Smoking: ☐ YES ☐ NO

7-Eduction level: ☐ Uneducated ☐ Elementary school ☐ Middle school ☐ High School ☐ Collage level or above

8-Family history of allergic rhinitis: ☐ YES ☐ NO

9-If the answer in previous question yes, which family side: ☐ Paternal ☐ Maternal

10- Pollen exposure or pet exposure: ☐ YES ☐ NO

11-Marrige: A-Duration.................B-Uses of oral contraceptive pills: ☐ YES ☐ NO

C-Consanguinity: ☐ YES ☐ NO E-Degree of relativity........................

12-Sleep time per night: ☐ <7 hours ☐ >7 hours

13-Stress level: ☐ NO stress ☐ Little stress ☐ Moderate stress ☐ Severe stress

14-Variation of symptoms: ☐ Seasonal ☐ All the year (perennial)

15-If it is seasonal in which season? ☐ Summer ☐ Atom ☐ Winter ☐ Spring

16-Timing of episodes of allergic rhinitis: ☐ Early morning ☐ Day time ☐ Evening

☐ Late night ☐ Post coital

17-Which month of the year most (you can chose more than one answer)

18-Persistence of symptoms per weeks ☐ <4 days ☐ >4 days

19-Persistence of symptoms ☐ <1 month ☐ >1month

20-Severity of symptoms: ☐ Mild ☐ Moderate to sever

21-Receiving medication: ☐ YES ☐ NO

If the answer in previous question yes is it: ☐ Regular ☐ On demand

Figure 1: Questionnaire.

As the consanguinity rate is very high in the Middle East countries, especially on Arab countries, it is highly important to investigate the morbidity patterns of allergic rhinitis in contagious marriages, and the extent, degree and pattern of the consanguinity in Saudi population suffering from atopic diseases like AR. It is of utmost importance to comprehend the correlation between contagious marriages and AR, for better management of such case, and to know the prevalence among male and female in Kingdom of Saudi Arabia.

So, our study aims to determine the effect of marriage as risk factor for allergic rhinitis, and to figure out the extent of consanguinity in the Saudi population and degree of impact on allergic rhinitis.

Material and Methods

Ethical consideration

The design of the study was approved by the Institutional Review Board of our institution

The study was conducted at the outpatient ENT clinic of King Faisal University polyclinic Center at the period from October 2015 to February 2016.

A random population based cross sectional study of 60 patients of age group 20-55 years old including both sex. The inclusive criteria were patients experienced symptoms related to out- door, indoor allergic rhinitis in the past 12 months. All of them were married and subjected to a questionnaire (Figure 1). It included 21 questions assessing symptoms of allergic rhinitis to verify the diagnosis, and its frequency and severity. It also included the marital details and patterns of consanguinity.

The data were collected anonymously and then results were analyzed statistically using SPSS Version 22. Chi-Square test was used.

Results

This study included 60 patients with age range (20-5) years. They were 31 females (51.7%) and 29 males (48.3%). Most of them had higher education (55=92%), employee (38=63%) and live in rural areas (48=80%). 17% of them were smokers and 18% usually expose to pollens. 48% have family history of allergic rhinitis in their parents. 70% sleep less than 7 h per day due to rhinitis. Most of the patients admitted having moderate stress in daily life (50%) and (23%) of them had little stress, while only (18%) were struggling with severe stress. 65% of our atopic patients experienced AR in special certain seasons, while 35% had AR all the months of the year. Table 1 shows seasons of affected patients. 35% of them have AR all the year.

	Frequency	Valid Percent
Valid Summer	8	13.3
Winter	11	18.3
Autumn	9	15
Spring	4	6.7
more options	7	11.7
All seasons	21	35
Total	60	100

Table 1: Numbers of affected patients per season.

Thirty-seven percent of our studied cases experienced allergic attacks in the early morning, followed by day time, followed by late night, then the least percent was for those who had it in the evening time (Table 2). Most of the affected patients (54%) had the frequency of attacks more than 4 days per week.

	Frequency	Valid Percent
Early Morning	22	36.7
day time	16	26.7
Evening	2	3.3
late night	4	6.7
more options	16	26.7
Total	60	100

Table 2: Time of attacks of allergic rhinitis per day.

Marriage and allergic rhinitis (Table 3)

The sixty patients were married for a period ranging from (1 month-38 years), third of them were relatives (35%). Only 10 females out of 31 used to take oral contraceptive pills (OCP) as a method of contraception. Seven female patients and 4 male ones admitted experience of post coital exacerbation of allergic rhinitis attacks (age of most of them less than 35 and family history of allergy, so possibility of allergic rhinitis is more than vasomotor rhinitis). There is a significant relationship between the degree of relatively and severity of symptoms with P value of 0.027.

Discussion

There is an increase in the prevalence of AR and in both developed and developing countries in the last decades [11]. This study may be the first one which addresses the correlation between marriage as a proposed risk factor and allergic rhinitis in Saudi population. We used a questionnaire to interview patients but there was a telephone survey carried out to obtain the prevalence and risk factors of AR in 6 European countries [12].

In this study we found a higher prevalence of AR in rural areas 80%, while one of the largest epidemiological studies in China showed the opposite where they had higher prevalence of AR in urban areas [1].

The current study reported the proportions of 35% were persistent and 65% were intermittent, Similarly, In China results which showed 13% of the subjects were identified as persistent AR while 87% as intermittent AR, indicating intermittent type accounts for the majority of AR [1]. In Northern Europe 24.8% were identified as having persistent AR versus 53.8% were intermittent type [1]. This variation of persistent and intermittent between Saudi Arabia, China and Europe could be attributed to climate factors and sensitization to allergens.

	Severity of symptoms		Chi-Sqare	P Value
Duration of Marraiage	Mild	Moderate to sever		
1 Month-1 Year	7	3	3.214	0.234
2 Year-20 Years	28	8		
21 Years-40 Years	11	3		
Uses of oral contraceptive pills	Severity of symptoms		Chi-Sqare	P Value

	Mild	Moderate to sever		
NO	14	7	4.228	0.121
YES	10	0		
NONE	22	7		
Total	46	14		
	Severity of symptoms		**Chi-Sqare**	**P Value**
Degree of relativity	**Mild**	**Moderate to sever**		
2nd	15	2	7.242	0.027*
3rd	1	3		
None	30	9		
Total	46	14		
	Postcoital period		**Chi-Sqare**	**P Value**
Gender	**No**	**Yes**		
Female	24	7	0.773	0.379
Male	25	4		
Total	49	11		
	Postcoital period		**Chi-Sqare**	**P Value**
Consanguinity	**No**	**Yes**		
No	30	9	1.67	0.196
yes	19	2		
Total	49	11		

Table 3: Marriage and rhinitis findings.

AR of shorter duration (less than 4 days per week) is more common than AR of longer duration (4 or more days per week) in a Korean study [13], while we found the opposite in our study 53% of our recruited cases experienced AR more than 4 days per week indicating higher allergen load or higher susceptibility in our patients.

On discussing some risk factors like smoking and exposure to pollen grains, we have found that 83% of our cases were non smokers, and 70% showed no exposure to pollen.

Our results showed intake of medications were as follows 66% of studied cases took medications and 56% of them only received it on demand, in contrast to the Chinese study, 45% of their cases took medications [1].

Cold air and cold weather are top inducing factors for AR in winter. The changes of temperature in cold weather affects stability of parasympathetic supply of the nose and the dry air increases the vascular stability of the nasal mucosa leading to its hypersensitivity. This was consistent with our results in eastern province in Saudi Arabia, 18% of our cases (the largest percentage) had the attacks in winter. We have proved in our study that most of the cases had the attacks in early morning time due to the presence of cold air in the early morning.

Recently Hyrkak et al. in 2014 underlined that cold weather-related respiratory symptoms could be thought to reflect functional changes in the airways, occurring as a result of either cooling of the skin or through the simultaneous cooling and drying of the nasal and airway mucosa on inhaling cold air [14]. Experimental studies have shown that these trigger responses such as congestion and rhinorrhea in the upper airways and bronchoconstriction in the lower airway.

These effects may be further intensified during exercise in the cold at high ventilation rates. Subjects with asthma may have an excess of cold-related respiratory symptoms because their capacity toward humidify the inspired air is reduced. In our study we found that more than 70% of our cases had mild type of AR rather than moderate to severe type. Higher stress levels increased the risk of AR in the present study.

Stress-related hypothalamic-pituitary-adrenal axis reacts to psychological stressors and triggers a cortisol response; this may explain our data in which 50% of our cases were having moderate stress which is may be related to the pathophysiology of AR development. This was also detected in a study done in Korea [13] who found the same results. In the same previously mentioned study short sleep duration have also been reported as risk factors for AR which was consistent with ours, where we found 75% of our cases did sleep less than 7 h per night.

The development of allergic rhinitis entails a complex interaction between genetic predisposition and environmental exposure to different factors, of which the most important is the implicated allergen. There is a clear hereditary component in allergic rhinitis that has been well corroborated by segregation studies and investigations in twins. From the strictly genetic perspective, it is believed that the disease may be the result of the interaction of different genetic alterations, each of which would contribute a small defect [15]. From this point arises the importance of studying family history of AR. A family history of AR was strongly associated with AR development in many studies. In agreement with previous reports, we found that a parental history of AR strongly influenced AR prevalence. A genetic predisposition to AR, or an environmental factor, may explain the high association between AR in parents and their children. Maternal AR symptom duration of over 1 month increases prevalence of AR in children as what was shown in a Korean study, in our study we have studied family history as one of the important risk factors for AR, 48% of our cases have positive family history and 20% of them from the mother's side.

On discussing the effect of marriage on appearance of allergic rhinitis symptoms, two previous studies could not find any prior description of an association between AR prevalence and marriage. One substantial study has connected marriage to positive physical and mental health outcomes [16]. Indeed, marriage exerted a protective effect on AR in the study done by An SY 2015 [13]. In contrast, unhappy marriage or dissatisfied marriage can put people under stress and health problems.

Thirty five percent of our study had positive contagious marriage, so consanguinity was statistically significant. It is well known that consanguinity marriage in the middle east and Arab countries is far much more than in the developed world. Such marriages are considered to be more stable, due to close similarities in social and cultural values between the couple, and the economic benefits of keeping wealth within the families.

It is well known that exogenous sex steroidal hormones (oral contraceptive pills) can influence the development of wheezes in the chest in females [17], our studied cases didn't show any statistical significance correlation (16% of P value of 0.121).

Little was published about study of the relationship between marriage and sexual activity with allergic rhinitis. Human seminal plasma allergy (HSPA), in women, is a rare phenomenon. It is usually caused by sensitization to proteins present in the seminal fluid, leading to immediate hypersensitivity manifestations during or soon after coitus. Symptoms can range from local pruritus to life-threatening anaphylaxis [5]. This rare disorder is most commonly thought to be mediated by the classical IgE-mediated pathophysiological mechanism, but usually these cases are overlooked. Shad and Sircar, presented in 1991 cases report of four patients had experienced postcoital exacerbation of asthma and allergic rhinitis in India. Here in our study we have reported 11 cases 7 females and 4 males having postcoital exacerbation of allergic symptoms. This postcoital rhinitis or honeymoon rhinitis is most probably due to emotional excitement or autonomic parasympathetic over activity with cholinergic release of mast cell mediators. We have found that 6 cases from 11 cases having positive postcoital phenomenon, having positive family history of AR, and positive postcoital AR as well. Spring was found the most common month to flare the postcoital attacks. Only 2 patients had positive consanguous marriage and positive postcoital AR.

However, we would like to stress that postcoital allergic rhinitis may be easily overlooked due to patient embarrassment or lack of awareness specially in our society, and hence it needs more detailed study to understand more about the pathophysiology and mechanisms which will lead to proper management and actual and adequate knowing of the prevalence of the disorder.

Conclusion

Allergic Rhinitis prevalence in Eastern province of Saudi Arabia is significantly higher in the rural areas than urban areas. Intermittent allergic rhinitis is the predominant type, and of the mild form. The main trigger factors and risk factors are genetic factors like family history, and environmental factors like pollen and smoking. It is more common in winter, at the early morning time.

Eighteen percent of cases experienced postcoital exacerbation of allergic rhinitis attacks. However, vasomotor rhinitis might be a possible diagnosis if the patient age is above 35 with no family history of allergies.

Acknowledgement

We would like to thank Anwar Sattam, medical student for her helpful work in datacollection. Our grateful thanks are also extended to Dr. Sayed Ibrahim Ali, Assistant professor of statistics for his assistances in the data analysis.

References

1. Li CW, Chen de HDH, Zhong JT, Lin ZB, Peng H, et al. (2014) Epidemiological characterization and risk factors of allergic rhinitis in the general population in Guangzhou city in China. PLoS One 9: e114950.
2. Wang DY (2005) Risk factors of allergic rhinitis: Genetic or environmental? Ther Clin Risk Manag 1: 115-123.
3. Ma Y, Tan G, Zhao Z, Li W, Huang L, et al. (2014) Therapeutic effectiveness of endoscopic vidian neurectomy for the treatment of vasomotor rhinitis. Acta Otolaryngol 134: 260-267.
4. Lieberman P, Meltzer EO, LaForce CF, Darter AL, Tort MJ (2011) Two-week comparison study of olopatadine hydrochloride nasal spray 0.6% versus azelastine hydrochloride nasal spray 0.1% in patients with vasomotor rhinitis. Allergy Asthma Proc 32: 151-158.
5. Bernstein JA (2009) Characteristics of nonallergic vasomotor rhinitis. World Allergy Organ J 2: 102-105.
6. Shah A, Sircar M (1991) Postcoital asthma and rhinitis. Chest 100: 1039-1041.
7. Falliers CJ (1976) Sexercise-induced asthma. Lancet 2: 1078-1079.
8. Shah A (2001) Asthma and sex. Indian J Chest Dis Allied Sci 43: 135-137.
9. Bell RA, Daly JA, Gonzalez MC (1987) Affinity-maintenance in marriage and its relationship to women's marital satisfaction. Journal of Marriage and the Family 49: 445-454
10. Bernstein IL, Englander BE, Gallagher JS, Nathan P, Marcus ZH (1981) Localized and systemic hypersensitivity reactions to human seminal fluid. Ann Intern Med 94: 459 465.
11. Sly RM (1999) Changing prevalence of allergic rhinitis and asthma. Ann Allergy Asthma Immunol 82: 233-248.
12. Bauchau V, Durham SR (2004) Prevalence and rate of diagnosis of allergic rhinitis in Europe. Eur Respir J 24: 758-764.
13. An SY, Choi HG, Kim SW, Park B, Lee JS, et al. (2015) Analysis of various risk factors predisposing subjects to allergic rhinitis. Asian Pac J Allergy Immunol 33: 143-151.
14. Hyrkas H, Jaakkola MS, Ikaheimo TM, Hugg TT, Jaakkola JJ (2014) Asthma and allergic rhinitis increase respiratory symptoms in cold weather among young adults. Respiratory Medicine 108: 63-70.
15. Dávila I, Mullol J, Ferrer M, Bartra J, del Cuvillo A, et al. (2009) Genetic aspects of allergic rhinitis. J Investig Allergol Clin Immunol 1: 25-31.
16. Meyler D, Stimpson JP, and Peek MK (2007) Health concordance within couples: A systematic review. Social Science & Medicine 64: 2297-2310.
17. Salam MT, Wenten M, Gilliland FD (2006) Endogenous and exogenous sex steroid hormones and asthma and wheeze in young women. J Allergy Clin Immunol 117: 1001-1007.

16

Juvenile Laryngeal Papillomatosis in Benin: Epidemiological, Diagnostic, Therapeutic and Evolutionary Aspects

Lawson Afouda Sonia[1*], Hounkpatin Spéro[2], Avakoudjo François[1], Brun Luc[3] and Adjibabi Wassi[1]

[1]*Ear Nose Throat Department at Hubert Koutoukou Maga National Teaching Hospital of Cotonou, Benin*

[2]*Ear Nose Throat Department at Borgou Regional Teaching Hospital, Benin*

[3]*Pathology Department at Borgou Regional Teaching Hospital, Benin*

[*]**Corresponding author:** Lawson Afouda Sonia, Ear Nose Throat Department at Hubert Koutoukou Maga National Teaching Hospital of Cotonou, Box: 0 3 BP 3196 Cotonou, France; E-mail: olatundeother@yahoo.fr

Abstract

Introduction: To describe the epidemiological profile of patients with laryngeal papillomatosis, to identify diagnostic aspects and evolution after treatment.

Method: This was a retrospective study over 16 years, from May 1995 to April 2011, in the ear nose throat in Hubert Koutoukou Maga, National Teaching Hospital of Cotonou. It was based on descriptive analysis of medical record together with operation report of patients.

Results: We have sampled 18 patients, 1.12 case/year. The sample included 10 males and 8 females with a frequency of 0.55 in favor of males. The average age was 6.95 year old and children in school or about to be in school were 14. The time-frame between the beginning of symptoms and consultation was 1.17 years. During the endoscopy, the lesions in grains or clusters sometimes obstructive acting as seat on the larynx were confirmed at pathologic check-up.

The treatment consisted of peeling all of them with an average of 4.6 (1-23) associated with the local whitewashing by mitomycin in 3 cases. A tracheotomy rescue had to be performed urgently (12 cases). The monitoring was effective in 14 cases over an average of 14.85 months (3 months-175 months). Ten (10) patients had both normal voice and breathing. In 3 cases the patients had suprasternal draw supine and intermittent dysphonia after decanulation. In a case the weaning could not be achieved. The complications were related to the peeling, to tracheotomy, and to the presence of the cannula.

Conclusion: Laryngeal papillomatosis is a common pathology in children. It is easy to diagnose this pathology, but this raises recurrent therapeutic problems such as education disruption and budget burden. The functional and vital prognosis can be involved, hence the need for early consultation.

Keywords: Juvenile laryngeal papillomatosis; Epidemiology; Diagnosis; Treatment; Complications

Introduction

Laryngeal papillomatosis is a benign squamous papillary tumor proliferation developed at the expense of the laryngeal mucosa in 90% of cases [1]. Broadly observed in children, though relatively rare it is the most common benign tumors of the larynx. Prevalence of the juvenile laryngeal papillomatosis is 0.7 to 3 [2,3]. The pathogenesis is poorly known evoking intricate theories that are caused by hormones, viral and traumatic. The latter is the only one to date that allows the isolation of the human papillomavirus (HPV) type HPV6 and HPV11. Currently, there is no cure which makes treatment difficult. The clinical course is unpredictable: evolutionary pursuit with a risk of asphyxiation and death, often enamelled healing recurrence with or without an extension to various parts of the respiratory tree. The degeneration is possible but rare and occurs most often in the adulthood [4]. The aim of this study was to describe the epidemiological profile of laryngeal papillomatosis, to identify diagnostic aspects, and to determine the evolutionary aspects after treatment.

Method

This is a retrospective study we conducted based on patients' medical record in ear nose throat department at Hubert Koutoukou Maga National Teaching Hospital of Cotonou from May 1995 to April 2011. The study covered patients with ages ranging between 0 and 17 year old and for whom the diagnosis of laryngeal papillomatosis was done based on anamnestic, clinical and paraclinical arguments. The examination indicated firstly a chronic dysphonia evolving for more than three weeks before then secondarily a dyspnea, and at indirect or direct laryngoscopy clusters blackberrys aspect in supraglottic, glottic or glotto-subglottic stage. We have received some patients at dyspnea stages as classified by Pineau and Chevalier Jackson (Table 1).

A rescue tracheotomy with an operation of a cannula was essential when the subject had a stage 3 dyspnoea of this classification. All patients underwent surgical treatment of papillomas with forcep peeling on bi-weekly average. The pathological examination after biopsy confirmed the diagnosis of laryngeal papillomatosis. This was followed by a painting with mitomycin site where the lesion was exuberant or recurrent. When the laryngeal was absorptive then the decannulation was made after weaning by gradual light reduction of the material in use. The parameters studied were frequency, sex, age, consultation period, reasons for consultation with or without associated signs, the location of lesions, treatment and evolution.

	Stage 1	Stage 2	Stage 3	Stage 4
Draw	Discreet	Moderate	Major Diffuse	low
Staining of integument	Normal	Vultuous	+/- Cyanosis	Cyanosis
Pulse rate	+/- Normal	+/- Increased	Increased	Collapsed
Arterial tension	+/- Normal	+/- Increased	Increased	Collapsed
State of consciousness	Normal	Agitation	Anguish	+++Disorders

Table 1: Classification of Pineau and Chevalier Jackson.

Results

Over the 16 years study period, 18 patients were consulted with a rate of 1.12 cases per year. The sample included of 10 males/18 with a frequency of 0.55 and an average age of 6.95 years (21 months-16 years). 14 children were in school or at age to be.

		Number (frequency)
Aspects of lesions	Grains of papillomas	02 (11%)
	papilloma clusters	03 (17%)
	Florida *	13 (72%)
Localisation	Supra glottis +glottis **	05 (28%)
	Glottis	04 (22%)
	Glottis+sub glottis	06 (33%)
	Supra glottis+glottis +subglottis	03 (17%)
Total		18 (100%)

*Over13 presenting a florida aspect 10 lesions were obstructive.

**In the localisation related to the first 2 stages of the larynx, one case spread over to the oropharynx.

Table 2: Distribution of patients by endoscopic examination.

Clinically, the consultation period was 1.17 years (1 week-5 years). 1/3 consulted for dysphonia drawling, another 1/3 dysphonia association and dyspnea without signs of decompensation and the remaining one 1/3 for dyspnea stage 3. Table 2 summarizes the distribution of patients according to the results of the endoscopic review. Clamp peeling with an average of 4.6 (1-23) was treatment opted for in our series. Mitomycin was applied 1 to 4 times by brushing after surgery in 3 patients. In an emergency, a tracheotomy rescue was necessary in 12 cases and in total during the study period, this act was performed 15 times with an average of 1.25 (1-3). Pathological examination of samples has proved laryngeal papillomatosis. 04 patients underwent additional consultations in emergency way; in a case there were 2 readmissions and 1 readmission in 3 cases.

The evolution was assessed in 14 patients over an average of 14.85 months (3 months-175 months) on the quality of the voice, breathing and the occurrence of complications (Table 3). Ten (10) patients had both normal breathing and voice. We noted the impossibility of decanulation in 1 case and in 3 cases the patients had suprasternal draw supine and intermittent dysphonia after decanulation.

		Number (frequency)
Peeling	functional complications	08/18 (44%)
	changing mucosa /dysplasia	01/18 (06%)
Tracheotomy	Emphysema facial-cervical-thoracic	02/12 (17%)
	Vicious cervical scar	01/12 (08%)
cannula	lobar Pneumonia	01/12 (08%)
	pericanular Purulent secretions	01/12 (08%)
	Tracheal-throat fistula	01/12 (08%)
	Granuloma	03/12 (25%)

Table 3: Distribution of patients according to the complications. All 18 patients were peeled -12 underwent emergency tracheotomy and wore a canula.

Discussion

We consulted 18 patients over 16 years with a rate of 1.12 cases per year. The sample included 10 males with a frequency of 0.55 in favour of males and an average age of 6.95 years. The consultation period was 1.17 years (1 week-5 years). 1/3 consulted for dysphonia drawling, another 1/3 dysphonia association and dyspnea without signs of decompensation and the remaining on third for dyspnea stage 3. Clamp peeling with a mean of 4.6 (1-23) was the treatment opted for in our series. Mitomycin was applied 1 to 4 times by brushing after surgery in 3 patients. In an emergency, a tracheotomy rescue was necessary in 12 cases and in total during the study period, this act was performed 15 times with an average of 1.25 (1-3). The evolution was assessed in 14 patients over an average of 14.85 months (3 months-175 months) on the quality of the voice, breathing and the occurrence of complications.

Epidemiologically, laryngeal papillomatosis is a benign and occasional disease which variable incidence is 0.2 to 0.7 cases per 100,000 population [5,6]. The number of new cases per year of the juvenile laryngeal papillomatosis is 0.7 to 3 [3] while it was 1.12 in our series. If the male predominance is for Ndiaye [3], laryngeal papillomatosis is more common in children and regardless of gender with an average age ranging from 6 to 10 years [7,8].
The diagnosis is often delayed because of the long use of consultation up to 5 years. Indeed, dysphonia first sign of laryngeal papillomatosis may be laryngitis or an asthmatics status differential diagnosis [9,10]. This is not the case in the series of Traissac [11], where 90% of cases were consulted at the stage of dysphonia. In our series, patients were

consulted in 2/3 of cases at the stage of dyspnea. This is a laryngeal dyspnea faster or slower type inspiratory bradypnea with draw and wheezing.

The review to nasofibroscopy or direct laryngoscopy under A/G achieves clinical assessment by objectifying in a mobile larynx lesions pink or greyish as grains, clusters, sometimes florid, obstructive or not. The lesions extended to the 3 floors of the larynx and oropharynx in one case. As for the tracheobronchial tree, it has not been explored due to limited technical facilities in our work environment.

The pathological examination was performed in all cases to confirm the benign lesions.

Therapeutically, the delay in consultation, sometimes multistage extension of the larynx and the obstructive nature of lesions required a tracheotomy first in 12/18 cases. This gesture would be saving an aggravating factor as it would favor the extension of lesions throughout the respiratory tract [1,12,13]. Peeling was the only surgical treatment for all patients because the gesture is simple, easily accessible and inexpensive.

In evolutionarily, 14/18 patients were reviewed. Recurrences were frequent with the need to resume peelings every 2 weeks. Apart from these controls set, 4 patients were received emergency in an array of dyspnea stage 3. During the monitoring period, the average peelings was 4.6 (1-23). The complications were related to emergency tracheotomy and residence of the cannula. The facial-cervical-thoracic emphysema can be explained by tight stitches on both sides of the incision instead of tracheotomy or too small tracheostomy tube allowing fuser upstream and downstream of the air. As for tracheal mucosa, it produces in contact with the tracheostomy tube of secretions which at long term gets over infected and goes down to the lower airways. Similarly mini friction of the cannula can create irritation, then a oeso-tracheal fistula and a granuloma. The sequelae of peeling are firstly a bad voice quality probably due to a lack of confrontation of the vocal cords after fibrosis or poor healing of the laryngeal mucosa and also observed the occurrence of dysplasia one patient by the mucosa redesign.

Conclusion

Laryngeal papillomatosis is a common pathology of the child. It is fairly easy to diagnose but poses therapeutic difficulties. The development is toward recurrence and education disruption of the child. The functional and vital prognosis can be involved, hence an early consultation is needed.

References

1. Conessa C, Herve S, Roguet E, Gauthier J, Poncet JL (2005) Chirurgie des tumeurs bénignes du larynx. Elsevier, Paris.
2. Snoeck R, Wellens W, Desloovere C, Van Ranst M, Naesens L, et al. (1998) Treatment of severe laryngeal papillomatosis with intralesional injections of cidofovir [(S)-1-(3-hydroxy-2-phosphonylmethoxypropyl)cytosine]. J Med Virol 54: 219-225.
3. Cristensen PH, Jorgensen K, Grontved A (1984) Juvenile papillomatosis of the larynx. 45 years follow up from county of Funen. Acta oto-laryngol 412: 37-39.
4. Bomholt A (1988) Juvenile laryngeal papillomatosis. An epidemiological study from the Copenhagen region. Acta Otolaryngol 105: 367-371.
5. Ondzotto G, Galiba J, Kouassi B, Ehouo F (2002) [Laryngeal papillomatosis: value of early diagnosis, apropos of 7 cases diagnosed at the University Hospital Center in Brazzaville, Congo]. Med Trop (Mars) 62: 163-165.
6. Ndiaye M, Ndiaye IC, Itiere OFA, Tall A, Diallo BK, et al. (2008) Papillomatose laryngée de l'enfant. Fr ORL 94: 379-382.
7. Timbo SK, Konipo-Togola F, Mohamed AA, Keita MA, Sacko HB, et al. (2002) [Laryngeal papillomatosis in Mali. Apropos of 19 cases collected at the Gabriel Touré Hospital of Bamako]. Bull Soc Pathol Exot 95: 31-33.
8. Maliki O, Nouri H, Ziad T, Rochdi Y, Aderdour L, et al. (2012) La papillomatose laryngée de l'enfant : aspects épidémiologiques, thérapeutiques et évolutifs. Journal de pédiatrie et de puériculture 25: 237-241.
9. Diouf R, Ouaba K, Ndiaye I, Diop EM, Diop LS (1989) [Laryngeal papillomatosis: report of 27 cases]. Dakar Med 34: 102-106.
10. Mohamed A, Timbo SK, Konipo-Togola F (1996) Papillomatose du larynx: réflexions à propos de 6 cas récents. Med Afr Noire 43: 630-632.
11. Traissac L, Devars F, Petit J, Portmann D, Papaxanthos M, et al. (1987) [Result of the treatment of juvenile papillomatosis of the larynx. Apropos of 158 cases]. Rev Laryngol Otol Rhinol (Bord) 108: 221-224.
12. Bauman NM, Smith RJ (1996) Recurrent respiratory papillomatosis. Pediatr Clin North Am 43: 1385-1401.
13. Cathelineau L, Pages C, Aubier F, Guimbaud P, Narcy P (1988) [Development of laryngeal papillomatosis in children. Apropos of 17 cases]. Arch Fr Pediatr 45: 387-392.

Mucosal Immune Responses Associated with NKT Cell Activation and Dendritic Cell Expansion by Nasal administration of α-galactosylceramide in the Nasopharynx

Shingo Umemoto, Satoru Kodama*, Takashi Hirano, Kenji Noda and Masashi Suzuki

Department of Otolaryngology,Oita University Faculty of Medicine 1-1 Idaigaoka, Hazama-cho, Yufu, Oita 879-5593, Japan

Abstract

Objective: Intranasal immunization is an effective method to induce mucosal immune responses in the upper respiratory tract.α-galactosylceramide (α-GalCer) is considered as one of the most potent candidates for a mucosal adjuvant. In the present study, mucosal immune responses in the nasopharynx associated with NKT cell activation by nasal administration of α-GalCer were examined for inducing protective immunity in the nasopharynx, with the ultimate goal of developing a mucosal vaccine for preventing upper respiratory infectious diseases.

Methods: Mice were administered α-GalCer intranasally as a ligand for NKT cells, without any antigen, weekly total three times. One week after the final administration of α-GalCer, mice were killed, and nasal immune responses were examined. Dendritic cells (DCs) in nasal-associated lymphoid tissue (NALT), a mucosal inductive site, were examined by immunohistochemistry. DCs, NKT cells, and B cells in NALT and nasal passage (NP) were examined by flow cytometry. Cytokine-producing CD4+ T cells were also examined by flow cytometry. Quantification of immunoglobulin (Ig)-producing cells was examined by enzyme-linked immunospot (ELISPOT) assay. In addition, bacterial challenges with live *Haemophilus influenzae* (Hi) and *Streptococcus pneumoniae* (Sp) were performed, and bacterial clearance from nasopharynx was examined.

Results: After nasal immunization of α -GalCer, DCs increased in NALT. Antibody-producing cells, mainly those that produce IgA, significantly increased in the NP, a mucosal effector site. Interleukin (IL)-17-producing Th 17 cells were also induced in the NP. Bacterial challenges with live Hi and Sp resulted in enhanced clearances of both bacterial species from the nasopharynx. It is interesting that bacterial clearance was impaired by IL-17 neutralization.

Conclusion: Nasal vaccination is effective for the induction of protective immunity against upper respiratory infection. The results of the present study demonstrated that nasal administration of α-GalCer could activate NKT cells in the nasopharynx, followed by the maturation of DCs, B cells, and some cytokine-producing CD4+ T cells. These findings suggest that the activation of NKT cells by nasal administration of α-GalCer induced protective immunity in the nasopharynx, possibly involving the interaction with DCs and induction of Th17 cells.

Keywords: α-GalCer; NKT cell; Dendritic cell; Th17; Mucosal immunity; Nasal vaccine; Haemophilus influenza; Streptococcus pneumoniae

Introduction

Mucosal surfaces such as those of the respiratory, gastrointestinal, and genital tracts, are the main entry site of most environmental antigens (Ags) or pathogens, and thus act as the first line of defense. Many studies have focused on developing mucosal vaccines capable of effectively inducing both mucosal and systemic immune responses [1-4]. Intranasal immunization is an effective method to elicit mucosal immune responses in the upper respiratory tract, and has shown efficacy in enhancing bacterial clearance from the nasopharynx, lungs, and other organs [5-7].

NKT cells are a specific subset of immune regulatory cells that express an invariant antigen receptor α-chain encoded by a Vα14-Jα28.1 rearranged gene segment in mice and Vα14-Jα28 in humans [8]. Glycolipids such as α-galactosylceramide (α-GalCer) presented via CD1d can directly activated NKT cells [9]. Upon activation, NKT cells rapidly produce both Th1 and Th2 cytokines, including interferon (IFN)- γ and interleukin (IL)-4, which contribute to the upregulation of both cellular and humoral immune responses [10].

Nontypeable *Haemophilus influenzae* (NTHi) and *Streptococcus pneumoniae* (Sp) are major pathogens of upper respiratory tract and cause infectious diseases including otitis media (OM) and rhinosinusitis [11-14]. Since colonization of these pathogens in the nasopharynx is important in the pathogenesis of OM, inhibition of bacterial colonization is effective for preventing upper respiratory infections. Due to recent increases in antibiotic-resistant NTHi or Sp strains, the development of a mucosal vaccine is considered an important public health goal. Previously, we showed that α-GalCer is one of the most potent candidates for a mucosal adjuvant [15,16]. Nasal vaccination with P6 outer membrane protein, which is common to all NTHi strains, and α-GalCer induced P6-specific immunoglobulin (Ig)A and Th1/Th2 immune responses in the nasopharynx, and nasal vaccination with P6 and α-GalCer induced NTHi-specific protective

***Corresponding author:** Satoru Kodama, Department of Otolaryngology, Oita University Faculty of Medicine, 1-1 Idaigaoka, Hazama-cho, Yufu, Oita 879-5593, Japan; E-mail: satoruk@oita-u.ac.jp

immunity, enhancing bacterial clearance from the nasopharynx [15,16]. Recently, it was shown that the co-administration of α-GalCer with ovalbumin (OVA) can induce full maturation of dendritic cells (DCs), thereby generating functional Ag-specific Th1-type CD4+ and CD8+ T cells that are resistant to OVA-expressing tumors [17]. In addition, α-GalCer administration triggers the *in vivo* maturation of mesenteric DCs. This contributes to T cell division *in vitro* and blocks the tolerance induced by both high and low doses of oral OVA [18]. It is also known that α-GalCer can serve as an effective adjuvant for a nasal vaccine that induces substantial protective immune responses against viral infections and tumor growth [19].

In this study, we investigated the efficacy of NKT cell activation by nasal administration of α-GalCer for inducing protective immunity in the nasopharynx, with the ultimate goal of developing a mucosal vaccine for preventing upper respiratory infectious diseases.

Materials and Methods

Animals

Specific pathogen-free (SPF) BALB/c mice (6 weeks old) were used in this study, and mice were maintained under SPF conditions throughout all experiments. The study was approved by the Committee on Animal Experiments of Oita University, Oita, Japan, and was performed according to local guidelines for animal experiments.

Administration of α-GalCer

α-GalCer (KRN7000, Kirin Pharma Co., Tokyo), was used for nasal immunization and activating nasal NKT cells. Mice were immunized intranasally on days 0, 7, and 14 with 10 μl phosphate-buffered saline (PBS) containing 2 μg of α-GalCer (α-GalCer group). Control mice were administered PBS without antigen (control group). Mice were killed on day 21, and nasal passages (NPs) and nasal-associated lymphoid tissue (NALT) were collected.

Immunohistochemistry

For histological analysis, mice were killed under deep anesthesia on day 21 and then perfused transcardially with PBS, followed by 10% neutral buffered formalin. Heads were immersed in the same fixative for 6 h and decalcified with 0.12 M EDTA for 2 weeks. After dehydration, tissues were embedded in paraffin. To detect CD11c+ DCs in NALT, a mucosal inductive site in the upper respiratory tract, 12-μm-thick serial and horizontal paraffin sections were prepared for light microscopic examination. Specimens were dehydrated through a graded series of ethanol and treated with 3% H2O2 in absolute methanol for 20 min. Sections were exposed to a 5% normal mouse serum in PBS for 30 min and then incubated for 24 h with biotinylated goat anti-mouse CD11c antibody. After rinsing with PBS, sections were incubated with ABC reagent for 1 h and developed in 0.05% 3,3'-diaminobenzidine-0.01% H2O2 substrate medium in 0.1 M phosphate buffer for 8 min.

Flow cytometry for DCs, NKT cells, and B cells

Mononuclear cells (MNCs: 1 x 10^6 cells) were isolated from NALT and NP, and the number of CD11c+ DCs, as well as the expression of functional markers on DCs, and NKT cells in NALT were analyzed by flow cytometry as described previously [20,21]. The number of B cells in NALT and NP were also analyzed by flow cytometry. The following monoclonal antibodies (mAbs) were used in this study: fluorescein isothiocyanate (FITC)-conjugated anti-mouse CD11c (HL3), phycoerythrin (PE)-conjugated anti-mouse CD11b (M1/70), Cy-Chrome-conjugated anti-mouse CD8α (53-6.7), Cy-Chrome-conjugated anti-mouse CD11c (HL3), FITC-conjugated anti-mouse MHC class I (H-2Kb, AF6-88.5), FITC-conjugated anti-mouse MHC class II (I-A/I-E, 2G9), FITC-conjugated anti-mouse CD80 (B7-1; 16-10A1), FITC-conjugated anti-mouse CD86 (B7-2; GL1), FITC-conjugated anti-mouse αβ (TCR β chain, H57-597), FITC-conjugated anti-mouse CD45R/B220 (RA3-6B2), PE-conjugated anti-mouse CD5 (53-7.5), PE-conjugated anti-mouse CD1d tetramer, and CyChrome-conjugated anti-mouse anti-mouse CD45R/B220 (RA3-6B2). These mAbs were purchased from BD Pharmingen (San Diego, CA). PE-conjugated mouse CD1d tetramer was purchased from BMC (Nagoya, Japan), and CD1d tetramer was loaded with α-GalCer according to the manufacturer's instructions. MNCs were incubated with various combinations of mAbs, and samples were analyzed by FACS Calibur (Becton Dickinson, Sunnyvale, CA).

Quantification of Ig-producing cells

MNCs were isolated from the NP and NALT, and the numbers of total Ig-producing cells were determined using an enzyme-linked immunospot (ELISPOT) assay, as previously described [15,20]. Briefly, 96-well plates (MultiScreen; Millipore) were coated with goat anti-mouse Ig (H+L) UNLD (1.0 μg/well) and incubated overnight at 4°C. Plates were washed and then blocked with complete medium for 1 h. Test cells were added at varying concentrations and were cultured at 37°C, 5% CO_2 for 4 h. After washing, horseradish peroxidase (HRP)-labeled goat anti-mouse IgM, IgG, or IgA was added (SBA). After overnight incubation at 4°C, the plates were washed and the spots developed at room temperature with 100 μl AEC (Moss) after incubation for 30 min.

Flow cytometry of cytokine-producing CD4+ T cells

MNCs (1 x 10^6 cells) from the NP were incubated with 100 μg/mL phorbol myristate acetate and 2 μg/mL ionomycin (Sigma, St. Louis, MO, USA) for 12 h in the presence of Golgi plug (BD Pharmingen). After fixing and permeabilization with Perm/fix solution (BD Pharmingen), cells were incubated with 1 μg/mL Fc Block (BD Pharmingen) for 15 min, and then stained with following mAbs: CyChrome-conjugated anti-mouse CD4 (H129.19), FITC-conjugated anti-mouse IFN-γ (XMG1.2), PE-conjugated anti-mouse IL-17 (TC11-18H10; BD Pharmingen) or PE-conjugated anti-mouse IL-22. After intracellular staining, samples were analyzed by FACS Calibur [21].

NTHi and Sp clearance from the nasopharynx

On day 21, bacterial challenge was performed and bacterial clearance was examined, as previously described [15,20]. Briefly, NTHi (strain 76) and Sp were cultured on chocolate agar plates and blood agar plates alternately overnight at 37°C in 5% CO_2, collected by scraping, and then resuspended in PBS (10^{10} CFU/ml) for nasal challenge. A 10-μl aliquot (10^8 CFU) of the live NTHi (NTHi group) or Sp (Sp group) suspension was injected intranasally. Then, 24 h after nasal challenge, mice were killed and nasal wash samples were collected. Aliquots from each sample were serially diluted 10-fold with sterile PBS, and 10-μl aliquots of the diluted samples were spread on chocolate agar plates (NTHi group) or blood agar plates (Sp group) for quantification of live bacteria. After overnight incubation at 37°C in 5% CO_2, the bacterial colonies were counted.

Neutralization of nasal IL-17 and IL-22 was performed to clarify the role of Th17 cells in protective immunity. To neutralize IL-17 and IL-22 in the nasopharynx, mice were twice intranasally administered 10 μg anti-mouse IL-17 mAb (50104; R&D Systems) and/or IL-22 mAb (142928; R&D Systems) in 10 μl PBS on days 16 and 20 [16].

Bacterial clearance was then examined, as described above (groups: control, α-GalCer, α-GalCer+anti-IL-17, α-GalCer+anti-IL-22, and α-GalCer+anti-IL-17+anti-IL-22).

Statistical analysis

Mann-Whitney U-test was used to compare data. P-values less than 0.05 were considered significant.

Results

DCs and NKT cells in NALT

The number and frequency of NKT cells were investigated by flow cytometry. The control group contained 1.49×10^2 cells of NKT cells in the NALT per mouse. The number and frequency of α-GalCer-CD1d tetramer-positive NKT cells increased in the NALT of the α-GalCer group (Table 1 and Figure 1). The α-GalCer group contained 3.88×10^2 cells of NKT cells in the NALT per mouse.

Immunohistochemical analysis showed that CD11c+ DCs were present in NALT of the α-GalCer group, with fewer CD11c+ DCs in NALT of the control group. Following nasal immunization with α-GalCer, CD11c+ DCs were evident in NALT of the α-GalCer group (Figure 2). The increase in DCs was confirmed by flow cytometry. The control group contained 1.07×10^3 cells of DCs in the NALT per mouse. The number of CD11c+ DCs increased in NALT of the α-GalCer group. The α-GalCer group contained 1.99×10^4 cells of DCs in the NALT per mouse. Statistical significant difference was detected between the control group and immunized group (Table 1). Among the increased DCs in NALT of the α-GalCer group, the expression of MHC class II, and B7-1 was markedly enhanced, when compared with those of the control group (Figure 3).

Group	CD11c+ DC †		NKT cell †	
	frequency (%)‡	number (cells)§	frequency (%)‡	number (cells)§
α-GalCer	3.33 ± 0.15*	1.99×10^4*	0.11 ± 0.032	3.88×10^2
Control	2.20 ± 0.12	1.07×10^3	0.06 ± 0.017	1.49×10^2

† Nasal-associated lymphoid tissue (NALT) cells were analyzed by three-color flow cytometry. NKT cells were determined as α-GalCer-CD1d tetramer-positive cells among $B220^-$, $CD4^+$ cells.
‡ Frequency of $CD11c^+$ dendritic cells (DCs) and $B220^-$ NKT cells in NALT mononuclear cells. Values are expressed as mean ± SE.
§ Absolute number of $CD11c^+$ DCs and NKT cells in NALT per mouse. Values were calculated according to the absolute number of isolated lymphocytes and the mean frequency of $CD11c^+$ DCs or NKT cells.
* $p<0.05$ compared with control group.

Table 1: Dendritic cells and NKT cells in NALT.

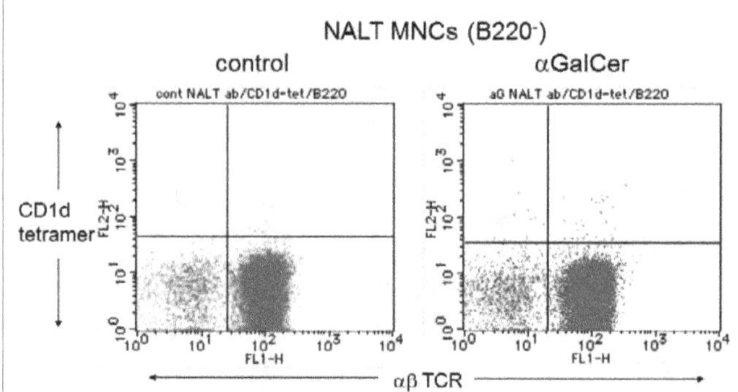

Figure 1: Flow cytometry of NKT cells in NALT. The number and frequency of α -GalCer-CD1d tetramer-positive NKT cells increased in the NALT of the α -GalCer group.

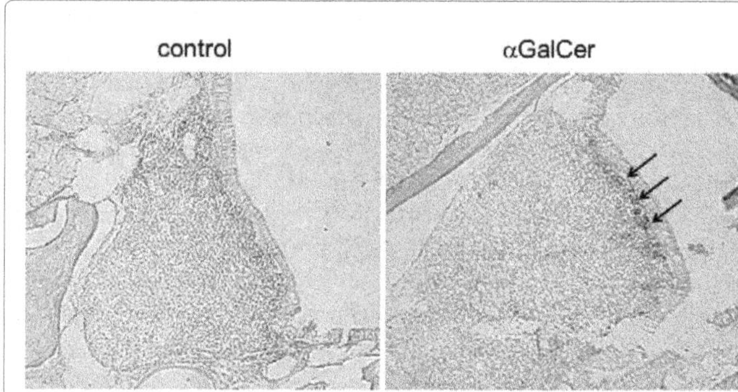

Figure 2: Immunohistochemistry of NALT. Appearance of $CD11c^+$ cells in NALT of the control and α -GalCer groups. $CD11c^+$ DCs (black arrows) were evident in NALT of the α -GalCer group. Magnification x100.

B cells in NALT and NP

The number of B cells was also confirmed by flow cytometry. The control group contained 2.49×10^5 cells of B220high, B-2 B cells in the NP per mouse. Following nasal immunization with α-GalCer, B220high, B-2 B cells were predominantly increased in the NP, a mucosal effector site. The α-GalCer group contained 3.27×10^5 cells of B220high, B-2 B cells in the NP per mouse. Statistical significant difference was detected between the control group and immunized group (Table 2 and Figure 4).Whereas no significant changes were detected in NALT, a mucosal inductive site.

Antibody-producing cells

The number of antibody-producing cell was determined by ELISPOT assay. A small number of antibody-producing cells was detected in the NP and NALT of the control group. Following nasal immunization with α-GalCer, the number of IgA-producing cells significantly increased in the NP of the α-GalCer group (Figure 5). Fewer IgA-producing cells were evident in NALT than in the NP. We also found no significant difference in IgG- and IgM-producing cells between the groups. This result shows that nasal immunization with α-GalCer induced B-cell activation and mucosal IgA production in the mucosal effector site (the NP).

Cytokine-producing CD4+ T cells in the NP

The number of cytokine-producing CD4+ T cells in the NP was also confirmed by flow cytometry. The control group contained 9.47×10^2 cells of IL-17-producing T cells in the NP per mouse. Following nasal immunization with α-GalCer, IL-17-producing T cells were increased in NP. The α-GalCer group contained 2.52×10^3 cells of IL-17-producing T cells in the NP per mouse. Statistical significant difference was detected between the control group and immunized group (Table 3). There was no significant difference in the number of IL-22-producing T cells between the control group and immunized group. As Th17 is the typical T cell that produces IL-17 and IL-22, this result seems to indicate that Th17 is involved in host defense in the upper respiratory tract induced by nasal immunization with α-GalCer.

NTHi and Sp clearance from the nasopharynx

Bacterial clearance from the nasopharynx was investigated according to live NTHi or Sp numbers in the nasal wash. After the bacterial challenges, a large number of NTHi or Sp was detected in the nasal wash of the control group. After nasal immunization, clearance of both NTHi and Sp was significantly enhanced in mice immunized with

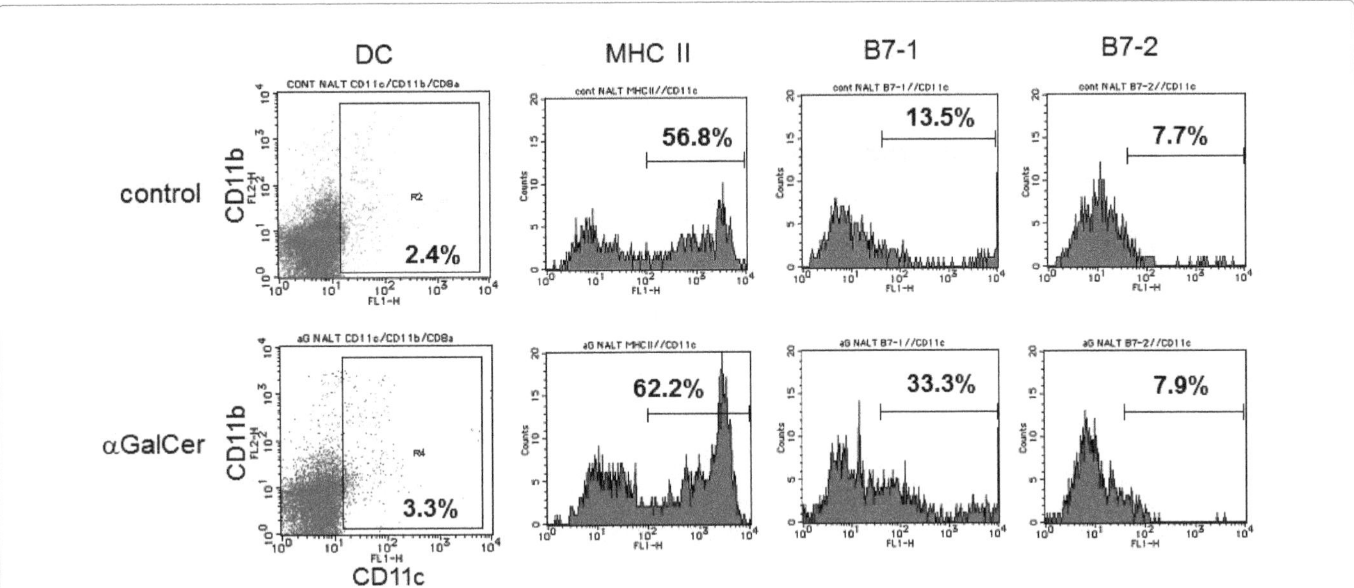

Figure 3: Flow cytometry of DCs in NALT. The number and frequency of DCs markedly increased in NALT of the α -GalCer group. The expression of MHC II, B7-1, and B7-2 was also enhanced.

Group	NP†		NALT†	
	frequency (%)‡	number (cells)§	frequency (%)‡	number (cells)§
α-GalCer	40.1 ± 0.50 *	3.27 x 10^5 *	53.3 ± 0.63	4.60 x 10^5
Control	30.6 ± 1.03	2.49 x 10^5	58.4 ± 0.19	3.63 x 10^5

† Nasal passage tissue cells and nasal-associated lymphoid tissue cells were stained to detect B220 expression to distinguish B2 B cells ($B220^{high}$) from B1 B cells ($B220^{low}$) and analyzed by flow cytometry.
‡ Frequency of B2 B cells. Values are expressed as mean ± SE.
§ Absolute number of B2 B cells in NP per mouse. Each value was calculated in according to the absolute number of isolated lymphocytes and the mean frequency of B2 B cells.
* $p<0.05$ compared with control group.

Table 2: B cells in the NP and NALT.

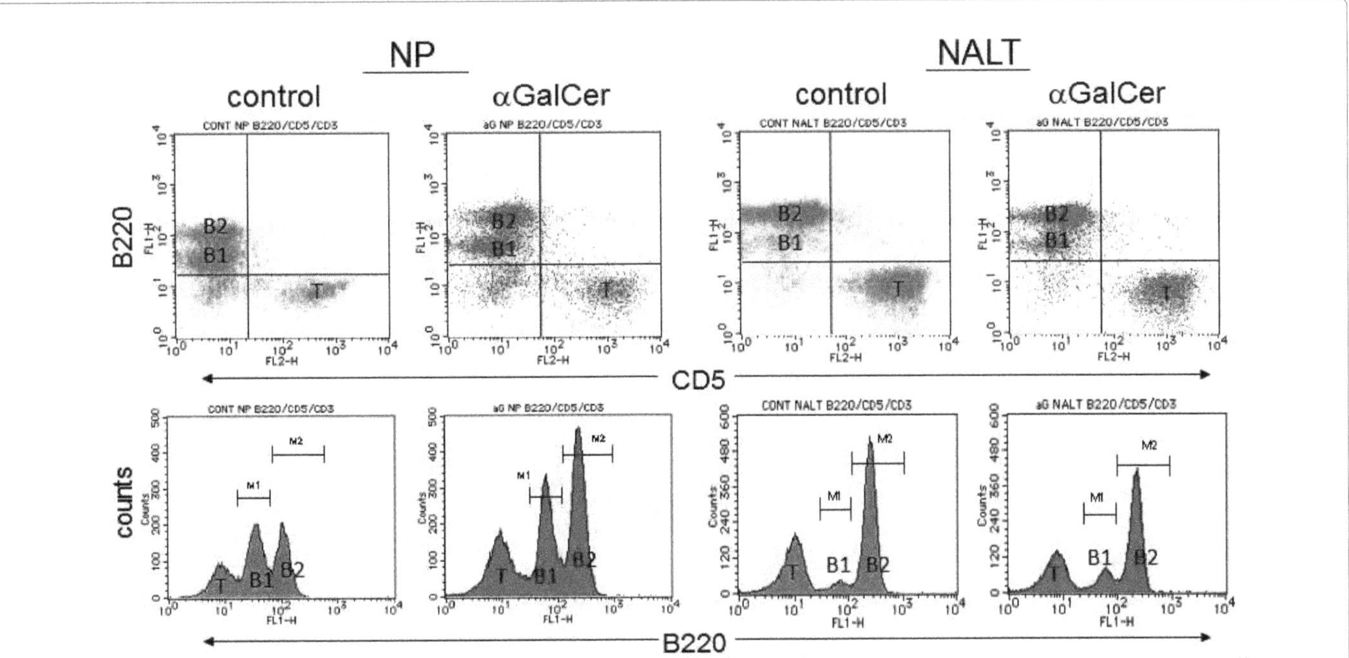

Figure 4: Flow cytometry of B cells in NALT and NP. $B220^{high}$, B-2 B cells were predominantly increased in the NP of the α -GalCer group, whereas no significant changes were detected in NALT.

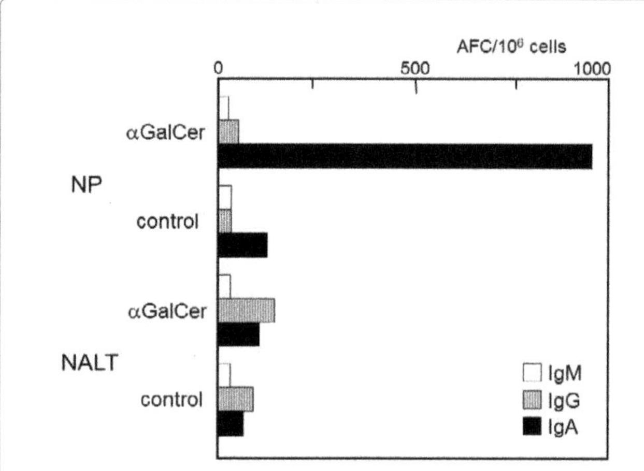

Figure 5: Number of antibody producing cells in the NP and NALT determined by the ELISPOT assay. IgA-producing cells significantly increased in the NP of the α -GalCer group. AFC, antibody-forming cell. Each experiment was performed with 5 mice per group.

Group	cytokine†	frequency (%)‡	number (cells)§
α-GalCer	IL-17	2.02 ± 0.02*	2.52×10^3*
	IL-22	1.02 ± 0.03	1.25×10^3
Control	IL-17	0.85 ± 0.07	9.47×10^2
	IL-22	1.03 ± 0.02	1.02×10^3

† NP cells were subjected to intracellular cytokine staining, and cytokine-producing cells were analyzed by flow cytometry.
‡ Frequency of IL17⁺, or IL-22⁺ CD4⁺ T cells in whole CD4⁺ T cells. Each value is expressed as the mean ± SE.
§ Absolute number of cytokine-producing CD4⁺ T cells in NP per mouse. Each value was calculated in according to the absolute number of isolated lymphocytes and the mean frequency of IL17⁺, or IL-22⁺ CD4⁺ T cells.
* p<0.05 compared with control group.

Table 3: Cytokine-producing CD4⁺ T cells in the NP.

α-GalCer, as indicated by the reduced live NTHi and Sp numbers in nasal washes of the α-GalCer group, respectively. Statistical significant differences in the clearance of both NTHi and Sp were detected between the control group and immunized group (Figure 6).

To investigate the role of IL-17 and IL-22 in protective immunity, bacterial clearance was also examined after neutralization of IL-17 and/or IL-22. Of interest, impaired Sp clearance was observed in the mice administered α-GalCer after additional intranasal administration of anti-IL-17 mAb and after administration of both anti-IL-17 and anti-IL-22. Statistical significant differences were detected between the α-GalCer group and IL-17-neutralization groups (α-GalCer+ anti-IL-17, and α-GalCer+ anti-IL-17+anti-IL-22; Figure 6). Whereas neutralization of IL-17 and/or IL-22 did not affect NTHi clearance enhanced by nasal immunization with α-GalCer. In protective nasopharyngeal immunity, a difference in key cytokines was observed in Sp and NTHi infections. This difference might depend on whether the pathogen is an extracellular or intracellular parasite, because the Th17 response facilitates the clearance of extracellular pathogens [22]. This result indicates that Th17 cells contribute partially to non-specific protective immunity, especially against extracellular parasites, induced by nasal administration of α-GalCer.

Discussion

Nasal vaccination is considered to be effective for the induction of protective immunity against upper respiratory infectious diseases, including OM and rhinosinusitis. [6,20,23-26]. The results of the present study demonstrated that nasal administration of α-GalCer alone could activate NKT cells in the nasopharynx, followed by the maturation of DCs, B cells, and some cytokine-producing CD4+ T cells. In our previous study we demonstrated that nasal immunization with P6 protein of NTHi and α-GalCer is effective in eliciting Ag-specific secretory IgA in the nasopharynx and specific IgG responses in the systemic compartment. Nasal vaccination with 10 μg P6 and 2

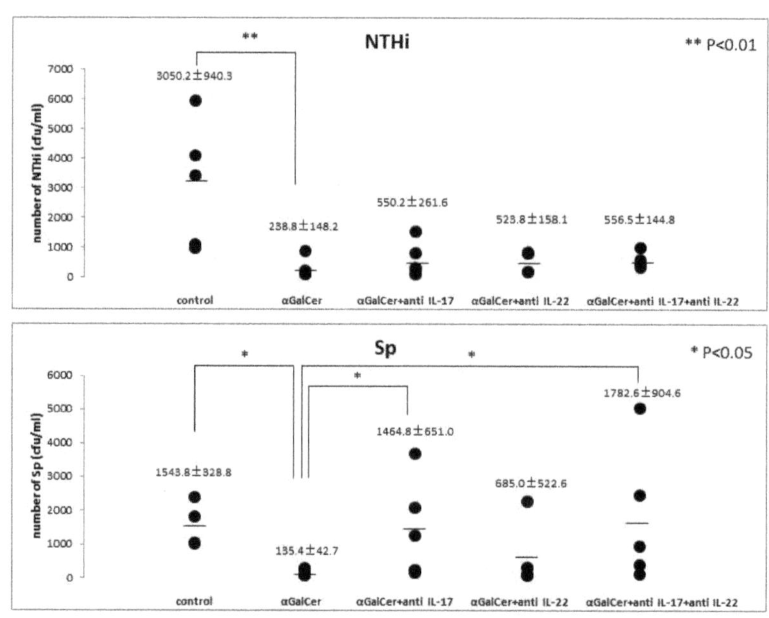

Figure 6: Bacterial clearance from the nasopharynx according to live NTHi or Sp numbers in the nasal wash. NTHi or Sp concentration was expressed as colony forming units (CFU) per milliliter of nasal wash. Enhanced NTHi and Sp clearance was observed in the α -GalCer group. NTHi and Sp clearance was impaired by the neutralization of IL-17. Values are expressed as mean ± SE. Each experiment was performed with 5 mice per group and was performed at least three times to verify results. *p<0.05, **p<0.01.

μg α-GalCer successfully induced NTHi-specific protective immunity, enhancing bacterial clearance from the nasopharynx [15,16]. In this study, the clearance of Sp as well as NTHi was partially enhanced by nasal administration of 2 μg α-GalCer alone, without bacterial Ags, since nasal immunization with bacterial Ags and α-GalCer could induce more effectively Ag-specific immune responses. Although the level of expansion in NKT cells and DCs in the present study was lower than in our previous study [15-16], certain immune responses against pathogenic bacteria were induced by nasal administration of α-GalCer. Thus, in the present study we demonstrated that the activation of NKT cells by nasal administration of α-GalCer induces broadly protective immunity in the upper respiratory tract. These responses were characterized by increased local IgA-producing cells and protection against NTHi or Sp challenge. To our knowledge, this is the first study to show the protective effect of NKT cells against both NTHi and Sp by nasal administration of α-GalCer (without any antigen).

α-GalCer is a ligand of NKT cells and thus can directly activate them when presented by CD1d. NKT cells both directly and indirectly modulate the functions of many other cell types, including NK cells and T cells. These interactions are bidirectional, as NKT cells receive signals from antigen-presenting cells (APCs), such as DCs, and *vice versa* [27]. Activation of NKT cells through recognition of α-GalCer-CD1d complexes results in the rapid production of Th1 and Th2 cytokines, such as IFN-γ and IL-4 [9,28], and the increased expression of the CD40 ligand [29], which induces DC maturation [30,31]. Interaction of NKT cells and DCs is also known to be important for the induction of protective immunity [10,15,18]. In the present study, although these mucosal immune responses were activated without Ag exposure under SPF but not germ-free conditions, the clearance of NTHi and Sp might have been enhanced because of cross-reactive antibodies, antimicrobial peptides, a proliferation-inducing ligand (APRIL) and/or induction of B-cell activating factor (BAFF), by activation of DCs and NKT cells in the nasal mucosa. The mucosal microenvironment and interaction with commensal bacteria are also essential for the development and maintenance of mucosal IgA and homeostasis [32]. Protective mucosal IgA against pathogenic bacteria could be induced by the activation of mucosal DCs carrying commensal bacteria [33]. Thus, the activation of nasal NKT cells by α-GalCer administration resulted in DC expansion and maturation in the nasal mucosa, and might contribute to the induction of nasopharyngeal protective immunity under SPF but not germ-free condition. In addition, activation of innate immune cells such as natural killer cells, or another immune pathway via Th17 cells might also be involved, and further investigation might be necessary to clarify this mechanism and to develop a broadly effective vaccine in the clinical setting.

For the pathway involving Th17 cells, the interaction between NKT and Th17 cells was examined by measuring Th17 cytokine-producing CD4+ T cells. Following nasal immunization with α-GalCer, IL-17-producing cells were increased in NP, so this result seems to indicate that Th17 cells are involved in host defense against Sp and NTHi in the upper respiratory tract. Although Th17 cells were originally identified as pro-inflammatory mediators of autoimmune disease [34], emerging data suggest that they play crucial roles in immune defense against extracellular and intracellular pathogens, including bacterial and fungal species, especially at mucosal surfaces [35,36]. Th17 cells contribute to protection by functioning as antimicrobial peptides, enhancing neutrophil recruitment, and modulating DC function [37,38]. Recently, nasal immunization has been shown to preferentially promote Th17 immune responses [39]. Furthermore, vaccine-induced Th17 cells have been shown to improve immune protection against Sp in the upper and lower respiratory tract [40,41]. Regarding the response against NTHi, we also previously demonstrated the involvement of Th17 cells in the response induced by nasal vaccination in the nasopharynx [16]. In conclusion, the results of the present study indicate that the activation of NKT cells by nasal administration of α-GalCer might positively modulate the mucosal immune system, possibly involving interaction with DCs and Th17 cells, in the nasopharynx.

References

1. Czerkinsky C, Anjuere F, McGhee JR, George-Chandy A, Holmgren J, et al. (1999) Mucosal immunity and tolerance: relevance to vaccine development. Immunol Rev 170: 197-222.
2. Belyakov IM, Derby MA, Ahlers JD, Kelsall BL, Earl P, et al. (1998) Mucosal immunization with HIV- peptide vaccine induces mucosal and systemic cytotoxic T lymphocytes and protective immunity in mice against intrarectal recombinant HIV-vaccinia challenge. Proc Natl Acad Sci 95: 1709-1714.
3. Berzofsky JA, Ahlers JD, Belyakov IM (2001) Strategies for designing and optimizing new generation vaccines. Nat Rev Immunol 1: 209-219.
4. Kozlowski PA, Neutra MR (2003) The role of mucosal immunity in prevention of HIV transmission. Curr Mol Med 3: 217-228.
5. Wu HY, Nahm MH, Guo Y, Russel MW, Briles DE (1997) Intranasal immunization of mice with PspA (pneumococcal surface protein A) can prevent intranasal carriage, pulmonary infection, and sepsis with Streptococcu pneumoniae. J Infect Dis 175: 839-846.
6. Sabirov A, Kodama S, Hirano T, Suzuki M, Mogi G (2001) Intranasal immunization enhances clearance of nontypeable Haemophilus influenzae and reduces stimulation of tumor necrosis factor alfa production in the murine model of otitis media. Infect Immun 69: 2964-2971.
7. Kurono Y, Yamamoto M, Fujihashi K, Kodama S, Suzuki M, et al. (1999) Nasal immunization induces Haemophilus influenzae-specific Th and Th2 responses with mucosal IgA and systemic IgG antibodies for protective immunity. J Infect Dis 180: 122-132.
8. Kronenberg M (2005) Toward an understanding of NKT cell biology: progress and paradoxes. Annu Rev Immunol 23: 877-900.
9. Kawano T, Cui J, Koezuka Y, Toura I, Kaneko Y, et al. (1997) CD1d-restricted and TCR-mediated activation of valpha14 NKT cells by glycosylceramides. Science 278: 1626-1629.
10. Taniguchi M, Seino K, Nakayama T (2003) The NKT cell system: bridging innate and acquired immunity. Nat Immunol 4: 1164-1165.
11. Murphy TF (2003) Respiratory infections caused by non-typeable Haemophilus influenzae. Curr Opin Infect Dis 16: 129-134.
12. Lynch JP 3rd, Zhanel GG (2010) Streptococcus pneumoniae: epidemiology and risk factors, evolution of antimicrobial resistance, and impact of vaccines. Curr Opin Pulm Med 16: 217-225.
13. O'Brien KL, Wolfson LJ, Watt JP, Henkle E, Deloria-Knoll M, et al. (2009) Hib and pneumococcal global burden of disease study team. burden of disease caused by Streptococcus pneumoniae in children younger than 5 years: global estimates. Lancet 374: 893–902.
14. Levine OS, Knoll MD, Jones A, Walker DG, Risko N, et al. (2010) Global status of Haemophilus influenzae type b and pneumococcal conjugate vaccines: evidence, policies, and introductions. Curr Opin Infect Dis 23: 236-241.
15. Noda K, Kodama S, Umemoto S, Abe N, Hirano T, et al. (2010) Nasal vaccination with P6 outer membrane protein and α-galactosylceramide induces nontypeable Haemophilus influenzae-specific protective immunity associated with NKT cell activation and dendritic cell expansion in nasopharynx. Vaccine 28: 5068-5074.
16. Noda K, Kodama S, Umemoto S, Nomi N, Hirano T, et al. (2011) Th17 cells contribute to nontypeable Haemophilus influenzae-specific protective immunity induced by nasal vaccination with P6 outer membrane protein and α-galactosylceramide. Microbiol Immunol 55: 574-581.
17. Fuji S, Shimizu K, Smith C, Boifaz L, Steinman RM (2003) Activation of natural killer T cells by α-galactosylceramide rapidly induces the full maturation of dendritic cells in vivo and thereby acts as an adjuvant for combined CD4 and CD8 T cell immunity to a coadministered protein. J Exp Med 198: 267-279.

18. Chung Y, Chang WS, Kim S, Kang CY (2004) NKT cell ligand alpha-galactosylceramide blocks the induction of oral tolerance by triggering dendritic cell maturation. Eur J Immunol 34: 2471-2479.

19. Ko SY, Ko HJ, Chang WS, Park SH, Kweon MN, et al. (2005) α-Galactosylceramide can act as a nasal vaccine adjuvant inducing protective immune responses against viral infection and tumor. J Immunol 175: 3309-3317.

20. Kodama S, Hirano T, Noda K, Abe N, Suzuki M (2010) A single nasal dose of fms-like tyrosine kinase receptor-3 ligand, but not peritoneal application, enhances nontypeable Haemophilus influenzae–specific long term mucosal immune responses in the nasopharynx. Vaccine 28: 2510-2516.

21. Hiroi T, Iwatani K, Iijima H, Kodama S, Yanagita M, et al. (1998) Nasal immune system: distinctive Th0 and Th1/Th2 type environments in murine nasal-associated lymphoid tissues and nasal passage, respectively. Eur I Immunol 28: 3346-3353.

22. Siciliano NA, Skinner JA, Yuk MH (2006) Bordetella bronchiseptica modulates macrophage phenotype leading to the inhibition of CD4+ T cell proliferation and the initiation of a TH17 immune responce. J Immunol 177: 7131-7138.

23. Kodama S, Suenaga S, Hirano T, Suzuki M, Mogi G (2000) Induction of specific immunoglobulin A and Th2 immune responses to P6 outer membrane protein of nontypeable Haemophilus influenzae in middle ear mucosa by intranasal immunization. Infect Immun 68: 2294-2300.

24. Kiyono H, Fukuyama S (2004) NALT- versus Peyer's-patch-mediated mucosal immunity. Nat Rev Immunol 4: 699-710.

25. Abe N, Kodama S, Hirano T, Eto M, Suzuki M (2006) Nasal vaccination with CpG oligodeoxynucleotide induces protective immunity against nontypeable Haemophilus influenzae in the nasopharynx. Laryngoscope 116: 407-412.

26. Bertot GM, Becker PD, Guzman CA, Grinstein S (2004) Intranasal vaccination with recombinant P6 protein and adamantylamide dipeptide as mucosal adjuvant confers efficient protection against otitis media and lung infection by nontypeable Haemophilus influenzae. J Infect Dis 189: 1304-1312.

27. Cerundolo V, Silk JD, Masri SH, Salio M (2009) Harnessing invariant NKT cells in vaccination strategies. Nat Rev Immunol 9: 28-38.

28. Spada FM, Koezuka Y, Porcelli SA (1998) CD1d-restricted recognition of synthetic glycolipid antigens by human natural killer T cells. J Exp Med 188: 1529-1534.

29. Vincent MS, Leslie DS, Gumperz JE, Xiong X, Grant EP, et al. (2002) CD1-dependent dendritic cell instruction. Nat Immunol 3: 1163-1168.

30. Fujii S, Liu K, Smith C, Bonito AJ, Steinman RM (2004) The linkage of innate to adaptive immunity via maturing dendritic cells in vivo requires CD40 ligation in addition to antigen presentation and CD80/86 costimulation. J Exp Med 199: 1607-1618.

31. Hermans IF, Silk JD, Gileadi U, Salio M, Mathew B, et al. (2003) NKT cells enhance CD4+ and CD8+ T cell responses to soluble antigen in vivo through direct interaction with dendritic cells. J Immunol 171: 5140-5147.

32. Macpherson AJ, Uhr T (2004) Induction of protective IgA by intestinal dendritic cells carrying commensal bacteria. Science 303: 1662-1665.

33. Macpherson AJ, McCoy KD, Johansen FE, Brandtzaeg P (2008) The immune geography of IgA induction and function. Mucosal Immunol 1: 11-22.

34. Bettelli E, Korn T, Oukka M, Kuchroo VK (2008) Induction and effector functions of T(H)17 cells. Nature 453: 1051-1057.

35. O'Connor W Jr, Zenewicz LA, Flavell RA (2010) The dual nature of T(H)17 cells: shifting the focus to function. Nat Immunol 11: 471-476.

36. Mucida D, Salek-Ardakani S (2009) Regulation of TH17 cells in the mucosal surfaces. J Allergy Clin Immunol 123: 997-1003.

37. Khader SA, Bell GK, Pearl JE, Fountain JJ, Rangel-Moreno J, et al. (2007) IL-23 and IL-17 in the establishment of protective pulmonary CD4+ T cell responses after immunization and during Mycobacterium tuberculosis challenge. Nat Immunol 8: 369-377.

38. Bai H, Cheng J, Gao X, Joyee AG, Fan Y, et al. (2009) IL-17/Th17 promote type T cell immunity against pulmonary intracellular bacterial infection through modulating dendritic cell function. J Immunol 183: 5886-5895.

39. Zygmunt BM, Rharbaoui F, Groebe L, Guzman CA (2009) Intranasal immunization promotes th17 immune responses. J Immunol 183: 6933-6938.

40. Zhang Z, Clarke TB, Weiser JN (2009) Cellular effectors mediating Th17-dependent clearance of pneumococcal colonization in mice. J Clin Invest 119: 1899-1909.

41. Lu YJ, Gross J, Bogaert D, Finn A, Bagrade L, et al. (2008) Interleukin-17A mediates acquired immunity to pneumococcal colonization. PLoS Pathog 4: e1000159.

Naopharyngeal Notochondroma- A Case Report and Literature Review

Bibek Gyanwali[1], **Hongquan Wu**[1], **Bunu Karmacharya**[2], **Meichan Zhu**[1] **and Anzhou Tang**[1*]

[1]*Department of Otolaryngology-Head and Neck Surgery, The First Affiliated Hospital of Guangxi Medical University, Nanning Guangxi,People's Republic of China*

[2]*Department of Radiology, The First Affiliated Hospital of Guangxi Medical University, Nanning Guangxi, People's Republic of China*

[*]**Corresponding author:** Anzhou Tang, Department of Otolaryngology-Head and Neck Surgery, The First Affiliated Hospital of Guangxi Medical University, 06# Shuangyong Road,Nanning Guangxi, People's Republic of China; E-mail: tazgxmu@163.com

Abstract

Background: Nasopharyngeal notochordoma is a rare congenital low-grade malignant tumor which is very rarely seen in clinical practice. We describe a case of nasopharyngeal notochondroma, the patient admitted in our department for surgery for fifth time.

Case report: The patient complained of left sided nasal obstruction, snoring, with left fronto-temporal headache and progressive decline of vision especially of left eye for 2 months. She had been performed surgery for the removal of nasopharyngeal notochodroma for four times. Every time she was performed surgery postoperative imaging examination showed no any residual tumor mass. But unfortunately there was always recurrence of mass. This time (fifth time) the patient was admitted for surgery, latter after the CT scan and MRI examination, showed bone destruction so patient denied for surgical treatment.

Conclusion: In this study we describe the clinical features, diagnostic evidence, treatment and discuss the possible reason of recurrence. Nasopharyngeal notochondroma is impossible to remove completely by surgery so other radiotherapy will help to increase prognosis and survival rate. As clinical feature of nasopharyngeal notochondroma is quite similar to nasopharyngeal carcinoma so it should not be confused in diagnosis and treatment.

Keywords: Notochondroma; Congenital; Malignant tumor; Recurrence

Introduction

Notochondromas are low-grade malignant tumors arising from embryonic remnants of notochord in craniopharyngeal axis, usually sccro-coccygeal and spino-occipital region. Remnants of notochord form the nucleus pulpous of the intervertebral disks in adult. A remnant of notochord persists in skull base, sacro-cccygeal area and body of vertebra. Nasopharyngeal notochondroma is a rare case in otolaryngology department, so it is often misdiagnosed as other diseases. It exhibits slow invasive growth and locally destructive nature. Because nasopharyngeal notochandromas present with new growth of mass in nasopharynx, done destruction of skull base so sometime it may be misdiagnosed as nasopharyngeal carcinoma especially in those reason where nasopharyngeal carcinoma is common. We describe the uncommon case of recurrent nasopharyngeal notochondroma.

Case Report

A 22 years old female, without any obvious inducing factors patient complained about left sided nasal congestion, snoring, with left fronto-temporal headache and progressive decline in vision especially left eye for 2 months, no nasal bleeding, no purulent nasal discharge, no bloody sputum, no eye movement abnormalities, no dysphasia, no limbs movement disorder. Six months ago she underwent resection of nasopharyngeal chordoma in our hospital. For the further diagnosis and treatment, patient come to out–patient department of our hospital, diagnosed as "post-operative recurrence of nasopharyngeal chordoma?" Since the onset of the disease, the general mental state, sleep and appetite is normal, no significant changes in body weight. From 2000-2014 4 times surgery was performed. Four previous surgeries in 2000 March; performed endoscopic naspharyngeal norochondroma resection surgery, in 2007 January and 2009 September performed combined endoscopic palatal approach notochordoma resection surgery, and in June 2014 performed endoscopic trans-sphenoidal approach nasopharyngeal notochondroma resection which was not performed in our hospital. This time when she was admitted in our department, all the preoperative tests were normal. Nasopharynx computed tomography scan (CT scan) (2015-1-20) (Figure 1A, B and C) and magnetic resonance image (MRI) (2015-1-23) (Figure 2A, B and C) revealed postoperative changes in skull base notochordoma, recurrence?

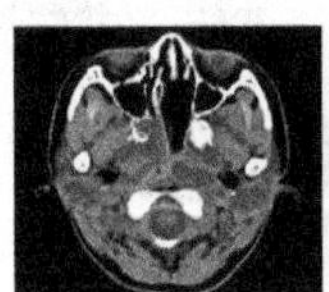
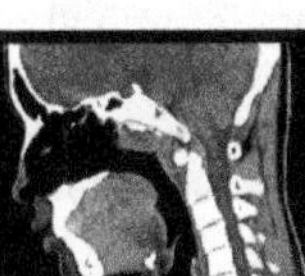
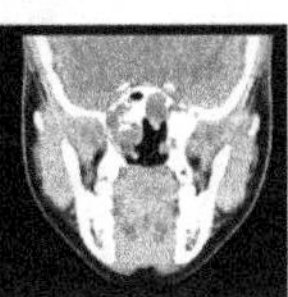

Figure 1: CT scans of fifth time preoperative (2015-1-20). (A) Axial (B) Sagittal (C) Coronal.

During routine nasopharyngeal endoscopy examination found polypoidy growth in nasopharynx (Figure 3) biopsy of that mass showed inflammatory polyps (Figure 3). Patient was planned for surgery again after the discussion with the patient's family member and consultation with department of radiotherapy, patient denied to perform surgery this time but rather try local radiotherapy and the patient was discharged from our department.

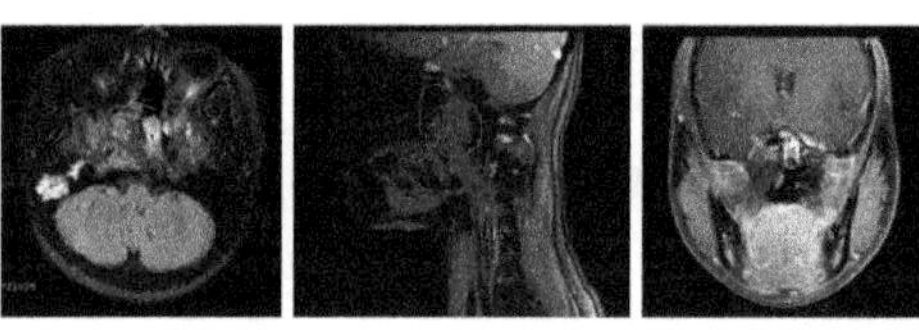

Figure 2: MRI of fifth time preoperative(2015-1-23). (A) Axial T1weighted (B) Sagittal T1-weighted (C) Coronal T1-weighted.

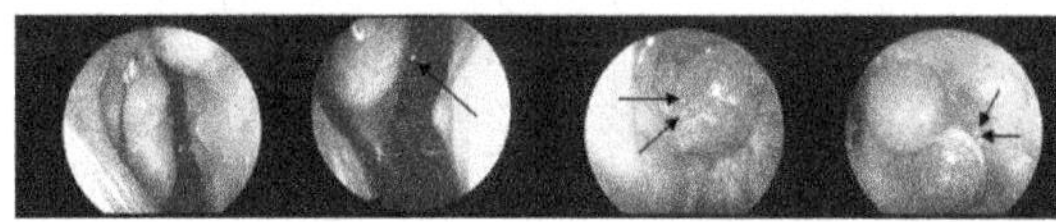

Figure 3: Nasopahryngeal endoscopic examination, showing polypoid mass in the nasopharynx.

Discussion

Nasopharyngeal notochordomas are slow-growing, can continue to grow for several years to more than 10 years. Nasopharyngeal chordoma occurs mainly in nasopharynx (basisphenoid or basiocciput or tissue around eustachian tube orifice), but also invade to the middle cranial fossa, saddle area, clivus, pterous apex and parasella [1]. Chordoma can occur at any age. Which can range from 1 year to 80 years old, but mostly occurred in the 40s. Male sexes are predominant, between the ages of 40-60 [2]. Nasopharyngeal chordoma usually presents with nasal obstruction, purulent nasal discharge, decreased sense of smell, nasal obstruction, snoring, tinnitus, hearing loss, decline of vision, headache, and sometimes may have nose bleeding and difficult in swallowing [3].

In our case the patient also complain of left sided nasal obstruction, snoring, with left fronto-temporal headache and progressive decline of vision especially left eye. Form 200-2014 the patient had been operated for 4 times with different surgical approach but there was reoccurrence of the tumor. Figure 4(A) showed the MRI preoperative images which were taken before the surgery for second time, mass in the skull base can be seen. After the surgery postoperative MRI Figure 5(b) showed no any remaining mass in the surgical area. Figure 1(c) showed the MRI take 6 months after the second time surgery the tumor reoccur, the skull base mass can be seen. Similarly in the Figure 2(A) mass can be seen but after surgery Figure 2(B) the nasopharynx seemed to be free of mass, seemed to be tumor is completely resected. But unfortunately this time when patient was admitted in our hospital with the complain of left sided nasal obstruction, snoring, with left fronto-temporal headache and progressive decline of vision, CT scan and MRI was performed showed the mass in the skull base and bone destruction confirming the reoccurrence of the mass. Every time the patient underwent surgery postoperative CT scan or MRI showed tumor free, but the mass reoccur again and again within few months.

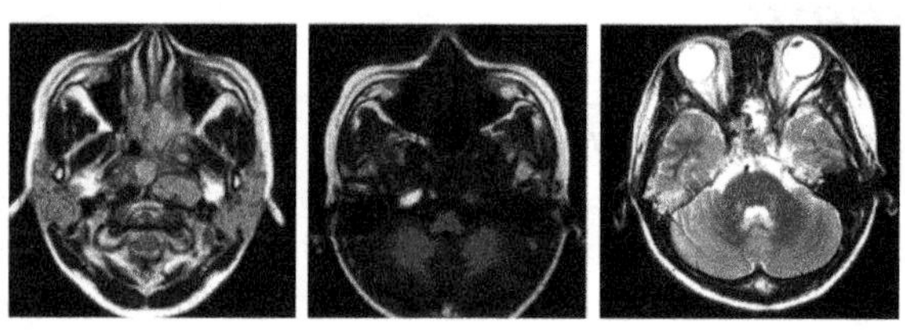

Figure 4: (A) Second time preoperative image (2007 January) of skull base notochondroma axial T1-weighted MRI. (B) Second time postoperative image (2007 January) axial T1-weighted MRI (C) Second time post-operative axial T2-weighted MRI after 6 months of second surgery.

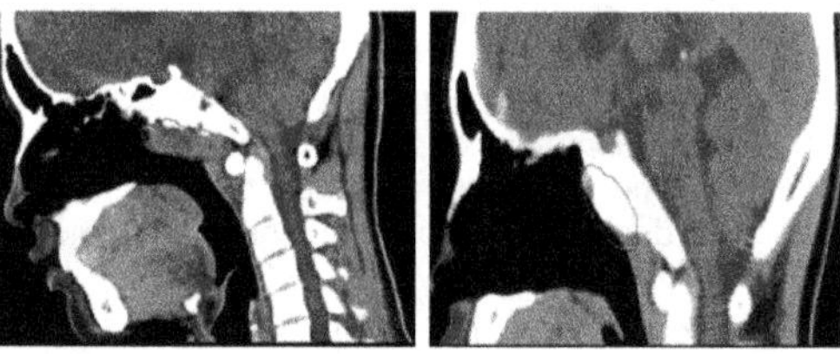

Figure 5: Sagittal CT scans (A) Third time preoperative (2009 September) (B) Third time postoperative(2009 September).

In addition to the history and physical examination, diagnosis is made mainly by pathological examination, but should rule out intracranial infection. Radiographs of the skull base, nasopharynx CT or MRI scan, can show nasopharyngeal mass and bone destruction. The principle treatment option is surgical resection of the nasopharyngeal mass, combined with postoperative radiotherapy and chemotherapy. Surgical resection of nasopharyngeal chondroma is still difficult. There are several common surgical approach, each revealed the extent of surgery, according to the the radiological findings, pathological changes and specific circumstances of the patient and lesion, selection of surgical approach is decided.

Confirming the location and extent of tumor by preoperative CT and MRI and other tests there are different surgical approaches [4]. Rong, et al. in 79 skull base neoplasms mentioned the use of eleven surgical approaches including midfacial degloving, frontal coronal discission, nasal eversion, maxillary swing, partial maxillary resection, total resection of orbit, mandibular swing, combination of front, temple, preauricular, post aureum, neck, and transoral approaches to resect the tumor[5]. In a study by George, et al. in 136 notochordomas treated and followed up over 20 years (1972–2012), mentioned that the delay before recurrence, metastasis and death is always better for the skull base notochordomas, quality of resection is the major factor of prognosis with 20.5% of deaths and 28% of recurrences after total resection resection as compared to 52.5% and 47.5% after subtotal resection. Adding proton therapy to a total resection can still improve the results. Protontherapy only improves the overall survival; the adjunct of proton therapy after total resection is clearly demonstrated [6].

In generally it is believed that notochordomas are less sensitive to radiotherapy, but is also increasingly used as postoperative treatment which has better effect than the surgery alone.

Skull base notochordomas sometime could be very challenging and, frustrating tumors to treat because of their critical location, invasive nature and reoccurrence rate. Ossama Al-Mefty and Luis Borba suggested both radical surgical removal and high-dose radiation therapy, particularly proton beam therapy, reportedly are effective in tumor control and improve survival rates. The mean disease-free interval was 14.4 months [7].

Nasopharyngeal chondroma when invade the surrounding tissue complete resection of the tumor become difficult. Most of the tumor most should be treated with radiotherapy (RT). It is believed that the risk of severe late complications and occurrence are low and cure rate high. Proton beam therapy alone or combined photon - proton beam therapy offers the advantage of improved dose distribution and the ability to treat the tumor to a higher dose without exceeding normal tissue tolerance. The 10-year local control rate after proton/photon RT is approximately 40% to 50% [8].

In another study by Feigl GC in 13 patients with 15 tumors first underwent maximal tumor resection. Within 2 to 10 months after surgery they were treated with Gamma knife surgery, GKS (mean treatment dose was 17 Gy and the mean dose was 52%), after the follow up for 17 months only one reoccurrence was at the radiation margin so he encouraged the use treatment combining surgery and early GKS [9].

Prognosis of Nasopharyngeal notochordoma depends largely on the extent of surgical resection, postoperative recurrence is common, and so the prognosis is poor. In a study conducted by Georges Noël, Jean-Louis Habrand et al. in 67 consecutive patients chordoma and chondrosarcoma of the skull base and the cervical spine treated with irradiation combined high-energy photons and protons. Photons represented two thirds of the total dose and protons one third. The median total dose delivered within gross tumor volume was 67 Cobalt Gray Equivalents (CGE; range: 60–70 CGE), found that within a median follow-up the 3-year local control rates was 71% for chordomas the 3-year overall survival rate was 88% [10]. Complete resection is very difficult to achieve, reoccurrence rate and metastasis after surgery is high. Complete resection is difficult to achieve due to tumor size, infiltrative nature, central location, and proximity to vital structures. Residual tumor is often unavoidable and invariably leads to recurrence. Tumor slippage during surgery is another cause of recurrence and may metastasis to lymph nodes, skin, lungs, liver and bones [2]. Nasopharyngeal notochordoma is a low-grade malignant tumor, selective postoperative radiotherapy is an effective method to increase the time interval to recurrence, radiation therapy offers excellent chances of cure.

Conclusion

Naospharyngeal notochondroma is a rare disease in the department of otolaryngology. Because of it clinical features and site of occurrence is similar to nasopharyngeal carcinoma so some time the disease may be miss diagnosed so otolaryngologist should pay attention to this disease. The main stay of treatment is believed to be surgery although complete surgical resection of mass is difficult to achieve. In order to resect the tumor completely and reduce the complication and possible malformation, according to the radiological findings, pathological changes and area involved different surgical approaches must be designed. Skull base chordoma is a rare neoplasm that is rarely cured after surgery alone. So to get better prognosis after surgery the surgeon should design the shortest approach, avoid damaging the important nasopharyngeal and intracranial structure, and resecting the total mass as possible.

From the above literature review and case report study we derived a conclusion that nasopharyngeal notochondroma are not completely resectable so the best possible treatment method should be surgical resection of mass along with radiotherapy (such as GKS or proton radian therpay, etc).

Acknowledgement

The authors have no information to disclose in relation to use of any writing assistance.

The authors would like to acknowledge Department of Radiology, First affiliated Hospital of Guangxi Medical University for the image courtesy.

Financial Support

All authors have not received any financial support from any person or organization for this study.

Conflict of Interest

The authors have no financial and personal relationship with other people or organization that could inappropriately influence this submission.

References

1. Perzin KH, Pushparaj N (1986) Nonepithelial tumors of the nasal cavity, paranasal sinuses, and nasopharynx. A clinicopathologic study. XIV: Chordomas. Cancer 57: 784-796.
2. Zhan J, Zhen Y, Feng Li (2009) Medical Journal of Defending Force in South West China 19: 1121-1122.
3. Notochondroma, Jiakong W, Zhou L, Tang A (2010) Otolaryngology-Head and Neck Surgery,Beijing,Peoples Medical Publishing House 2: 385-386.
4. Vougioukas V, Hubbe U, Schipper J, Spetzger U (2003) Navigated transoral approach to the cranial base and the craniocervical junction: technical note. Neurosurgery 52: 247-250.
5. Rong BG, Chen WL, Ding YP, Xie G, Chen Y, et al. (2005) [Surgical approaches to the skull base neoplasms]. Zhonghua Er Bi Yan Hou Tou Jing Wai Ke Za Zhi 40: 291-294.
6. George B, Bresson D, Bouazza S, Froelich S, Mandonnet E, et al. (2014) [Chordoma]. Neurochirurgie 60: 63-140.
7. al-Mefty O, Borba LA (1997) Skull base chordomas: a management challenge. J Neurosurg 86: 182-189.
8. Mendenhall WM, Mendenhall CM, Lewis SB, Villaret DB, Mendenhall NP (2005) Skull base chordoma. Head Neck 27: 159-165.
9. Feigl GC, Bundschuh O, Gharabaghi A, Safavi-Abassi S, El Shawarby A, et al. (2005) Evaluation of a new concept for the management of skull base chordomas and chondrosarcomas. J Neurosurg 102 Suppl: 165-170.
10. Georges Noal, Jean-Louis Habrand, Eric Jauffret, Renaud de Crevoisier, Sygon Dederke, et al. (2003) Radiation Therapy for Chordoma and Chondrosarcoma of the Skull Base and the Cervical Spine. Strahlentherapie und Onkologi 179: 241-248.

Nutritional Management for Patients with Head and Neck Cancer: The Second Step of an Italian Survey

Marianna Trignani[1*], Melissa Laus[2], Valentina Mastronardi[2], Olga Leone[2], Marilina De Rosa[2], Giulio Campitelli[2], Angelo Di Pilla1, Giuseppe Santarelli[3], Albina Allajbej[1], Ambra Pamio[4], Domenico Genovesi[1] and Adelchi Croce[2]

[1]*Department of Radiation Oncology, G. DAnnunzioUniversity of Chieti, SS. Annunziata Hospital, Chieti, Italy*

[2]*Department of Otorhinolaryngology, G. DAnnunzio University of Chieti, SS. Annunziata Hospital, Chieti, Italy*

[3]*Department of Nutrition, SS. Annunziata Hospital, Chieti, Italy*

[4]*Department of Hygiene and Public Health, G. DAnnunzio University, Chieti, Italy*

[*]**Corresponding author:** Marianna Trignani, Department of Radiotherapy, SS Annunziata Hospital, Via Dei Vestini, 66100 Chieti, Italy;
E-mail: marianna.trignani@unich.it

Abstract

Background: The purpose of this study was to survey the opinion of Italian otolaryngologist about nutritional management in patients with head and neck tumors.

Materials and Methods: A survey of 10 questions was e-mailed to 100 Italian centers of Otolaryngology.

Results: A total of 27 surveys were filled in. Nutritional supplementation in preventive phase was used by 37% respondents. The majority of respondents (88.3%) stated to use percutaneous endoscopic gastrostomy (PEG) in a reactive phase. Nutritional counselling before starting treatment was performed "rarely" by 33.3% of respondents while "always" by 29.6% of respondents; however 85.2% of respondents stated that medical nutritionist assessment should represent a standard procedure before starting an oncologic treatment.

Conclusions: Current practice about nutritional management for head and neck tumors is wide heterogeneous. Early or reactive approaches remain questionable, though otolaryngologists agree on the use of PEG in a reactive phase.

Keywords: Endoscopic gastrostomy; Survey; Nutrition; Head and neck cancer

Introduction

Growing evidence shows that more aggressive therapeutic regimens improve survival outcome of patients with head and neck cancers (HNC) [1]. However these better treatment outcomes are associated with increased morbidity worsening quality of life of the patient [2-14]. HNC patients are more likely to experience nutritional deficiencies during all phases of disease [15-23]. Studies show that nearly 40-50% of HNC patients have a markedly impaired nutritional status at the time of diagnosis, 55% have a negative energy balance throughout the course of the disease; severe weight loss has been documented in 58% of patients without enteral nutritional support [17-20].

It has been demonstrated that pre-treatment weight loss is the strongest independent predictor of survival and that malnutrition is associated with poor treatment outcomes [24-27]. Nutritional support, oral supplements and enteral tube feeding such as nasogastric tube (NGT), percutaneous endoscopic gastrostomy (PEG) and percutaneous fluoroscopic gastrostomy (PFG), are often required for HNC patients and its can be employed in different phases of oncologic management (before, during or after the primary oncologic treatment). To date, due to a lack of relevant guidelines and scientific evidences, the debate over the better choice between PEG or NGT and over the timing of their placement persists; furthermore nutritional support strategy in HNC remains nonstandard and extremely variable for different centres and physicians [28].

In view of this, we explored the opinion of otolaryngologists concerning nutritional management of HNC patients, with particular regard to PEG placement. In this study, we report the results of our survey, the first Italian survey directed to Otolaryngologists about the management of nutritional support in patients with HNC. This survey represents the second step of a project aimed to search for a point of view of experts dedicated to HNC (radiotherapists and otolaryngologists), in order to establish common guidelines [29].

Materials and Methods

A questionnaire focused on the different points of view of management of nutritional support in HNC (Table 1) was sent to 100 Italian centres of Otolaryngology. It was an online questionnaire of 10 multiple-choice questions, approved by a multidisciplinary team (MDT) composed by otolaryngologists, radiotherapists and nutritionists. The survey was prepared on the Survey Monkey online interface (www.SurveyMonkey.com). Starting from 1 April 2014 personalized e-mail invitations with direct links to the survey were sent to the Directors of the selected Italian centres of Otolaryngologists (the same questionnaire had sent to 106 Italian centres of radiation oncology) [29]. No compensation was offered to participating. Responses were collected over a 2-month period (until 30 June 2014).

We performed a descriptive analysis consisting in frequencies and percentage automatically calculated by Survey-Monkey; in addition one sample Chi-squared test was performed to determine the difference in frequency respect to uniform distribution a priori hypothesized.

Results

A total of 27 of 100 questionnaires (27%) sent to Italian centres of Otolaryngology were filled in, respondents answered all questions. Most otolaryngologists' respondents (66.7%) affirmed to treat less than 10 HNC patients per month. The three sites most frequently treated were: larynx (51.9%), oropharynx (29.6%) and oral cavity (22.2%). The majority of otolaryngologists respondents (33.3%) claimed to rarely make the nutritional counselling before surgery and 29.6% claimed to always make the nutritional counselling (p=0.535). While 29.6% of respondents do not use any nutritional supplement before surgical treatment, most respondents (37%) affirmed to use "other" nutritional supplements such as oral supplements and parenteral administration of nutrients (p=0.161). About the question "when do you use PEG?" 11.1% of the otolaryngologists respondents reported to place PEG in a prophylactic way, while 88.9% in a reactive phase; 92.6% of otolaryngologists said that PEG before starting treatment should not be a standard procedure (p<0.001). Tumor stage and site were considered as criteria for placement of PEG by 85.2% of otolaryngologists respondents (p<0.001). About nutritional counseling, 85.2% otolaryngologists stated that medical nutritionist assessment before starting an oncologic treatment should represent a standard procedure (p<0.001). At today it is assumed that a multidisciplinary approach is necessary for a proper nutritional management of HNC and in reference to this, 92.6% Otolaryngologists said to evaluate patients with HNC within a MDT.

Questionnaire	A1	A2	A3	A4
1. How many patients with H&N cancers are monthly treated in your department?	<10	20-Oct	>20	-
2. What is the site most frequently treated?	Larynx	Oral cavity	Oropharynx	Other
3. What is the second site most frequently treated?	Larynx	Oral cavity	Oropharynx	Other
4. Do you perform nutritional counseling before starting surgical treatment?	Rarely	Never	Always	Almost always
5. Which is the preferred route for prophylactic administration of nutritional supplements in patients with head and neck region?	Not use	NG tube	PEG	Other
6. In your experience, what are the criteria for PEG placement?	Stage	Site	Stage and Site	Other
7. When do you use PEG?	Prophylactic phase	Reactive phase	-	-
8. In your opinion, prophylactic PEG placement should be a standard procedure?	Yes	No	-	-
9. In your opinion, nutritional counseling before starting surgical treatment should be a standard procedure?	Yes	No	-	-
10. Do you work within a multidisciplinary team?	Yes	No	Other	
A: Answer				

Table 1: Questionnaire.

Discussion

Nutritional management is one of the most important problems in HNC patients. Several factors affect nutritional status in these patients during all phases of disease: locally advanced disease at diagnosis, anatomic location of the tumor mass, low socioeconomic status, older age, tobacco and excessive alcohol intake, treatments performed on primary tumor [15,16,21-23,30-34]. Studies show that nearly 40-50% of HNC patients have a markedly impaired nutritional status at the time of diagnosis [17,18]. Severe weight loss has been documented in 58% of patients without enteral nutritional support and it has been shown that 55% of patients could experience an additional 10% or more weight loss during both radiation therapy and chemotherapy [20,35-36]. It was demonstrated by several authors that malnutrition is associated with poor treatment outcomes, in terms of surgical site infections, wound dehiscence, morbidity, cancer recurrence, mortality and quality of life [26,27] therefore it is very important to prevent, to recognize and to treat malnutrition in an early phase of HNC treatment.

Initial nutritional intervention often involves food enrichment and oral nutrition supplements and there are several enteral feeding strategies, such as NGT, PEG and PFG, used to improve the nutritional status of patients, but up till now there has been no consistent evidence about which method is the optimal one [30,33,37,38]. NGT and PEG are the preferred strategies for enteral support, both of them have been demonstrated to be effective in achieving nutritional intake in HNC patients undergoing radiation therapy or concurrent radio-chemotherapy [37,39,40]. NGT is easy to place but poorly tolerated for prolonged periods of feeding, because it is associated with frequent ulceration, esophageal reflux and general discomfort; however PEG is better tolerated, with a lower rate of acute complications if compared with other tubes, and quality of life is potentially improved [41]. The debate over the use of PEG and NGT in HNC patients is still open and it involves considerations about modality and timing of tube feeding positioning, particularly in patients whose nutritional status is intact [31,32,34,37,39,42]. Furthermore, best practice nutrition management guidelines recommend that specialized nutritionist should be part of the MDT, together with surgeon, radiotherapist and oncologist.

This survey showed the opinions of Italian otolaryngologists regarding the role of nutritional supplementation and early placement of PEG in HNC patients. 27 out of 100 Italian Centres of otolaryngology responded to the survey, showing a poor response rate (27%) but coherent with rates recorded in other similar investigations with otolaryngologists [43,44]. The majority of Italian otolaryngology centres rarely perform nutritional counselling (33.3%) and do not use preventive nutritional supplements (29.6%), but we found no statistically significant differences in these recorded responses ($p=0.535$). Otolaryngologists agree with placing PEG in reactive phase (88.9%), in fact only 11.1% of otolaryngologists place PEG in prophylactic phase ($p<0.001$). Indeed 92.6 % of physicians affirmed that the placement of PEG before starting treatment should not be a standard procedure, confirming their common clinical practice ($p<0.001$). Dedicated MDT, in Italy, represents a consolidated reality (92.6% of the interviewed otolaryngologists reported to work within a MDT) and 85.2% of otolaryngologists interviewed consider that medical nutritionist assessment before starting treatment should represent a standard procedure, but only 29.6% declared to perform it always, suggesting that medical nutritionist is not steady part of the MDT. This latter result appeared to be statistically significant ($p<0.001$). This survey showed results partially conflicting in respect to the best practice management guidelines recommending the nutritionist within a dedicated MDT, while it is in agreement with other evidences in relation to the enteral feeding (both about type and timing of placement) [28].

Despite this study showed that the nutritionist is a ghost figure, the importance of nutritional evaluation in clinical practice is largely demonstrated and several authors observed a smaller weight loss, a better nutritional status and global quality of life in HNC patients when an intensive nutritional counselling is performed [45-50]. Regarding enteral nutrition, 92.6% of Italian otolaryngologists believes that prophylactic feeding should not represent a standard procedure, in agreement with a great part of literature, showing consensus that prophylactic feeding doesn't give benefits on nutritional or therapeutic outcomes if compared to reactive feeding. The present survey has as major limitation, namely the low participation rate. As in other surveys addressed to surgeons, response rates are often unsatisfying; however, in our opinion, this failing result is a starting point to encourage otolaryngologists discuss and share their practice using tools such as surveys, as well. We do not claim to provide recommendations nor strong scientific evidence from this survey, but it is clear that there is no uniformity in the nutritional management of HNC; furthermore, personal opinion and clinical experience often affect decision making more than recommendation and guidelines. Further researches are required in order to establish the optional nutritional approach and standard guideline for a common nutrition management in HNC patients. Finally, we believe that participation in the surveys should be encouraged in order to better use the information that this tool can provide.

References

1. Forastiere AA, Trotti A (1999) Radiotherapy and concurrent chemotherapy: a strategy that improves locoregional control and survival in oropharyngeal cancer. J Natl Cancer Inst 91: 2065-2066.
2. Trotti A (2000) Toxicity in head and neck cancer: a review of trends and issues. Int J Radiat Oncol Biol Phys 47: 1-12.
3. Logemann JA, Pauloski BR, Rademaker AW, Lazarus CL, Gaziano J, et al. (2008) Swallowing disorders in the first year after radiation and chemoradiation. Head Neck 30: 148-158.
4. Bonner JA, Harari PM, Giralt J, Azarnia N, Shin DM, et al. (2006) Radiotherapy plus cetuximab for squamous-cell carcinoma of the head and neck. N Engl J Med 354: 567-578.
5. Mendenhall WM, Parsons JT (1998) Altered fractionation in radiation therapy for squamous-cell carcinoma of the head and neck. Cancer Invest 16: 594-603.
6. Parsons JT, Mendenhall WM, Cassisi NJ, Isaacs JH Jr, Million RR (1988) Hyperfractionation for head and neck cancer. Int J Radiat Oncol Biol Phys 14: 649-658.
7. Garden AS, Asper JA, Morrison WH, Schechter NR, Glisson BS, et al. (2004) Is concurrent chemoradiation the treatment of choice for all patients with Stage III or IV head and neck carcinoma? Cancer 100: 1171-1178.
8. Cohen EE, Lingen MW, Vokes EE (2004) The expanding role of systemic therapy in head and neck cancer. J Clin Oncol 22: 1743-1752.
9. Brizel DM, Albers ME, Fisher SR, Scher RL, Richtsmeier WJ, et al. (1998) Hyperfractionated irradiation with or without concurrent chemotherapy for locally advanced head and neck cancer. N Engl J Med 338: 1798-1804.
10. Pignon JP, Bourhis J, Domenge C, Designé L (2000) Chemotherapy added to locoregional treatment for head and neck squamous-cell carcinoma: three meta-analyses of updated individual data. MACH-NC Collaborative Group. Meta-Analysis of Chemotherapy on Head and Neck Cancer. Lancet 355: 949-955.
11. Fu KK, Pajak TF, Trotti A, Jones CU, Spencer SA, et al. (2000) A radiation therapy oncology group (RTOG) phase III randomized study to compare hyperfractionation and two variants of accelerated fractionation to standard fractionation radiotherapy for head and neck squamous cell carcinomas: first report of RTOG 9003. Int J Radiat Oncol Biol Phys 48: 7-16.
12. Bernier J, Domenge C, Ozsahin M, Matuszewska K, Lefèbvre JL, et al. (2004) Postoperative irradiation with or without concomitant chemotherapy for locally advanced head and neck cancer. N Engl J Med 350: 1945-1952.
13. Lazarus CL, Logemann JA, Pauloski BR, Rademaker AW, Larson CR, et al. (2000) Swallowing and tongue function following treatment for oral and oropharyngeal cancer. J Speech Lang Hear Res 43: 1011-1023.
14. Lazarus CL, Logemann JA, Pauloski BR, Colangelo LA, Kahrilas PJ, et al. (1996) Swallowing disorders in head and neck cancer patients treated with radiotherapy and adjuvant chemotherapy. Laryngoscope 106: 1157-1166.
15. (2006) Clinical trials: oral complications of cancer therapies. National Institutes of Health.
16. Bassett MR, Dobie RA (1983) Patterns of nutritional deficiency in head and neck cancer. Otolaryngol Head Neck Surg 91: 119-125.
17. Tisdale MJ (1997) Cancer cachexia: metabolic alterations and clinical manifestations. Nutrition 13: 1-7.
18. Westin T, Jansson A, Zenckert C, Hällström T, Edström S (1988) Mental depression is associated with malnutrition in patients with head and neck cancer. Arch Otolaryngol Head Neck Surg 114: 1449-1453.
19. Hammerlid E, Wirblad B, Sandin C, Mercke C, Edström S, et al. (1998) Malnutrition and food intake in relation to quality of life in head and neck cancer patients. Head Neck 20: 540-548.
20. Raykher A, Russo L, Schattner M, Schwartz L, Scott B, et al. (2007) Enteral nutrition support of head and neck cancer patients. Nutr Clin Pract 22: 68-73.
21. Mangar S, Slevin N, Mais K, Sykes A (2006) Evaluating predictive factors for determining enteral nutrition in patients receiving radical radiotherapy for head and neck cancer: a retrospective review. Radiother Oncol 78: 152-158.

22. Ravasco P, Monteiro-Grillo I, Vidal PM, Camilo ME (2003) Nutritional deterioration in cancer: the role of disease and diet. Clin Oncol (R Coll Radiol) 15: 443-450.

23. Lees J (1999) Incidence of weight loss in head and neck cancer patients on commencing radiotherapy treatment at a regional oncology centre. Eur J Cancer Care (Engl) 8: 133-136.

24. Heimburger DC, Ard JD (2006) Handbook of Clinical Nutrition (4th edn.), MO: Mosby, St Louis.

25. Mick R, Vokes EE, Weichselbaum RR, Panje WR (1991) Prognostic factors in advanced head and neck cancer patients undergoing multimodality therapy. Otolaryngol Head Neck Surg 105: 62-73.

26. Brookes GB, Clifford P (1981) Nutritional status and general immune competence in patients with head and neck cancer. J R Soc Med 74: 132-139.

27. van Bokhorst-de van der Schuer, van Leeuwen PA, Kuik DJ, Klop WM, Sauerwein HP, et al. (1999) The impact of nutritional status on the prognoses of patients with advanced head and neck cancer. Cancer 86: 519-527.

28. Findlay M, Bauer J, Brown T (2011) Evidence based practice guidelines for the nutritional management of adult patients with head and neck cancer. Sydney, Australia: Clinical Oncological Society of Australia.

29. Trignani M, Di Pilla A, Taraborrelli M, Perrotti F, Caponigro G, et al. (2015) Early percutaneous endoscopic gastrostomy and nutritional supplementation for patients with head and neck cancer: an Italian survey of head and neck radiation oncologists. Support Care Cancer 23: 3539-3543.

30. Langius JA, Zandbergen MC, Eerenstein SE, Van Tulder MW, Leemans CR, et al. (2013) Effect of nutritional interventions on nutritional status; quality of life and mortality in patients with head and neck cancer receiving (chemo)radiotherapy; a systematic review. Clinical Nutrition 32: 671-678.

31. Salas S, Baumstarck-Barrau K, Alfonsi M, Dique L, Baggary D, et al. (2009) Impact of the prophylactic gastrostomy for unresectable squamous cell head and neck carcinomas treated with radio-chemotherapy on quality of life: a prospective randomized trial. Radiother oncol 93: 503-509.

32. van den Berg MG, Rütten H, Rasmussen-Conrad EL, Knuijt S, Takes RP, et al. (2014) Nutritional status, food intake, and dysphagia in long-term survivors with head and neck cancer treated with chemoradiotherapy: a cross-sectional study. Head Neck 36: 60-65.

33. Magné N, Marcy PY, Foa C, Falewee MN, Schneider M, et al. (2001) Comparison between nasogastric tube feeding and percutaneous fluoroscopic gastrostomy in advanced head and neck cancer patients. Eur Arch Otorhinolaryngol 258: 89-92.

34. Capuano G, Grosso A, Gentile PC, Battista M, Bianciardi F, et al. (2008) Influence of weight loss on outcomes in patients with head and neck cancer undergoing concomitant chemoradiotherapy. Head Neck 30: 503-508.

35. Ng K, Leung SF, Johnson PJ, Woo J (2004) Nutritional consequences of radiotherapy in nasopharynx cancer patients. Nutr Cancer 49: 156-161.

36. Silver HJ, Dietrich MS, Murphy BA (2007) Changes in body mass, energy balance, physical function, and inflammatory state in patients with locally advanced head and neck cancer treated with concurrent chemoradiation after low-dose induction chemotherapy. Head Neck 29: 893-900.

37. Wang J, Liu M, Liu C, Ye Y, Huang G (2014) Percutaneous endoscopic gastrostomy versus nasogastric tube feeding for patients with head and neck cancer: a systematic review. J Radiat Res 55: 559-567.

38. Ogino H, Akiho H (2013) Usefulness of percutaneous endoscopic gastrostomy for supportive therapy of advanced aerodigestive cancer. World Journal of Gastrointestinal Pathophysiology 4: 119-125.

39. Sadasivan A, Faizal B, Kumar M (2012) Nasogastric and percutaneous endoscopic gastrostomy tube use in advanced head and neck cancer patients: a comparative study. J Pain Palliat Care Pharmacother 26: 226-232.

40. Koyfman SA, Adelstein DJ (2012) Enteral feeding tubes in patients undergoing definitive chemoradiation therapy for head-and-neck cancer: a critical review. Int J Radiat Oncol Biol Phys 84: 581-589.

41. Löser C, Aschl G, Hébuterne X, Mathus-Vliegen EM, Muscaritoli M, et al. (2005) ESPEN guidelines on artificial enteral nutrition--percutaneous endoscopic gastrostomy (PEG). Clin Nutr 24: 848-861.

42. Nugent B, Parker MJ, McIntyre IA (2010) Nasogastric tube feeding and percutaneous endoscopic gastrostomy tube feeding in patients with head and neck cancer. J Hum Nutr Diet 23: 277-284.

43. Russi EG, Sanguineti G, Chiesa F, Franco P, Succo G, et al. (2013) Is there a role for postoperative radiotherapy following open partial laryngectomy when prognostic factors on the pathological specimen are unfavourable? A survey of head and neck surgical/radiation oncologists. Acta Otorhinolaryngol Ital 33: 311–319.

44. Sylvester DC, Carr S, Nix P (2013) Maximal medical therapy for chronic rhinosinusitis: a survey of otolaryngology consultants in the United Kingdom. Int Forum Allergy Rhinol 3: 129-132.

45. Isenring EA, Capra S, Bauer JD (2004) Nutrition intervention is beneficial in oncology outpatients receiving radiotherapy to the gastrointestinal or head and neck area. Br J Cancer 91: 447-452.

46. Isenring E, Capra S, Bauer JD (2004) Patient satisfaction is rated higher by radiation oncology outpatients receiving nutrition intervention compared with usual care. J Hum Nutr Diet 17: 145-15.

47. Arends J, Bodoky G, Bozzetti F, Fearon K, Muscaritoli M, et al. (2006) ESPEN Guidelines on Enteral Nutrition: Non-surgical oncology. Clin Nutr 25: 245-259.

48. Isenring EA, Bauer JD, Capra S (2007) Nutrition support using the American Dietetic Association medical nutrition therapy protocol for radiation oncology patients improves dietary intake compared with standard practice. J Am Diet Assoc 107: 404-412.

49. Bossola M (2015) Nutritional interventions in head and neck cancer patients undergoing chemoradiotherapy: a narrative review. Nutrients 7: 265-276.

50. Valentini V, Marazzi F, Bossola M, Miccichè F, Nardone L, et al. (2012) Nutritional counselling and oral nutritional supplements in head and neck cancer patients undergoing chemoradiotherapy. J Hum Nutr Diet 25: 201-208.

Otosclerosis Surgery: Contribution of Imaging in Surgical Failures and Labyrinthine Complications Diagnosis

Myriam Jrad[1*], Asma Ben Mabrouk[1], Aymen Ben Othmen[1], Jihene Marrakchi[2], Anis Zaidi[1], Rym Zainine[2], Ghazi Besbes[2] and Habiba Mizouni[1]

[1]*Department of Radiology, La Rabta Hospital, Jabberi 1017, Tunis, Tunisia*

[2]*Department of ENT, La Rabta Hospital, Tunis, Tunisia*

[*]**Corresponding author:** Myriam Jrad, MD, Clinical Chief, Departement of Radiology, La Rabta Hospital, Jabberi 1017, Tunis, Tunisia;
E-mail: myriamjrad@gmail.com

Abstract

Objective: The purpose of this study was to review the role of post-operative imaging and to illustrate with a rich iconography the main causes of surgical failures and post-operative complications of otosclerosis.

Subjects and methods: This a retrospective study of 49 ears having otosclerosis and undergoing middle ear surgery. CT scan was performed in the postoperative assessment when post-operative complication or unsatisfactory surgical results were suggested.

Results: Surgical failures were noticed in 28 ears (57%): Hearing loss was the most frequent symptom (89%).Tinnitus was found in 21 cases and vertigo in three cases. Audiometric exploration found 21 cases of conductive hearing loss, six cases of mixed type and one case was a sensorineural type. The causes of surgical failure were erosion of the long process of the incus in four cases, uncudo-mallear dislocation in one case, displacement of the prosthesis in five cases and fibrosis of the oval window in one case. Progression of otosclerosis was noticed in 13 cases. Labyrinthine complication was retained in 21 ears of our study. The causes of labyrinthine complication were intravestibular protrusion of the prosthesis (15 cases), intravestibular footplate dislocation (1 case), perilymphatic fistula (1 case), ossificans labyrinthitis (1 case), infectious labyrinthitis (1 case) and intravestibular granulation tissue (1 case). In one case, no abnormities was retained in CT and MRI

Conclusion: After this study, to ensure maximum efficiency in the postoperative monitoring and the management of complications and post-operative failures, the clinician is required to take into account both the functional findings, results audiometric and radiological data.

Keywords: Ostosclerosis; Scanner; Surgery; Complications; Prosthesis

Introduction

Otosclerosis is a primitive osteodystrophy of endochondral layer of the otic capsule. It is responsible for conductive hearing loss and sometimes mixed hearing loss. Clinical incidence varies from 0.1 to 2% worldwide. In Tunisia, its prevalence ranges from 0. 4% to 0.8% [1]. Its therapeutic management is most often the fate of the surgery which aim is usually to correct conductive component of deafness. It is therefore necessary for functional surgery patient prognosis. A significant hearing improvement is achieved in most surgical patients. However, a small proportion of patients may have persistent or recurrent deafness and sometimes signs of labyrinthisation. Imaging then finds its indications. The CT scan is realized in first intention, completed with MRI if radio-clinical discrepancy or labyrinthisation signs [2]. The purpose of this study is to review the role of post-operative imaging and to illustrate the main causes of surgical failures and post-operative complications of otosclerosis.

Material and Methods

This was a retrospective study on patients diagnosed with otosclerosis that received surgery (stapedectomy or stapedotomy) attended at the otology department of La Rabta Hospital between 1995 and 2015. A post-operative clinical assessment was made of all the patients at two months, six months and every one year after surgery. Persistent or recurrent hearing loss, tinnitus or vertigo was noticed. Postoperative audiometry was performed at 3, 6, 9, 12, 18 and 24 months and then annually. Air conduction (AC), bone conduction (BC), post-operative air bone gap (ABG) and net decibel (dB) gain of each ear was detected. Tonal audiometry of AC and BC was undertaken at frequencies of 500, 1.000 and 2.000 Hz. Hearing improvement was defined as air-bone gap closure to 10 dB or less and/or AC improvement of 20 dB or more. CT scan was performed when surgical failure or labyrinthine complication were suggested. The temporal bone CT Scan was performed using a 64 channels multidetector scanner General Electric GE. The exploration was conducted in the standard axial plan with helicoidal technique and volumetric acquisition (120 kv, 200 mA, rotation time of 0.5 s, thickness of the section of 0.5 mm, matrix 512 × 512). The head of the patient was located in a neutral position and the time of study was of 4 to 6 s. The data analysis was performed in an Advantage® work station. The temporal bones were visualized in three basic plans (axial, sagital and coronal), reconstructed in isometric way (with the same resolution as the original acquisition) every 0.6 mm. In addition, there were performed 2D reconstructions multiplanar and oblique curves, and Maximum Intensity Projections (MIP), according to the structure of clinical interest or as the findings: Ossicular chain, round and oval windows, the cochlea, vestibular aqueduct, semi-circular canals and facial nerve canal.

MRI was performed using a GE 1.5 Tesla or Siemens 3Telsa system. The following scan parameters were used for the T2-weighted TSE sequence (FOV 130 × 130 × 24 mm, 0.6 mm isotropic voxels, TR/TE/TSE factor 2400 ms/200 ms/73 and 80 sections, resulting in an acquisition time of approximately 6 min) 3D Volumetric CISS in axial plan with coronal and sagittal reformation and MIP reconstruction. Oblique sagital reformatted images in perpendicular plan to 7th and 8th nerve in internal auditive conducts were performed.

Imaging records were retrospectively evaluated by a senior radiologist, and radiology resident. Statistical analyses were performed with software package: Statistical Package for the Social Sciences. Clinical and audiological data were correlated to CT and MRI findings. These correlations were analyzed with linear and binary logistic regression model (Pearson test): p-value<0.05 was considered to indicate a statistically significant difference.

Results

A total of 326 patients diagnosed with otosclerosis that received surgery were initially identified from the department of otology clinical records. Thirty five of 326 (10.7%) had developed post-operatively clinical symptoms suggested surgical failure or labyrinthine complication. Fourteen patients were operated bilateraly a total of 49 ears; 7 (20 %) were males and 28 (80%) were females (sex ratio=0.25). Their ages were between 24 years and 80 years; the mean age was 49.7 years. Patients were underwent stapedotomy with vein graft interposition and reconstruction with either a Teflon piston in 14 cases (29%), a bucket handle prosthesis in 23 cases (47%), or a total prosthesis in 12 cases (24%).

Surgical Failure

Surgical failures were noticed in 28 ears (57%). They were an early procedural failure (<6 months) in four cases and a failure occurred during follow-up in 24 cases over a period ranging from 6 months to 26 years with a mean of 7.8 years.

Clinical data

In this group of patients, the hearing loss was the most the commonest presenting symptoms described in 25 cases (89% of failure). In three cases, it was persistent deafness in early postoperative (less than three months). In the remaining 22 cases (79%), there was a recurrence of deafness after a temporary improvement postoperative period, which was of variable duration ranging between 1 and 26 years. Tinnitus was found in 21 cases (75%), always associated with one or more other clinical features. Vertigo was found in three cases (11%). In one case, it appeared in immediate postoperative period.

Audiological finding (Figure 1a)

In 4 cases (14%), hearing loss was developed in early postoperative. They were about, in all cases, conductive type. The ABG was about 41.1 dB. In late post-operative, we noticed 21 cases of mixed hearing loss, 2 cases of conductive type, 1 case of sensorineural hearing loss and no cases of postoperative deafness. The ABG was about 45.7 dB.

CT finding

The deadline for completion of the CT scan in late post-operative period and during follow-up was variable with an average of 8.1 years and extremes ranging from 9 months to 26 years. In the latter case, the scanner was indicated for mixed hearing loss progressively worsening with associated vertigo. The dose length product (DLP) averaged 571 milli gray (mGy) per centimeter with a range of 420-1213. Surgical failure was due to erosion of the long process of the incus in four cases (14%), incudo-mallear dislocation in one case (4%) and displacement of the prosthesis in 11 case (39%): Five cases of displacement of the lateral end of the prosthesis from the uncus, two cases of disconnected medial end (Figure 2) and four cases of complete dislocation of the prosthesis (Figure 3). In two case, CT showed a hypodensity of the ovale window due to fibrosis in one case (Figure 4) and a short prosthesis with a medial end does not comes into contact with the oval window in the other case. Progression of otosclerosis (Figure 5), compared to pre-operative imaging, was noticed in 13 cases (46%) associated with displacement of the prosthesis in three cases. No abnormalities were raised only in one CT scan.

MRI finding

MRI was performed in only two patients within a period not exceeding three months after practicing scanner. It was motivated by the result of CT showing a fibrosis of the oval window and a progression of otosclerosis with the presence of an exuberant hypodensity making suspect of an intravestibular extension. In the first case, no abnormality was raised. In the second case, MRI showed intra vestibular nodular lesion hypointense T2 enhanced after Gadolinum injection due to granulation tissue (Figure 6).

Labyrinthine complication

In 21 ears (43%) labyrinthine complications were retained. In these cases, patients showed signs of functional use in a subsequent period ranging from one to 21 years and an average of 6.6 years.

Clinical finding

Tinnitus was found in 8 cases (29%), associated in all cases with one or more other clinical symptom. Vertigo was found in 10 cases (36%). The hearing loss was described in 14 cases (50%). In the all cases, there was a recurrence of deafness after a temporary improvement over an average period of 7.3 years.

Audiological finding (Figure 1b)

In early postoperative, all patients of this group had ABG between 10 and 15 dB. We only collected the audiological data having been suspected diagnosis of labyrinthine complication, which was occurred after a mean of 6.6 years. During follow-up, 14 patients developed deafness: mixed type (12 ears), conductive hearing loss (1 ear) and sensorineural hearing loss (1 ear).

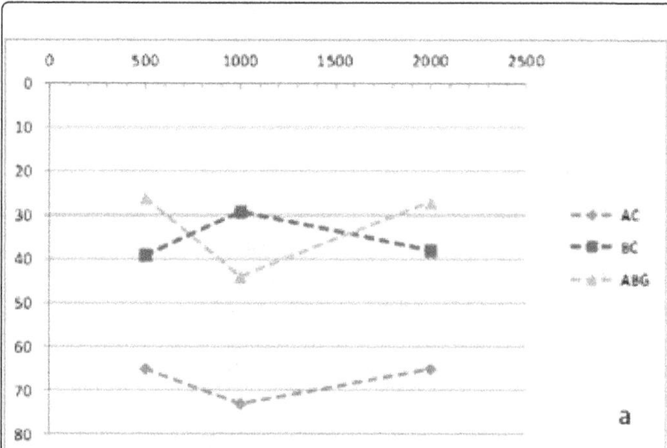

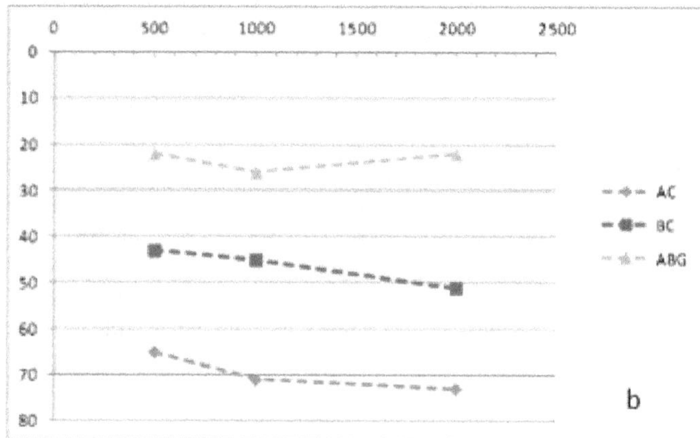

Figure 1: (1a) Audiological finding of patients with surgical failure and (1b) labyrinthine complication, AC=Air Conduction, BC=Bone Conduction.

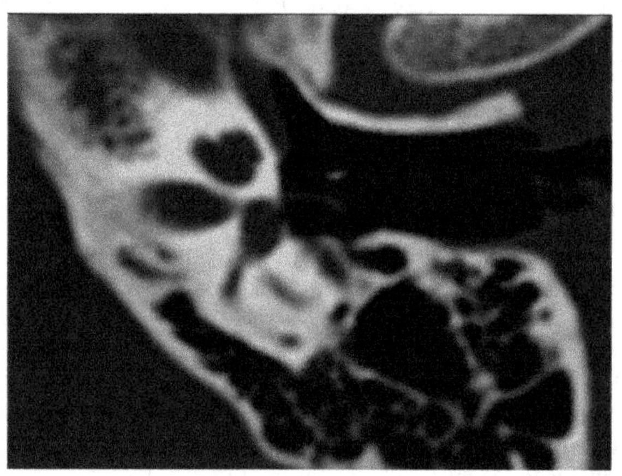

Figure 2: Axial oblique CT scan section: The proximal end of the prosthesis is in anterior footplate and extra status.

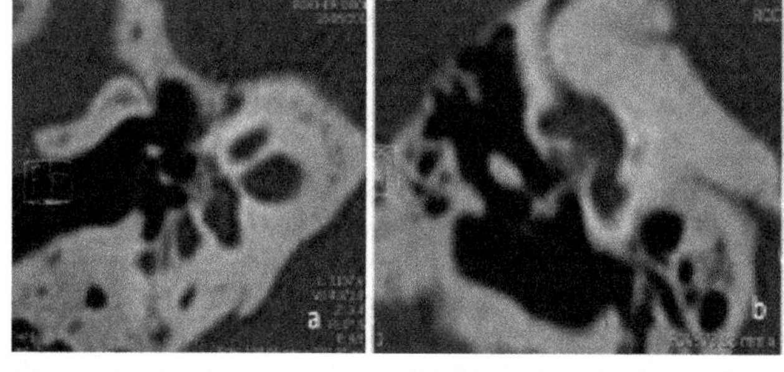

Figure 4: (a) CT scan of temporal bone: Oblique axial sections and (b) coronal oblique section a patient operated a year ago: Otosclerosis prestapedian home to exuberant development responsible for a total filling the niche of the oval window due to fibrosis of the oval window.

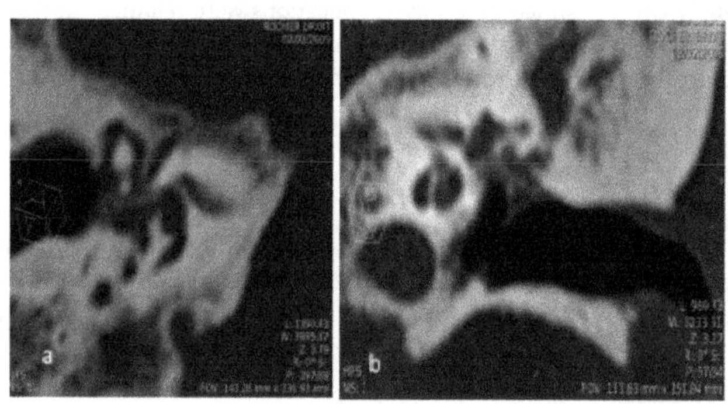

Figure 3: (a) Axial oblique section and (b) coronal oblique CT scan section: separation of the piston at its hook of the long process of the incus with subsequent rotation, the hook being turned back. The proximal end of the prosthesis is in anterior footplate and extra status.

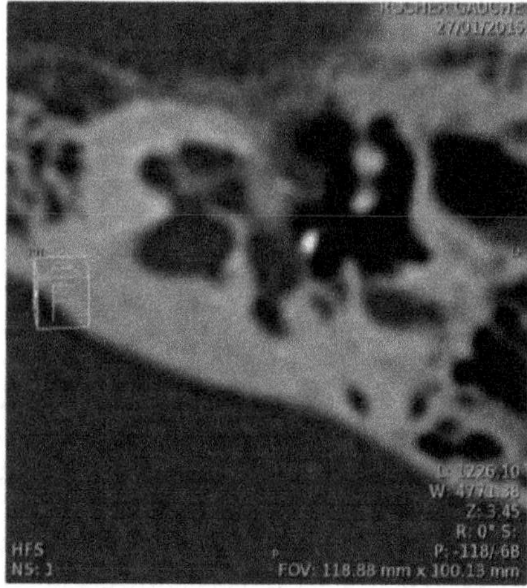

Figure 5: Prestapedian hypodensity coming in contact with the cochlea and vestibule related progressive pursuit of otosclerosis.

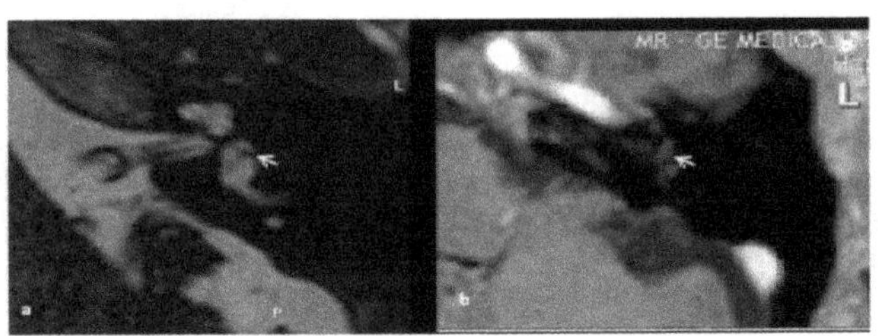

Figure 6: (a) Axial T2-weighted MR image, (b) Contrast-enhanced axial T1-weighted MR image shows intra vesibular nodular lesion hypointense T2 (a) enhanced after Gadolinum injection (b) due to postoperative intravestibular granuloma (arrow).

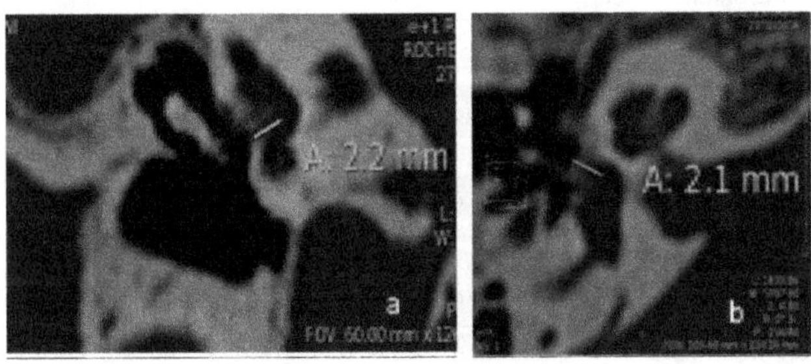

Figure 7: (a) Oblique coronal CT image and (b) oblique axial CT image: deep intravestibular postion of the prothesis reaching sensorineural area of the labyrinth.

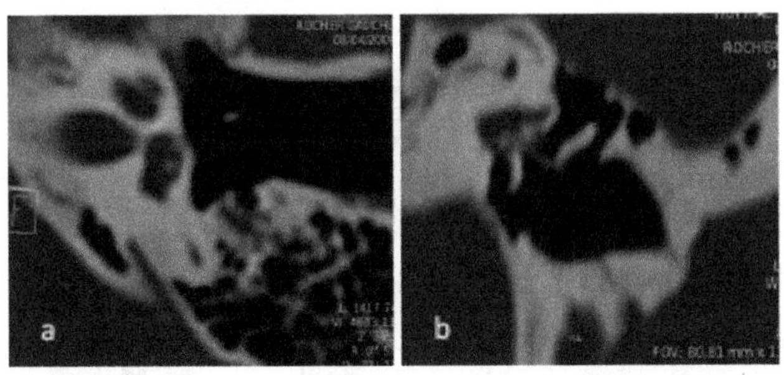

Figure 8: (a) Oblique axial CT image and (b) oblique coronal CT image: Patient operated 14 years ago: Transplatinaire prosthesis in normal posterior situation at the labyrinthine tank with depression of the rest of platinum in the vestibule correspondent to intravestibular footplate dislocation.

CT finding

In this group, the dose length product (DLP) averaged 665 milli gray (mGy) per centimeter with a range of 398-1242. CT showed a deep intavestibualr position of the medial end of the prosthesis exceeding the external half of the vestibule in 15 cases (71%) (Figure 7). In two cases CT showed a focal hyperattenuation in the vestibule one case due to intravestibular footplate dislocation (Figure 8). An extensive hyperattenuation in lateral semicircular canal was noticed in one case consistent with labyrinthine ossificans (Figure 9). Intravestibular granulation tissue was suspected in one case. CT was normal in two cases.

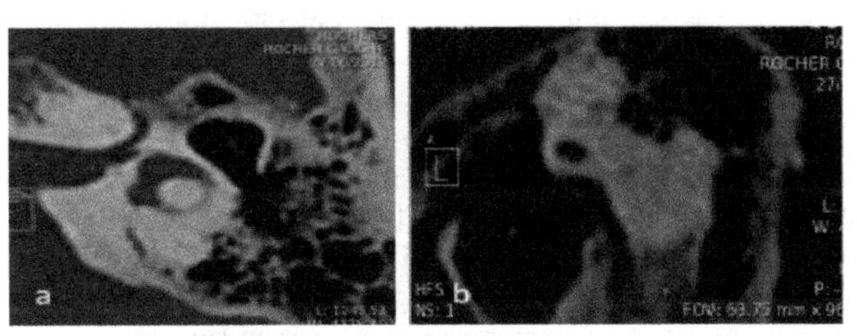

Figure 9: (a) Oblique axial CT image and (b) oblique sagital CT image: Extensive hyperdensity in lateral semicircular canal.

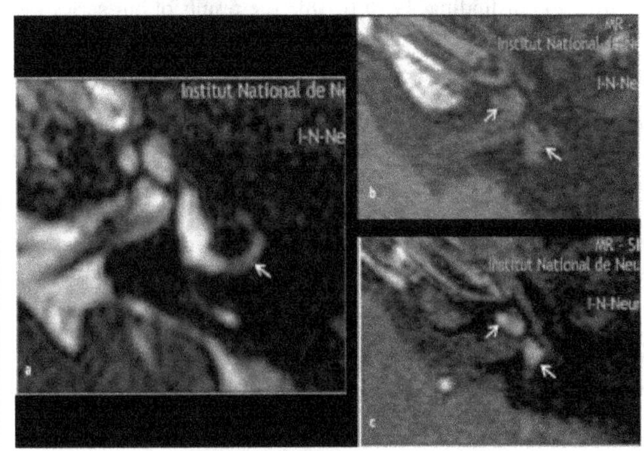

Figure 10: (a) Axial T2-weighted MR image, (b)Axial T1-weighted MR image, Contrast-enhanced axial T1-weighted MR image (c) shows shows abnormal hypointensity of the labyrinthine fluid (arrow) (a) enhanced after Gadolinum injection (b) due infectious labyrinthitis (arrow).

MRI Finding

In only three cases, MRI was performed. In two cases, no abnormalities were raised in CT scan conducted in first-line. MRI was requested to complement the research of any other cause that may explain the functional symptoms described showing an infectious labyrinthitis (Figure 10) in one case and no abnormalities in the other case. In the third case, the patient complained of recurrent hearing loss and vertigo. MRI confirmed perilymphatic fistula suspected on CT.

Discussion

The essential limitations of our study was the small number of patients included in our study and the lack of correlation of imaging results to the results of the surgery Failures and complications affect less than 10% of patients operated on for otosclerosis. Recurrent hearing loss or deafness after a period of improvement hearing is the most common symptom described in 91% of cases on average in the literature [3,4]. Persistent deafness has been described in average 21%. Tinnituses are associated in all cases reviewed in the literature [3] to another functional symptom. Recurrent deafness is often conductive type, but most often it degrades to become mixed type and even deafness. This evolution is variable over time with deadlines that can go up to 7 years and over in the literature [5]. Vertigo is infrequent and is only present in 10 to 20.1% of cases in literature [6]. In our study, hearing loss was found in 79% and vertigo in 25%. It was a recurrent hearing loss in 54.4%. The failures are the most common reasons for revision surgery. These failures are due to a displacement of the prosthesis, the progression of otosclerosis, lysis/erosion of the descending branch of uncus, fibrosis of the oval window and incudo-mallear dislocation. Several studies [7-11] examined the causes of failures found at the post-operative CT scan. Table 1 summarized their results comparing to our findings [11-15]. The labyrinthine complications are less common causes of revision surgery. The main causes of labyrinthine suffering are secondary to migration of the prosthesis from the center portion of the oval widow, peri-lymphatic fistula, reparative granuloma extending into the vestibule, labyrinthitis or bleeding intra-vestibular. Table 2 summarized their results comparing to our findings [9,10,16-18]. The results of our series were comparable with previously published studies. On suspicion of failure or post-operative complication, clinical and audiometric results conclude in some cases in suffering or a labyrinthine destruction without any etiological specificity. CT and MRI are extremely useful in the etiological diagnosis. Based on clinical results, audiometric and the imaging findings, retaining conclusion of complications and failures of the primary surgical treatment of otosclerosis may require medical treatment cochlear support and/or vestibular, recovery surgical or hearing aid fitting [19,20]. However, several studies have reported that the CT scan data were not always correlated with operative findings, especially in case of lysis of uncus or fibrosis of the oval window [21]: Ayache et al. about 26 cases of revision surgery, showed a discrepancy between the conclusions of the radiologist and surgeon observations in 50% of cases while the correlations were excellent in 37.5% of cases and partial in 12.5% of cases. However, the helical acquisition techniques and MPR reconstruction, which were not used in this series, significantly improve the reliability of imaging and used to dictate the surgical procedure or take medical treatment. Moreover, according to some articles [10,22], simple erosion of uncus, frequently observed during surgical revision regardless of the type of prosthesis is usually not detected on CT.

	Han et al. [16]	**Wiet et al. [10]**	**Lesinski [7]**	**Betsch et al. [9]**	**Lippy et al. [5]**	**Our study**
	n=74	**n=1147**	**n=279**	**n=73**		**n=49**
Displacement of prosthesis	17.5	45	81	37.1	58.1	24
Lysis/Erosion of uncus	43.2	23.6	31	8.5	-	8
Progression of otosclerosis	24.3	10.5	13.5	7.1	-	20
Fibrosis of oval window	44.6	2.9	-	32.8	2.7	2
Uncudo-mallear dislocation	-	0.8	4	5.7	-	4
Short prosthesis	20.3	4.5	5	5.7	-	0

Table 1: Underlying causes of surgical failures of our study comparing to litterature (p. 100).

	Han et al. [16]	**Wiet et al. [10]**	**Shea [18]**	**Lesinski [7]**	**Betsch et al. [9]**	**Our study**
	n=74	**n=1147**	**n=308**	**n=279**	**n=73**	**n=49**
Peri-lymphatic fistula	5.4	10	2	5.4	5.7	2
Intravestibular protrusion of prosthesis	1.4	0.4	0.8	2	5.7	22
Reparative granuloma extending into the vestibule	-	2.3	0.4	-	5.7	2
Labyrinthitis	-	-	-	-	-	4
Floating platinium	-	-	0.8	-	-	2

Table 2: Underlying causes of labyrinthine complications of our study comparing to litterature (p. 100).

Conclusion

To ensure maximum efficiency in the postoperative monitoring and the management of complications and post-operative failures, the clinician is required to take into account both the functional findings, results audiometric and radiological data. However, in some cases during the postoperative period, imaging may be insufficient in the search for an etiology for the patient's symptoms. In the future, technological advances in imaging and the confrontation between the imaging data and operative findings should help increase the reliability of imaging.

Conflicts of Interest

The authors declare that they have no conflicts of interest.

References

1. Ben Amor NR, Khelifa Z, Ben Gamra O, Zribi S, Hariga I, et al. (2013) Otospongiose: A Propos De 149 Cas. Joural Tunisien d'ORL 29.
2. Rangheard AS, Marsot-Dupuch K, Mark AS, Meyer B, Tubiana JM (2001) Postoperative complications in otospongiosis: Usefulness of MR Imaging. AJNR Am J Neuroradiol 22: 1171-1178.
3. Babighian GG, Albu S (2009) Failures in stapedotomy for otosclerosis. Otolaryngol Head Neck Surg 141: 395-400.

4. Naggara O, Williams T, Ayache D, Heran F, Piekarski JD (2005) Imaging of postoperative failures and complications in stapes surgery for otosclerosis. J Radiol 86: 1749-1761.

5. Lippy WH, Battista RA, Berenholz L, Schuring AG, Burkey JM (2009) Twenty-year review of revision stapedectomy. Otol Neurotol.

6. Bakhos D, Lescanne E, Charretier C, Robier A (2010) Révisions dans l'otospongiose: A propos de 89 cas. Ann fr ORL path maxillo-fac 127: 227-232.

7. Lesinski SG (2002) Causes of conductive hearing loss after stapedectomy or stapedotomy: A prospective study of 279 consecutive surgical revisions. Otol Neurotol 23: 281-288.

8. Lesinski SG (2003) Revision stapedectomy. Curr Opin Otolaryngol Head Neck Surg 11: 347-354.

9. Betsch C, Ayache D, Decat M, Elbaz P, Gersdorff M (2003) Revision stapedectomy for otosclerosis: Report of 73 cases. J Otolaryngol 32: 38-47.

10. Wiet RJ, Kubek DC, Lemberg P, Byskosh AT (1997) A meta-analysis review of revision stapes surgery with argon laser: Effectiveness and safety. Am J Otol 18: 166-171.

11. Veillon F, Williams M (2014) Imagerie des échecs et des complications du traitement chirurgical de l'otospongiose. Imagerie de l'oreille et de l'os temporal. Traumatologie, urgences, otospongiose. Lavoisier, pp: 879-888.

12. Bittermann AJ, Wegner I, Noordman BJ, Vincent R, van der Heijden GJ, et al. (2014) An introduction of genetics in otosclerosis: A systematic review. Otolaryngol Head Neck Surg 150: 34-39.

13. Lippy WH, Schuring AG (1984) Stapedectomy revision following sensorineural hearing loss. Otolaryngol Head Neck Surg 92: 580-582.

14. Kulakova LA, Poliakova EP, Bodrova IV, Lopatin AS (2014) The results of the surgical treatment of otosclerosis in the elderly subjects. Vestn Otorinolaringol 14: 17-19.

15. Bast F, Mazurek B, Schrom T (2013) Effect of stapedotomy on pre-operative tinnitus and its psychosomatic burden. Auris Nasus Larynx 40: 530-533.

16. Han WW, Incesulu A, McKenna MJ, Rauch SD, Nadol JB Jr., et al. (1997) Revision stapedectomy: Intraoperative findings, results, and review of the literature. The Laryngoscope 107: 1185-1192.

17. Lesinski SG (2002) Causes of conductive hearing loss after stapedectomy or stapedotomy: A prospective study of 279 consecutive surgical revisions. Otol Neurotol 23: 281-288.

18. Shea JJ Jr (1998) Forty years of stapes surgery. Am J Otol 19: 52-55.

19. Stone JA, Mukherji SK, Jewett BS, Carrasco VN, Castillo M (2000) CT evaluation of prosthetic ossicular reconstruction procedures: What the otologist needs to know. Radiographics 20: 593-605.

20. Silverstein H (2005) The future of stapes surgery. Ear Nose Throat J 84: 394-395.

21. Haberkamp TJ, Harvey SA, Khafagy Y (1996) Revision stapedectomy with and without the CO_2 laser: An analysis of results. Am J Otol 17: 225-229.

22. Ayache D, El Kihel M, Betsch C, Bou Malhab F, Elbaz P (2000) Revision surgery of otosclerosis: A review of 26 cases. Annales d'oto-laryngologie et de chirurgie cervico faciale: Bulletin de la Societe d'oto-laryngologie des hopitaux de Pari 117: 281-290.

21

Personal Music Devices: An Assessment of User Profile and Potential Hazards

Virangna Taneja[1,2,*], Shelly Khanna Chadha[2], Achal Gulati[2] and Ankush Sayal[2]

[1]*University Hospital Coventry and Warwickshire NHS Trust, Masonway, Birmingham B152EE, United Kingdom*

[2]*Department of Otolaryngology and Head, Neck Surgery MAM College and association LN Hospital, Delhi, India*

[*]**Corresponding author:** Virangna Taneja, University Hospital Coventry and Warwickshire NHS Trust, Masonway, Birmingham B152EE, United Kingdom; E-mail: virangnataneja@ymail.com

Abstract

Objectives: To profile the use of personal music devices (PMDs) in the study cohort, evaluate their output levels, and assess the users with regard to listening habits, symptomatology and hearing thresholds.

Study design: A randomised prospective study including 500 individuals aged between 16 and 30 years.

Methods: A questionnaire-based assessment included their demographic profile, PMD usage history and symptomatology and then they were classified into high (286) and low risk (214) groups.

Results: The average weekly usage of PMDs was 5.39 days/week, mean volume was 4.88, which increased to 5.9 in noisy areas, and average output used was 66.04 dB. Evaluation by pure tone audiometry (PTA) showed average hearing loss of 21.35 dB in the high risk group.

Conclusions: In total, 57.2% of the individuals included in this study demonstrated high risk behaviour for use of PMDs. Those with risky listening behaviour showed audiometric evidence of early noise-induced hearing loss (NIHL).

Keywords: Personal music devices (PMD); Noise-induced hearing loss (NIHL); Excessive noise

Introduction

Exposure to excessive noise is a major cause of hearing disorders worldwide. The World Health Organization programme for Prevention of Deafness and Hearing Impairment (WHO 1997,) stated [1]: Exposure to excessive noise is the major avoidable cause of permanent hearing impairment worldwide. Noise-induced hearing loss is the most prevalent irreversible industrial disease, and the biggest compensatable occupational hazard. According to WHO estimates, in 2005, there were 278 million people worldwide with bilateral moderate to profound hearing loss with two-thirds living in the developing world [2]. In addition to noise at the workplace, loud sounds at leisure times may also reach excessive levels, for instance, with Personal Music Devices (PMDs) and in discotheques. Over the two decades since the 1980s, the number of young people suffering from social noise exposure has increased and, in contrast, the number suffering from occupational noise exposure has decreased [3]. The increase in unit sales of PMDs has been phenomenal in Europe over the last 4 years [3].

According to one report, [4] 16% of disabling hearing loss in adults is attributed to occupational noise ranging from 7% to 21% in various sub-regions. Serra et al. [5] reported that sound levels of PMDs ranged between 75 and 105 dB and levels in discotheques ranged between 104.3 and 112.4 dB and that prolonged exposure to such levels leads to noise-induced hearing loss (NIHL). This can be prevented to a large extent by reducing exposure time and levels.

International Organization of Standardization (ISO) (1999) [6] and OSHA (Occupational Safety and Health Administration) guidelines [7] define a time-weighted average level of 85 dB for 8 h per day as the maximum permissible limit with a 3 dB increase between exposure time and sound level.

Over the last few years, there has been a trend towards an increasing population risk due to PMDs as their sound quality has improved and as they have been adopted by an increasing proportion of the population. In view of this increasing trend in PMD usage, our study was done to profile the use of personal music devices (PMDs) in the study cohort, evaluate their output levels, and assess the users with regard to listening habits, symptomatology and hearing thresholds.

Materials and Methods

This was a randomised prospective study conducted by the Department of Otorhinolaryngology and Head and Neck Surgery at Maulana Azad Medical College, New Delhi, India.

Study population

The study population included 500 individuals who were between 16 and 30 years of age without any history of ear disorder or systemic illness. Those with pre-existing ear disorders or hearing loss as well as those with associated confounding factors such as occupational exposure, or use of ototoxic medications were excluded from the study.

Following informed consent, a questionnaire was filled by each person. This included type of device, duration of usage, volume at which the device was commonly used, and any symptoms associated with persistent usage. Based on the survey, the subjects were divided into high and low risk groups.This division was done on the basis of the intensity and duration of exposure, and OSHA [7] guidelines for occupational exposure were followed. Those individuals who repeatedly exceeded the prescribed limits of exposure were assigned to the high risk group, whereas those whose exposure occasionally or never exceeded the prescribed limits were assigned to the low risk group.

Fifty individuals each from the high and low risk groups were then randomly selected and these 100 candidates underwent a detailed systemic examination, otoscopic examination and pure tone audiometry (PTA). The results were compared after taking the average of threshold levels at 0.5, 1, 2, 4 and 6 kHz. A separate analysis was carried out for the hearing threshold at 4 kHz.

Assessment of output of various devices

A total of 110 devices were assessed which included 90 mobile phones, 10 Apple iPods and 10 music players.

The output of all of the devices was calculated using an Affinity Interacoustics Sound Pressure Level (SPL) meter attached to computer software. The testing was done in a soundproof room. A B&K Sound Level Calibrator Type 4231 was used. The same pieces of music were used in each device.

The earphones of the device being tested were connected to the SPL meter and sealed to avoid sound dissipation. Two different pieces of music, one of high pitch and the other of low pitch were played each for duration of 30 s. The average of the outputs estimated during the 30 s was calculated for both pieces of music. The average of the levels of sound generated by the two different pieces was taken as the output level. The minimum and maximum outputs of the device, the output at the most commonly used volume and at the volume used in noisy areas were calculated in decibels.

Results and Analysis

A total of 500 healthy young individuals in the age group 16-30 years were included in the study, of which 286 were demonstrating high risk behaviour and 214 were showing low risk behaviour. Their mean age was 22.59 years; 54% of the high risk and 70% of the low risk individuals were in the age group 20–24 years. Of the 500 individuals, 273 were males. Of all individuals in our study group, 202 were undergraduates. In the high risk group, 64% were undergraduates compared to 74% in the low risk group. The majority (306) were cohabitating with their parents and siblings; 62% of the high risk users lived with their parents and siblings compared to 54% in the low risk group. This is significant as household members often warn the users against high risk usage of PMDs.

In the high risk group, most of the individuals were using both mobile phones as well as other devices as a source of music whereas in the low risk users, 68% were using only mobile phones as their personal music device; 451 were using earbud type earphones. None of the 500 individuals knew about the use of a noise limiter. In total, 410 were not being warned by anybody about the high risk use of PMDs.

Weekly usage of PMDs varied between 1 day and all 7 days per week with an overall mean weekly usage of 5.39 days. The mean was 6.88 days/week in the high risk group compared to 3.42 days/week in the low risk group and this turned out to be highly significant. The daily duration of usage varied between 0.2 h/day and 12 h/day with a mean of 2.034 h/day. The mean daily duration was 3.62 h/day in the high risk group with a constant usage for 1.5 h compared to 1.003 h/day in the low risk group with a constant duration for 0.45 h and the daily duration of usage was highly significant. The high risk users were listening music for more than 5yrs compared to low risk users who were listening for less than 1yr The volume at which PMDs were used varied from 1 to 10 with a mean volume of 4.88. The mean volume used by high risk users was 7 compared to 2.6 by low risk users. In noisy areas, volume commonly used was 8.2 in the high risk group, compared to 3.64 in the low risk group Table 1.

The outputs of all of the devices were measured using an Affinity Interacoustics SPL meter. The minimum and maximum outputs of all of the devices were of almost equal range but the output was significantly different in both the high and low risk groups in terms of volume commonly used. In the high risk group, the mean output at commonly used volume was 76.75 dB compared to 55.33 dB in the low risk group. Similarly, the output in noisy surroundings was 82.10 dB in the high risk group compared to 60.76 dB in the low risk group (p value being <0.001) Table 2.

Symptomatology was also assessed in both groups. Headache was a predominant complaint in 54% of the candidates indulging in high risk behaviour; 22% of the high risk candidates had to raise the volume of their TVs to hear properly compared to 8% of low risk individuals (p=0.05). In total, 16% of the relatives of high risk candidates felt that they had to talk loudly compared to 4% in the low risk group (p=0.04). When we compared the two groups for these symptoms, they were significantly more prevalent among the high risk subjects. Other symptoms were also assessed such as ringing sensation in the ears (p=0.153), complaints of hearing loss, difficulty in understanding speech, and difficulty in hearing the telephone bell/doorbell. All of these symptoms were not significant in the two groups. In total, 12% of the high risk candidates compared to 6% of the low risk individuals had to take a break from music as they felt that the sound became too loud with the continuous use of headphones. Some even had earache due to excessive use of their earphones.

Sub Group	N	Mean frequency of use (days/week)	Mean duration of use (h/day)	Mean volume used	Mean volume in noisy areas
High risk group	50	6.88	3.62	7.08	8.24
Low risk group	50	3.42	1.003	2.66	3.64
Total	100	5.15	2.312	4.87	5.94

Table 1: Usage pattern of PMDs in high and low risk groups.

Sub Group		Minimum (dB)	Maximum dB	Commonly used volume	Noisy surroundings
High Risk	N	50	50	50	50
	Minimum	48	74	54	54
	Maximum	58.5	102.5	102.5	102.5
	Mean	49.92	90.86	76.75	82.1
Low Risk	N	50	50	50	50
	Minimum	48	76	48	48
	Maximum	64.5	102.5	86	99
	Mean	50.09	88.46	55.33	60.76

Table 2: Output levels of PMDs in high and low risk groups.

Otoscopic examination revealed bilateral normal tympanic membrane in both groups.

Pure tone audiometry (PTA) findings were significantly different in both groups. These showed a hearing loss of 20.9 dB in the right ear with 19 dB at 4 kHz and 21.8 dB in the left ear with 21.5 dB at 4 kHz in the high risk group. The findings for the low risk group were 14.7 dB with 14.8 dB at 4 kHz for the right ear and 13.4 dB with 13.5 dB at 4 kHz for the left ear. The results of the chi square test were highly significant in terms of PTA findings at the consecutive frequencies of 1, 2, 4 and 6 kHz as well as at 4 kHz (p=0.000) Table 3.

Sub Group		PTA findings: HL at 1, 2, 4, 6 kHz, right ear	PTA findings: HL at 1, 2, 4, 6 kHz, left ear	HL at 4 kHz, right ear	HL at 4 kHz, left ear
High Risk	N	50	50	50	50
	Minimum	10	12.5	10	10
	Maximum	42.5	45	40	50
	Mean	20.9	21.825	19.05	21.5
Low Risk	N	50	50	50	50
	Minimum	10	10	10	10
	Maximum	20	25	20	20
	Mean	14.725	14.86	13.4	13.5

Table 3: Audiometric findings for right and left ear in high and low risk groups.

Discussion

The huge increase in popularity of PMDs has dramatically increased exposure to high sound levels amongst the youth. Studies have reported that increasing numbers of adolescents and young adults now experience symptoms indicative of poor hearing, such as distortion, tinnitus, hyperacusis or threshold shifts [8,9]. The present study analysed the behaviour and usage pattern of PMDs in individuals between 16 and 30 years of age. In 2009, Vogel et al. concluded that adolescents are much more likely to engage in risky behaviour in terms of usage pattern of PMDs [10]. In 2000, Smith et al. found that the numbers of young people with social noise exposure had tripled (to around 19%) since the early 1980s [11]. Agarwal et al. observed that, in 2003-4, 16.1% of US adults had hearing loss of which 8.5% was exhibited in the age group of 20-29 years and the prevalence seemed to be growing among this age group [12]. Studies done in the past by Niskar et al. [9] in 2001 and Chung et al. [8] in 2005 reported that a large number of adolescents and young adults are experiencing hearing loss.

In the present study, the usage pattern of PMDs was almost comparable amongst males and females but a greater number of males listened at high volume and for longer duration compared to females. This finding was different to that of Vogel et al. [10] who found that both males and females were likely to be at risk of hearing loss. In 2001, Niskar et al. [9] estimated the prevalence of noise-induced hearing threshold shift (NITS) among children aged 6-19 years in the Third National Health and Nutrition Examination Survey, 1988-1994 in USA. They found that 12.5% had NITS in one or both ears, with a higher prevalence in boys (14.2%) compared to girls (10.1%).

In the present study, undergraduate students demonstrated higher device usage compared to graduates and postgraduates. A study by Shah et al. [13] found that only 5% of undergraduates and 27% of graduates reported listening for less than 1 h/day and undergraduates were listening at higher volumes.

Parental monitoring is widely recognised as playing an important role in reducing an adolescent's risky health behaviour. We found that 62% of individuals having high risk habits of listening to PMDs were warned by their parents against the dangers of high volume music. The warnings by parents were heeded by most part of the time and ignored at other times.

None of the 500 individuals enrolled in our study knew about the use of a noise limiter. Several studies have shown that, even when individuals are aware of the risk of noise exposure, they are reluctant to use hearing protection [14]. A study by Vogel et al. [10] demonstrated that risky listening behaviour ranged between 33.2% and 93.2% and rates of protective listening behaviour ranged between 6.6% and 18.5%. They found that 32.8% were frequent users of PMDs, 48% listened at high-volume settings and 6.8% always or nearly always used a noise-limiter.

In the present study, we observed that most individuals were using mobile phones as a mode of listening to music but in the high risk group, the majority were using other sources of music along with their mobile phones. There has been a phenomenal increase in unit sales of portable audio devices including MP3 players in the EU over the last 4 years (2004-2007) [3]. A study by Shah et al. [13] on the type of PMD usage concluded that mobile phones were the most commonly used PMDs, followed by DVD players and iPods.

The usage of earphones has a significant impact on the damage caused by PMDs as their usage increases the amplitude of sound reaching the cochlea. Out of all 500 individuals in our study, 451(90.2%) were using earbud type earphones and results were similar in the high risk group. Studies by Vogel et al. [10] and by Shah et al. [13] have shown similar findings.

Regardless of socio-demographic characteristics, we found that weekly usage of PMDs varied between 1 day and all 7 days per week. The average duration and volume at which PMDs were being used was higher in the high risk group compared to the low risk group. The minimum and maximum outputs of all of the devices being used in our study were of almost equal range but the output varied with respect to the listening habits of the individual. In the high risk group, the mean outputs at commonly used volume and in noisy areas were both higher compared to the low risk group.

All of the enrolled individuals were evaluated for symptoms relating to hearing loss. We found that 28% of the high risk group occasionally suffered a ringing sensation in their ears, and 14% had difficulty in hearing; 22% of the high risk individuals had to raise the volume of their TVs to hear properly. Relatives of the candidates felt that the individuals talked loudly, and had difficulty in understanding speech, etc. Others received complaints from relatives who told them that they were speaking loudly (16%) and some had difficulty in understanding speech.

When assessed using PTA, the high risk group was found to have greater hearing loss at frequencies of 0.5, 1, 2, 4 and 6 kHz compared to the low risk group. We found that people listening to music at high volume and for longer durations were experiencing NIHL, which was documented by PTA.

Similar results were reported by Vogel et al. [10] who found that frequent users reported a much higher frequency of risky listening behaviour than infrequent users, ranging from twice as high to nearly five times as high. These users also reported a frequency of protective listening behaviour that was 2 to 3 times lower than that of infrequent users. A survey by Rice et al. [15] concluded that personal cassette player users suffering from post-exposure tinnitus or dullness of hearing should regard these symptoms as a sign of possible sensitivity to NIHL. Sometimes before subjective deafness becomes apparent to the individual, the changes can be picked up by audiometry.

In conclusion, we found that 57.2% of the individuals included in this study demonstrated a high risk behaviour (i.e. listening to music for >1 h/day and at high volume) for use of personal music devices. In the high risk group, individuals were listening to music with a mean weekly usage of 6.88 days/week, a mean daily usage of 3.62 h/day, and an average 1.5 h/day of continuous use. On a scale of 1–10, the average volume at which they were listening to music was 7, and 8 in noisy areas.

Risky listening behaviour can lead to the development of noise-induced hearing loss amongst exposed individuals, as demonstrated by the rise in audiometric hearing thresholds. It is essential that adolescents should be made aware of healthy listening habits and the potential risks of continued misuse or overuse of personal music devices.

References

1. World Health Organisation (1997) Prevention of noise-induced hearing loss: report of an informal consultation held at the World Health Organization, Geneva.
2. Nagapoornima P, Ramesh A, Lakshmi S, Suman R, Patricia PL, et al. (2007) Universal hearing screening. Indian J Pediatr 74: 545-549.
3. SCENIHR (Scientific Committee on Emerging and Newly Identified Health Risks) (2008) Scientific opinion on the potential health risks of exposure to noise from personal music players and mobile phones including a music playing function.
4. Nelson DI, Nelson RY, Concha-Barrientos M, Fingerhut M (2005) The global burden of occupational noise-induced hearing loss. Am J Int Med 48: 446-458.
5. Serra HR, Bussoni EC, Richter U, Minoldo G, Franco G, et al. (2005) Recreational noise exposure and its effects on the hearing of adolescents. Part I: An inter-disciplinary long term study. Int J Audiol 44: 65-73.
6. International Committee for Standardization (1990) Acoustics - Determination of occupational noise exposure and estimation of noise induced hearing impairment. ISO 1999: 1990, Geneva.
7. http://www.cdc.gov/niosh/98-126.html
8. Chung JH, Des Roches CM, Meunier J, Eavey RD (2005) Evaluation of noise induced hearing loss in young people using a web based survey technique. Paediatrics 108: 40-50.
9. Niskar AS, Kieszak SM, Holmes AE, Esteban E, Rubin C, et al. (2001) Estimated prevalence of noise-induced hearing threshold shifts among children 6 to 19 years of age: the Third National Health and Nutrition Examination Survey, 1988-1994, United States. Pediatrics 108: 40-43.
10. Vogel I, Verschuure H, van der Ploeg CPB, Brug J, Raat H (2009) Adolescents and MP3 players: Too many risks, too few precautions. Pediatrics 123: 953-958.
11. Smith PA, Davis A, Ferguson M, Lutman ME (2002) The prevalence and type of social noise exposure in young adults in England. Noise Health 2: 41-56.
12. Agarwal Y, Platz EA, Niparko JK (2008) Prevalence of hearing loss and differences by demographic characteristics among US adults. Data from the National Health and Nutrition Examination Survey, 1999-2004. Arch Intern Med 168: 1522-1530.
13. Shah S, Gopal B, Reis J, Novak M (2009) Hear today gone tomorrow: An assessment of portable entertainment player use and hearing acuity in a community sample. J Am Board Fam Med 22: 17-23.

22

Possibility for Allergy Immunotherapy with Long Synthetic Peptide of Bet V1

Motoharu Uehara[1*] **and Hiroyuki Hirai**[2]

[1]*Uehara Otolaryngology Clinic, showaminami-3-10-12, kushiro city, Hokkaido 0840909, Japan*

[2]*Advanced Medical Technology and Development Division, BML, Japan*

[*]**Corresponding author:** Motoharu Uehara, M.D., Doctor, Uehara Otolaryngology Clinic, showaminami-3-10-12, kushiro city, Hokkaido 0840909, Japan; E-mail: ueharaoto@jeans.ocn.ne.jp

Abstract

In allergy immunotherapy (AIT) using peptides, although the choice of T-cell epitope in consideration of the HLA type is important, application to all HLA types is difficult. We recently devised a new method to address this problem in AIT for white birch pollinosis, using long-chain synthetic peptides by dividing the sequence of Bet v1a, the major allergen in white birch pollen, into three peptides that overlap by 10 amino acid residues. Theoretically, these peptides contain all possible T-cell epitopes for any HLA type. Further, these peptides show weak allergenicity and are considered less prone to cause anaphylaxis because the three-dimensional structures differ significantly from the native Bet v1a. The combination of these three peptides of Bet v1a appears to provide an effective, safe form of AIT for white birch pollinosis. This method may thus be applicable to other allergens.

Keywords: White birch pollinosis; Bet v1; Allergy immunotherapy; Peptide; Basophil activation test

Introduction

Allergy immunotherapy (AIT) is a radical treatment for allergic rhinitis. This approach has a history of over 100 years and has been advancing with methods such as use of peptides, recombinant proteins and hypoallergens with the aim of improving safety in patients [1,2]. Traditional AIT is performed by subcutaneous injection (SCIT). As an alternative, sublingual immunotherapy (SLIT) has gained some traction because of an apparent reduction in adverse effects [3,4]. AIT has been reported to prevent sensitization for various allergens [4,5]. Nevertheless, AIT has not been popular in Japan for the following reasons: i) side effects include rare cases of fatal anaphylactic shock; ii) long-term treatment decreases adherence; and iii) unnecessary costs may be incurred as pre-treatment markers for identifying unresponsive patients are not yet available. The effectiveness and safety of AIT must therefore be improved to allow increased clinical application.

Allergic rhinitis is a typical type I allergic reaction. The mechanism begins when the allergen is deposited on the nasal epithelium and taken up by a submucosal antigen-presenting cell (APC). The allergen is then processed into peptides within the APC and after forming a complex with a major histocompatibility complex (MHC) class II molecule, is transported to the cell surface. In the presence of co-stimulatory signals, T cells recognize the MHC-peptide complex and a sequence of allergic reactions is initiated. Peptides recognized by T cells are known as T-cell epitopes. Due to the polymorphic nature of MHC molecules, every patient has different T-cell epitopes (Figure 1). Stimulated T cells produce various cytokines, in turn inducing B cells to differentiate into plasma cells producing immunoglobulin (Ig)E antibodies. These IgE antibodies bind to mast cells via Fc receptors found on the mast cell surface. This entire process is known as sensitization. When reintroduced, the allergen binds with IgE antibodies on mast cells and the cross-linking with the antibodies serves as a stimulus for secreting chemical mediators such as histamine from mast cells, triggering an isolated allergic reaction.

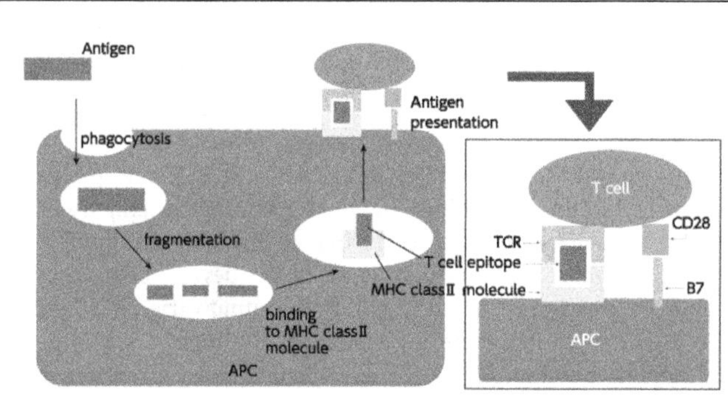

Figure 1: Mechanism for antigen presentation of T-cell epitopes. The allergic reaction begins when the allergen is taken up by submucosal APCs. The allergen is processed into peptides within the APC and after forming a complex with a MHC class II molecule, is transported to the cell surface. In the presence of co-stimulatory signals, T cells recognize the MHC-peptide complex. Peptides recognized by T cells are known as T-cell epitopes. MHC molecules are extremely polymorphic and exhibit varying binding specificities for peptides by MHC type. Each MHC type thus has different T-cell epitopes for any given antigen.

Since administration of allergens is involved, AIT is considered to induce the above allergy reactions. However, high doses of allergen administered in AIT can result in a shift in the Th1/Th2 balance immune to a Th1 predominance, accompanied by induction of T-regs and increased concentrations of the regulatory cytokines interleukin (IL)-10 and IL-27, although the underlying mechanisms remain unclear [6]. The specific IgG4 and IgA that can act to neutralize reactivity to the allergen are thus induced and the allergy is suppressed. Activating T cells therefore seems central to AIT.

IT of birch pollen allergy

Birch pollen allergy is one of the most prevalent hay fevers in Northern Europe and North America, as well as in Hokkaido and parts of Honshu in Japan. AIT is used primarily in Northern Europe [7,8], but its use in Japan has not yet been approved and only symptomatic treatment is available. In recent years, oral allergy syndrome (OAS), a condition related to birch pollinosis, has become increasingly problematic, as anaphylactic shock is known to occur on rare occasions [9]. While measures to address OAS are much needed, avoidance of trigger foods is the only measure that has been put in place in Japan at present. The onset of OAS is thought to be caused by the cross-reactivity of specific IgE to epitopes in birch pollen and trigger foods when the level of birch pollen-specific IgE increases with the progression of birch pollinosis. Preventing the onset of OAS may be possible if AIT is performed in the early stages of birch pollinosis [10].

Peptide immunotherapy

The IgE antibody binds to the epitope (known as the B-cell epitope) that is mainly present on the surface of the allergen. Since B-cell epitopes are dependent on the tertiary structure of allergen proteins, changing the tertiary structure through allergen modification, such as in peptide allergens, diminishes the binding strength of IgE to the allergen and may weaken the allergic reaction [11]. T-cell epitopes, however, were not impaired in peptide allergens [12,13]. Reduction of the side effects from AIT using peptides may permit the use of high concentrations of antigens and shorten the treatment period.

Conventional peptide immunotherapy has used peptides of about 15 amino acid residues, selected from several peptides of the allergen by determining T-cell epitopes. This method requires peptide selection for each patient due to the differences in MHCs, and is thus expensive. As one countermeasure, a peptide panel of major T-cell epitopes for each MHC has been reported [14].

On the other hand, longer peptides are able to reduce the number of total peptides and facilitate screening, although the synthesis of these longer peptides is more difficult. Short peptides with a T-cell epitope can bind with MHC molecules not only on professional APCs such as dendritic cells and B cells, but also on all cell surfaces that do not possess co-stimulatory molecules. Reports have indicated the possibility that T cells reacting with B cells are not activated, resulting in a state of anergy [15]. However, as long as T-cell epitope peptides cannot bind with MHC molecules on the B-cell surface, T-cell anergy is unlikely to occur. Most T-cell epitopes are taken up by dendritic cells and T cells are efficiently activated (Figure 2). As a risk of using long peptides, the peptide may become a B-cell epitope, and a previous study reported side effects associated with a 27-residue peptide [16].

Basophil activation test (BAT)

Long peptides in AIT carry a risk of inducing anaphylaxis as an allergen [16]. Therefore, to prevent the occurrence of side effects in peptide immunotherapy, testing the binding between patient IgE and the peptides to be administered is important. For this check, the application of ImmunoCAP^{TM} system, a method for quantitative determination of allergen-specific IgE, is considered. Addition of peptides to this system is able to check patient's IgE binding to the peptide as inhibition of their IgE binding to the antigen of ImmunoCAP, but this process is not simple. Alternatively, use of a BAT can be considered. The BAT is an allergy test to identify the causal allergen by assessing basophil activation in a flow cytometer using the CD203c or CD63 markers. BAT has been used as a diagnostic tool for food and pollen allergies and is highly useful due to its flexibility in terms of test allergens [17,18]. The BAT is thus suitable for pretesting peptides for AIT.

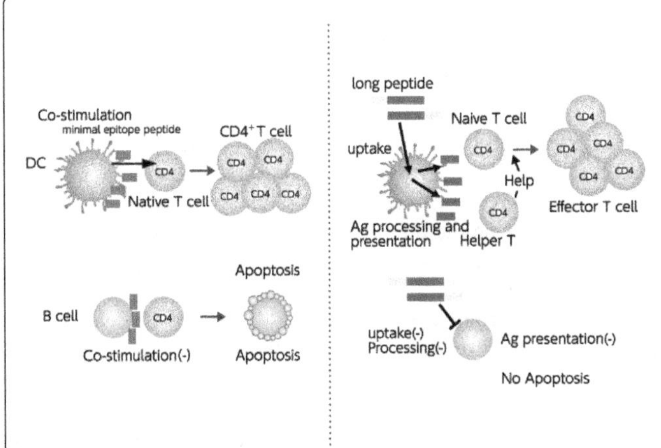

Figure 2: Differences in dendritic cells and B cells between long- and short-peptide immunotherapy.
Short peptides can bind directly to the MHC on various cells. DCs have co-stimulatory molecules, but unstimulated B cells do not. T cells reacting to the DC with peptide are activated, but do not activate in response to B cells with peptide, resulting in a state of anergy. Long peptides cannot bind to the MHC directly. DCs phagocytose the long peptides, which are then digested in a lysosome, and the resulting fragments bind to the MHC. However, on B cells, intake of an antigen requires recognition by the B-cell receptor. Peptides that are not recognized cannot be taken up by B cells for presentation to the MHC. T-cell anergy thus will not occur. AIT using long peptides thus activates T cells more efficiently.

AIT using Bet v1a long-chain synthetic peptide

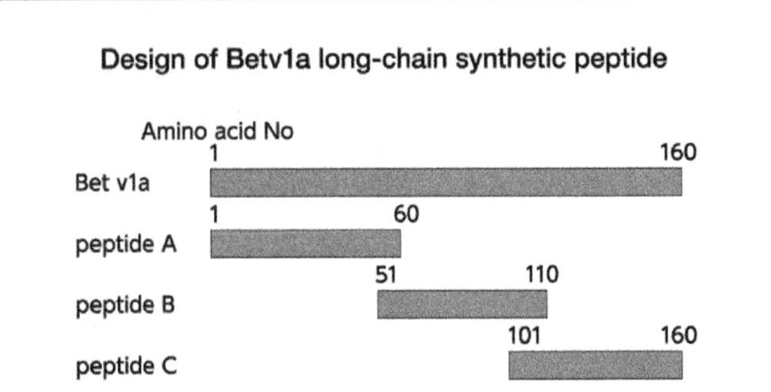

Figure 3: Design of Bet v1 long-chain synthetic peptide.
Based on the amino acid sequence of Bet v1a, each peptide was synthesized with 10-residue overlaps. The peptide comprising amino acid residues 1 to 60 from the N terminus was called Peptide A. Similarly, Peptide B contained residues 51 to 110 and Peptide C contained residues 100 to 160.

Long peptides of about 60 amino acid residues can be now synthesized, although synthesis of peptides containing multiple disulfide bonds is not easy.

Using long peptides for AIT is cheaper and allows easier purification than using recombinant protein. In our previous report [19], the full-length Bet v1a was divided into three parts and overlapping synthetic peptides were created (Figure 3).

None of the three peptides exhibited any reaction to the patient's basophils in the BAT (Figure 4). These three peptides were thus considered to have no B-cell epitopes. We confirmed this in an inhibition assay using the ImmunoCAP™ system with the CAP from white birch pollen. The results showed that none of the peptides were inhibited. In other words, these peptides were unable to bind with IgE antibodies. Furthermore, the lymphocyte stimulation test (LST) showed weak positive reactions with these peptides (Figure 5), demonstrating that the peptides have T-cell epitopes.

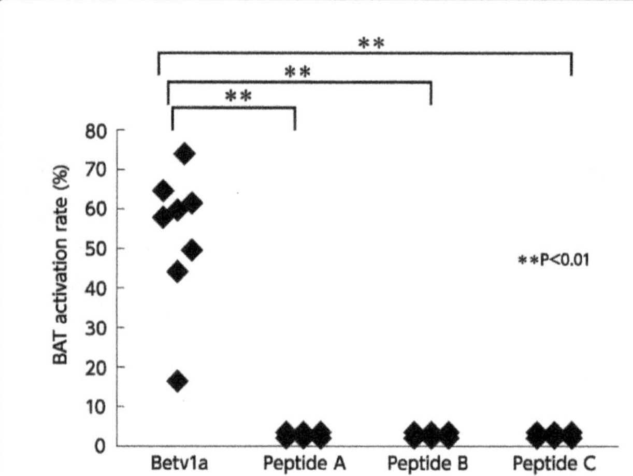

Figure 4: BAT of Bet v1a and the three synthetic peptides.
BAT was conducted using an Allergenicity Kit (Beckman-Coulter, Brea, CA) and a 10-fold dilution series from 1 μg/mL to 10 ng/mL for each antigen. Expression levels of CD203c on basophils were analyzed using a flow cytometer. The largest positive ratios (%) of CD203c in comparison with a negative control were plotted. Reactions of all peptides demonstrated a marked decline.

Since the present peptides are not short and contain the entire amino acid sequence of Bet v1a, immunotherapy using them is not limited to one specific MHC. These peptides seem likely to be applicable to all MHC and would thus be effective even in ethnically diverse populations. Furthermore, the antigen concentration could be increased within a short period of time and this therapy may shorten the treatment period, as B-cell epitopes are absent. In addition, BAT is likely to prove helpful in investigating whether serious allergic reactions can occur due to the inclusion of B-cell epitopes prior to peptide administration.

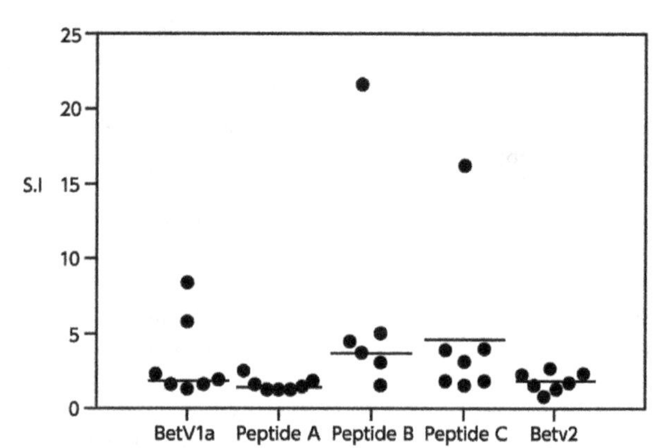

Figure 5: Lymphocyte stimulation test (LST) of Bet v1a, Bet v2 and the three synthetic peptides.

LST was conducted using a series of six 3-fold dilutions from 5 μg/mL of each antigen and 105 PBMCs from a 4 day culture. Uptake of 3H-thymidine in the final 24 h was measured. The largest relative values of the stimulation index compared to the control were plotted.

Conclusion

We have provided an outline of AIT using three long-chain synthetic peptides of 50-60 amino acid residues for white birch pollinosis. This AIT may offer advantages in term of effects, adaptations to different MHC, and reduced side effects in comparison to short peptides or whole proteins, although clinical study is needed for the confirmation. This method may also be applicable to other allergens.

References

1. O'Hehir RE, Prickett SR, Rolland JM (2016) T cell epitope peptide therapy for allergic diseases. Curr Allergy Asthma Rep 16: 14.
2. Marth K, Focke-Tejkl M, Lupinek C, Valenta R, Niederberger V (2014) Allergen peptides, recombinant allergens and hypoallergens for allergen-specific immunotherapy. Curr Treat Options Allergy 1: 91-106.
3. Mauro M, Russello M, Incorvaia C, Gazzola GB, Di Cara G, et al. (2007) Comparison of efficacy, safety and immunologic effects of subcutaneous and sublingual immunotherapy in birch pollinosis: A randomized study. Eur Ann Allergy Clin Immunol 39: 119-122.
4. Marogna M, Tomassetti D, Bernasconi A, Colombo F, Massolo A, et al. (2008) Preventive effects of sublingual immunotherapy in childhood: An open randomized controlled study. Ann Allergy Asthma Immunol 101: 206-211.
5. Schmitt J, Schwarz K, Stadler E, Wüstenberg EG (2015) Allergy immunotherapy for allergic rhinitis effectively prevents asthma: Results from a large retrospective cohort study. J Allergy Clin Immunol 136: 1511-1516.
6. Matsuoka T, Shamji MH, Durham SR (2013) Allergen immunotherapy and tolerance. Allergol Int 62: 403-413.
7. Khinchi MS, Poulsen LK, Carat F, Andre C, Hansen AB, et al. (2004) Clinical efficacy of sublingual and subcutaneous birch pollen allergen-specific immunotherapy: A randomized, placebo-controlled, double-blind, double-dummy study. Allergy 59: 45-53.
8. Grönlund H, Gafvelin G (2010) Recombinant Bet v1 vaccine for treatment of allergy to birch pollen. Hum Vaccin 6: 970-977.

9. Webber CM, England RW (2010) Oral allergy syndrome: A clinical, diagnostic, and therapeutic challenge. Ann Allergy Asthma Immunol 104: 101-108.

10. Bolhaar ST, Tiemessen MM, Zuidmeer L, van Leeuwen A, Hoffmann-Sommergruber K, et al. (2004) Efficacy of birch-pollen immunotherapy on cross-reactive food allergy confirmed by skin tests and double-blind food challenges. Clin Exp Allergy 34: 761-769.

11. O'Hehir RE, Young DB, Kay AB, Lamb JR (1987) Cloned human T lymphocytes reactive with Dermatophagoides farinae (house dust mite): A comparison of T- and B-cell antigen recognition. Immunology 62: 635-640.

12. Pellaton C, Perrin Y, Boudousquie C, Barbier N, Wassenberg J, et al. (2013) Novel birch pollen specific immunotherapy formulation based on contiguous overlapping peptides. Clin Transl Allergy 3: 17.

13. Spertini F, Perrin Y, Audran R, Pellaton C, Boudousquié C, et al. (2014) Safety and immunogenicity of immunotherapy with Bet v1-derived contiguous overlapping peptides. J Allergy Clin Immunol 134: 239-240.

14. Hirahara K, Tatsuta T, Takatori T, Ohtsuki M, Kirinaka H, et al. (2001) Preclinical evaluation of an immunotherapeutic peptide comprising 7 T-cell determinants of Cry j 1 and Cry j 2, the major Japanese cedar pollen allergens. J Allergy Clin Immunol 108: 94-100.

15. Norman PS, Ohman JL Jr, Long AA, Creticos PS, Gefter MA, et al. (1996) Treatment of cat allergy with T-cell reactive peptides. Am J Respir Crit Care Med 154: 1623-1628.

16. Wada H, Isobe M, Kakimi K, Mizote Y, Eikawa S, et al. (2014) Vaccination with NY-ESO-1 overlapping peptides mixed with Picibanil OK-432 and montanide ISA-51 in patients with cancers expressing the NY-ESO-1 antigen. J Immunother 37: 84-92.

17. Fujisawa T, Nagao M, Hiraguchi Y, Hosoki K, Tokuda R, et al. (2009) Biomarkers for allergen immunotherapy in cedar pollinosis. Allergol Int 58: 163-170.

18. Chinuki Y, Kaneko S, Dekio I, Takahashi H, Tokuda R, et al. (2012) CD203c expression-based basophil activation test for diagnosis of wheat-dependent exercise-induced anaphylaxis. J Allergy Clin Immunol 129: 1404-1406.

19. M Uehara, Y Abe (2013) Possibility for immunotherapy with long synthetic peptide of Bet v1. J Jpn Immunol Allergol Otolaryngol 31: 247-251.

Pregnancy and Dental Treatment

ABI AAD Lamia* **and Dany Joseph Daou**

Dental Public Health Department, Lebanese University, Hadath, Hadath Lebanon

***Corresponding author:** ABI AAD Lamia BDS, DESS in Community Oral Health and Epidemiology, Dental Surgeon, Dental Public Health Department, Lebanese University, Hadath, Hadath Lebanon; E-mail: lamiaabiaadlb@yahoo.fr

Abstract

Background: Pregnancy is accompanied with numerous physiological changes that present oral health consequences. Oral disease during pregnancy has been linked to pre- eclampsia, gestational diabetes, preterm birth, low birth weight and stillbirths. Despite evidence-based recommendations regarding the need for dental treatment and counselling of pregnant women, many dentists retain misconceptions regarding dental care during pregnancy and are reluctant in providing necessary dental preventive and curative services.

Aim: To assess the beliefs and practices of Lebanese dentists with respect to the dental care of pregnant women.

Methods: Self-administered questionnaires were answered by a sample of 195 dentists. Dentists' knowledge of oral disorders associated with pregnancy in addition to their practices with respect to the administration of radiographs and prescriptions of medications were assessed. Chi-square tests were used to test the association between selected demographic variables and pregnancy-related knowledge outcomes.

Results: Fifty-two percent of dentists believed anesthesia was risky for pregnant women and only 55% would take a radiograph when necessary. Only 56% recognized gingivitis as a consequence of pregnancy and 76% recognized the presence of gingival bleeding as a symptom. The majority prescribes analgesics, specifically acetaminophens (90.3%), 73.5% prescribe antibiotics and only 9.2% are willing to prescribe an anti-inflammatory drug. Female dentists ($p=0.05$) and dentists with greater years of experience ($p=0.04$) were more aware of the risk of gingival bleeding during pregnancy. Those holding degrees from Lebanese universities were more aware of the association between gingivitis and pregnancy ($p=0.03$).

Conclusion: The knowledge and practices of Lebanese dentists with respect to pregnant women are suboptimal. There is a need to re-assess the dental curriculum and consider the incorporation of training and re-training courses into continuing dental education programs.

Keywords: Pregnancy; Health; Oral health; Dental Treatment

Introduction

Oral health is a basic human right that is integral to general health and well-being [1]. Oral diseases such as dental caries, gingivitis and chronic periodontitis are common in all age groups and in vulnerable individuals, particularly in pregnant women who experience numerous physiological changes that present oral health consequences [2-4]. Common symptoms such as gastro-intestinal reflux (acidity), nausea and vomiting result in an acidic oral environment that promotes acid demineralization of tooth enamel and the growth of dental caries pathogens [5-8]. Rising circulation levels of estrogen and progesterone elicit an inflammatory response that predisposes women to a spectrum of pregnancy-related gingival manifestations, including gingivitis, periodontitis, gingival hyperplasia and pyogenic granuloma [5,7]. In fact, pregnancy gingivitis is recognized as a clinically proven reversible manifestation of pregnancy and is estimated to occur in 30 to 100 percent of pregnant women [9-11]. Moreover, the increased susceptibility to infections and reduced ability to repair soft tissue caused by hormonal fluctuations increases the risk of developing periodontitis [12]. Believed to affect 5 to 20 percent of pregnant women, untreated periodontitis results in the loss of alveolar bone and supporting structures and ultimately in tooth loss [13]. Finally, research is increasingly implicating oral disease during pregnancy in the development of complications beyond the pregnant woman's oral cavity. Periodontal disease, in particular, has been linked to pre-eclampsia (pregnancy hypertension that poses risk to mother and foetus), gestational diabetes, preterm birth, low birth weight and still births [14-23].

Rather than being a state of disease, pregnancy presents a normal physiological phase in a woman's lifetime and warrants – at the least – the routine preventive and emergency oral health care provided to other members of the general population.24 Beyond routine dental treatment, the particular relationship between pregnancy and oral health warrants for additional pregnancy-specific preventive care and oral health education [24]. The provision of dental treatment during pregnancy is not only safe, it is also an integral aspect of antenatal care and is advised by the American Congress of Obstetricians and Gynecologists and the American Academies of Periodontology and Pediatrics [25-30].

Research consistently highlights the fact that, globally, dentists remain to show hesitation and reluctance towards providing dental treatment to pregnant women despite the availability of detailed evidence-based guidelines [24,25,31-33]. Although there is reason to believe that dental attendance by pregnant women in Lebanon is deficient, there has been no investigation into the attitudes of Lebanese dentists with respect to providing dental care during pregnancy. The aim of this study was to assess the knowledge and attitudes of Lebanese dentists towards the provision of oral health care to pregnant women.

Materials and Methods

This survey was conducted between January and March 2016. It focused on the knowledge attitude and practices of Dentists in treating pregnant women. This methodology had a quantitative character. Based on a review of the literature, a self-administered questionnaire was developed and adopted after being tested on 15 dentists. The self-administered questionnaire used to collect data was composed of 14 questions organized into 4 categories:

- Demographic variables of the study sample
- Knowledge of dentists about the treatment of pregnant women
- Practices of dentists regarding the treatment of pregnant women
- Prescription of medicines related to dental treatments for pregnant women

The questionnaires were hand-distributed to a convenience sample of 215 dentists and 195 questionnaires were collected and included in the study. The approached dentists were given a choice of either and English or French language questionnaire and were asked to return the questionnaire after answering individually in order to avoid collective answers and peer influence. The questionnaires were anonymous to maintain confidentiality.

Statistical Analysis

Data entry was performed using the software Access (Microsoft Office). Descriptive statistics of the main exposure and outcome variables were generated for the data. The percent distributions of the demographic characteristics of the responding dentists, in addition to the outcomes assessing pregnancy-related knowledge and practices, were generated to present numbers and proportions. Bivariate analysis was used to test the association between selected demographic variables and pregnancy-related knowledge outcomes using Chi Square tests of association. The IBM® SPSS® version 20.0 statistical package was used to carry out all statistical analyses. Statistical significance was set at 0.05.

Results

Demographic characteristics of the study sample

The sample included 195 dentists. Out of a total of 215 distributed questionnaires, 195 were returned and were included in the study leading to a response rate of 90%. The sample of dentists was almost equally distributed between genders (51.3% females and 48.7% males). The majority had 10 years of experience or less (56.7%) and held local dental degrees (79.4%; Table 1).

Of all responding dentists, 69% reported to have ever received a pregnant woman in their practice and the majority of responding dentists (86.5%) selected the second trimester as the period of choice to provide dental interventions for pregnant women (Table 2). Opinions regarding the risk of anesthesia and radiographs during pregnancy were contradictory. Around half of the sample (52%) considered anesthesia risky for pregnant women and only 55% would take a radiograph when necessary. Although 76% recognized gingival bleeding as a consequence of pregnancy, only 56% acknowledged gingivitis as a symptom (Table 2).

Variable	N	%
Gender		
Female	100	51.30%
Male	95	48.70%
Total	195	100.00%
Years of experience		
10 years or less	110	56.70%
11-20 Years	40	20.60%
>20 Years	44	22.70%
Total	194	100.00%
Origin of diploma		
Lebanon	150	79.40%
West Europe	15	7.90%
East Europe	14	7.40%
Arab World	10	5.30%
Total	189	100.00%

Table 1: Demographic characteristics of dentists.

Variable	N	%
Months of choice to treat a pregnant woman		
1st trimester	12	6.50%
2nd trimester	160	86.50%
3rd trimester	13	7.00%
Total	185	100.00%
Is anaesthesia risky for pregnant women?		
Yes	101	51.80%
No	94	48.20%
Total	195	100.00%
Do you do X-rays for pregnant women when necessary?		
Yes	105	55.00%
No	86	45.00%
Total	191	100.00%
Oral manifestations during pregnancy*		
Caries risk	59	30.10%
Gingival bleeding	149	76.00%

Pregnancy gingivitis	110	56.10%
Epulis gravidic	41	20.90%
Dental fractures	11	5.60%
Canker (Aphthous ulcers)	18	9.20%
Dental sensitivity	15	7.70%
*Percentages in the manifestations during pregnancy may add to more than 100 % because more than one option is allowed		

Table 2: Knowledge and practice of dentists during pregnancy.

Prescription of medication

The vast majority of responding dentists would prescribe analgesics to a pregnancy woman (90.3%), the preference clearly being for acetaminophens (Paracetamol; 90.4%) (Table 3). Greater caution was apparent regarding the prescription of antibiotics (73.5%), but, when prescribed, the preferred antibiotic was a Betalactamin or Aminopenicillin (79%). The avoidance of anti-inflammatory drugs was clear, with only 9.2% willing to prescribe them during pregnancy (Table 3).

Medications	N	%
General Families		
Antibiotics	144	73.50%
Analgesics	177	90.30%
Anti-Inflammatory	18	9.20%
Antibiotics subtypes*		
Betalactamine/Aminopenicilline (with or wihout clavulonic acid)	114	79.20%
Other Antibiotics	17	11.80%
Based on gynecologist prescription	21	14.60%
Analgesics subtypes*		
Acetamenophene/Paracetamol	160	90.40%
Based on gynecologist prescription	6	3.40%
*The percentage of subtypes in both antibiotics and analgesics refers only to the dentists who prescribe the medicine in each category		

Table 3: Prescription of medicines.

Bivariate analysis

When compared to male dentists, a higher proportion of female dentists reported that they would mention to a pregnant woman the risks of anesthesia (p=0.03), especially the risk of malaise (p=0.02; Chart 1). They were also more aware of the risk of gingival bleeding during pregnancy (p=0.05; Chart 2).

Experience was a significant predictor of the recognition of gingival bleeding as a consequence of pregnancy, dentists with greater years of experience being more likely of this recognition (p=0.04; Chart 3). With respect to the acknowledgement of gravidic gingivitis, dentists holding diplomas from Lebanese dental universities were more likely to recognize the association between with pregnancy than those holding degrees from other countries (p=0.03; Chart 4).

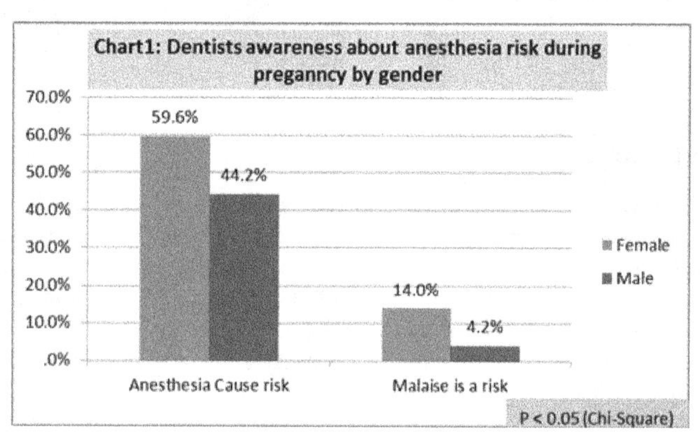

Chart 1: Dentists awareness about anesthesia risk during pregnancy by gender, Anesthesia: p=0.03; malaise: p=0.02.

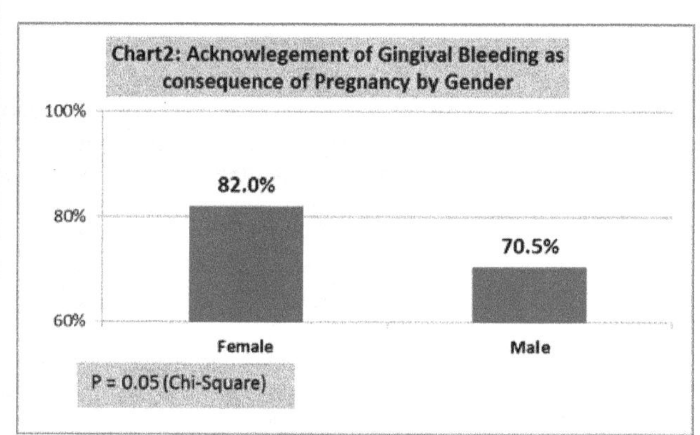

Chart 2: Acknowlegement of gingival bleeding as consequence of pregnancy by gender, p=0.05.

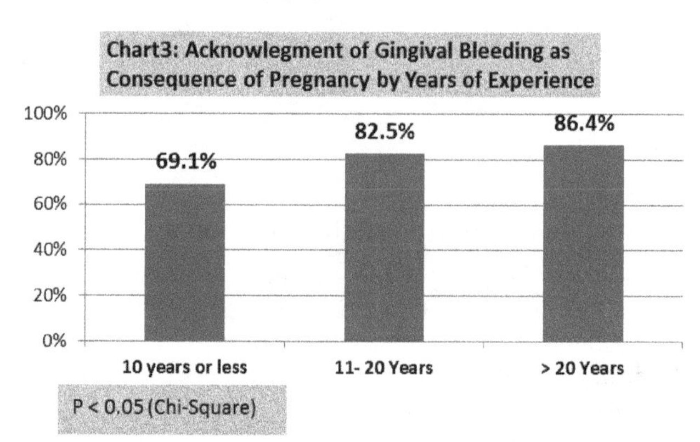

Chart 3: Acknowlegement of gingival bleeding as consequence of pregnancy by years of experience, p=0.04.

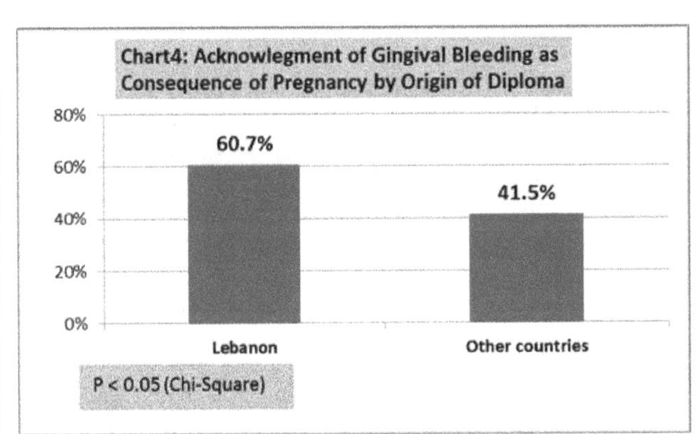

Chart 4: Acknowlegement of gingival bleeding as consequence of pregnancy by origin of diploma, p=0.03.

Discussion

The importance of maintaining good oral health during pregnancy is irrefutable. Early detection of oral pathology in pregnant women may contribute to the restriction of associated systemic diseases and thus the reduction of pregnancy and childbirth-related Complications [22,23]. Furthering the importance of maternal oral health care are the observations that preserving the expecting mother's oral health during pregnancy may promote the establishment of a solid foundation for maintaining good oral health for her child after birth and may reduce the risk of early childhood caries [34-36]. The significance of maternal prenatal dental care is therefore increasingly being recognized, with recommendations for preventive, routine and emergency dental care in addition to pregnancy-specific counselling and oral health education [24,25,37]. Unfortunately, there is substantial evidence that as many as half of pregnant women around the world do not seek dental assistance during their gestational period, even when experiencing oral problems [12,25,34,38-41]. While numerous factors are implicated in reducing the utilization of dental health care by pregnant women, poorly informed or unprepared dental healthcare professionals often pose an additional barrier to the provision of dental health care services to pregnant women [33].

The results of our study suggest that both the beliefs and the practices of Lebanese dentists are suboptimal with respect to the oral health care of pregnant women. Despite gingivitis being the most common oral change during pregnancy [3], a quarter of the responding dentists did not consider gingival bleeding a consequence of pregnancy, slightly less than half acknowledged gravidic gingivitis and only about one fifth acknowledged pregnancy epulis. These proportions are strikingly low when compared to various international reports from different countries, where the proportions of dentists acknowledging the association between pregnancy and bleeding gums, gingivitis or periodontal pathology exceeds 90% [42,43]. It is interesting to note that female dentists were more likely to be aware of the risk of gingival bleeding during pregnancy and were also more likely to mention the risks of anesthesia, especially malaise, to pregnant women. A similar observation of greater knowledge among female dentists has previously been reported [44], although in another study no differences in the level of knowledge were observed between male and female dentists [24]. It is positive to note that with greater years of experience, dentists in our sample were more likely to acknowledge the association between gingival bleeding and pregnancy. Interestingly, dentists holding diplomas from Lebanese dental universities were more likely to recognize the association between gravidic gingivitis and pregnancy than those holding degrees from other countries. However, it is impossible to say whether this association is truly related to the country of education or is confounded by another factor, for example gender or years of experience.

Dentist practices regarding the use of local anesthesia and radiology were below recommended standards. Even though the use of local anesthetics with vasoconstrictors is considered safe throughout pregnancy [45], 51.8% of the responding Lebanese dentists believed that local anesthesia poses a risk during pregnancy and 61% believed the major risk from anesthesia is due to the presence of vasoconstrictors. The reluctance to administer anesthesia with or without vasoconstrictor observed in our sample supports the presence of similar misconceptions in several other countries. In another study in the region, 48% of dentists practicing in Saudi Arabia either considered epinephrine to be unsafe or were unsure about its safety [46]. Similarly, results from several studies of dentist practices across Europe and South America suggest that between 41 and 46% of dentists avoid the use of vasoconstrictors in pregnant women [45-49].

Despite the fact that diagnostic radiographs are believed to be safe during pregnancy when used with the recommended neck (thyroid) collar and abdomen shields, 45% of the responding dentists reported not to use radiographs even when needed [50]. A similar perception has been reported in Saudi Arabia, with 42.5% of dentists refusing to take a radiograph even when needed for diagnosis [46]. Data from international research is more heterogeneous, the proportions of dentists believing radiographs to be unsafe ranging between 18.4% [44] and 56.7% [51,52] in the USA and between 10.7% and 71.5% of dentists refusing to take x-rays during pregnancy in various countries [5,24,53,54].

With respect to the prescription of drugs, the practices of Lebanese conformed to the US Food and Drug Administration (FDA) guidelines. Almost three quarters of Lebanese dentists reported willingness to prescribe antibiotics, of whom around 80% would select Betalactamine/Aminopenicillin. These results fall in the range reported by regional and international studies where between 58 and 96 percent of dentists in various countries would prescribe penicillin or amoxicillin [5,46,49,53-56]. The vast majority of surveyed dentists would also prescribe an analgesic when needed and the first choice for more than 90% would be acetaminophen, with less than 10% willing to prescribe the less favourable option of NSAIDS [5]. Although most international studies report that more than 75% of dentists would prescribe acetaminophen or paracetamol [5,46,53-55], few studies report that about 50% of dentists would not [24,56]. The literature also confirms the reluctance of dentists towards the prescription of NSAIDs, with only 11-31 percent of dentists willing to prescribe aspirin, ibuprofen or NSAIDs in general [24,49,55,56]. Despite some limitations inherent to the study design and data collection method, the results of our study demonstrate that both the knowledge and the practices of Lebanese dentists with respect to pregnant women are lacking. It must be noted that the questionnaire used was not formally validated and was rather tested for face validity and ease of understanding in a focus group discussion followed by pilot testing in 15 individuals. Additionally, the nature of our convenience sample prevents the ability to generalize our results to include all practicing dentists in Lebanon. On the other hand, the high response rate and moderate sample size provide strength to our results and suggest that, although the exact percentages cannot be generalized to the entire population of Lebanese dentists, our study does capture a truly existing and previously unreported phenomenon of misinformation and incorrect practices among dentists in Lebanon with regards to pregnant women. Our findings demonstrate a need to broaden the knowledge of dentists in Lebanon regarding the care of pregnant women. This may require curriculum changes in undergraduate courses in Lebanon, but also practical training in order to empower graduating dentists and ensure the translation of knowledge into clinical practice. The high proportion of Lebanese dentists receiving degrees abroad may suggest the need to involve the Lebanese Dental Association in developing regulations that ensure that the knowledge of these dentists is either assessed or reinforced through training courses prior to enrollment in the association. The results also emphasize the importance of continuing education in the form of training courses and pregnancy-specific conferences, especially in the presence of a significant proportion of currently practicing dentists with incorrect beliefs and concepts. Additionally, in a culture where a physician's opinion may sometimes be more valued by lay people than the opinion of a dentist, the importance of a multidisciplinary approach must be emphasized [38]. This requires the insurance that general physicians, gynecologists, obstetricians and midwives pose no barrier to the utilization of health care by pregnant women and that they become integral to the pathway of referral to dental care and counseling in early during pregnancy rather than a source of dissemination and strengthening of already existing misconceptions regarding dental care during pregnancy [38].

Conclusion

Our study illustrates clear deficiencies in the beliefs and the practices of Lebanese dentists with respect to the oral health care of pregnant women. While practices regarding the prescription of antibiotics, analgesics and NSAIDs conform to international guidelines, evidence-based knowledge regarding the association between pregnancy and gingivitis, in addition to the safe use of local anesthesia and radiology are all lacking. The data support the need for a comprehensive approach to strengthen the knowledge of all dentists practicing in Lebanon with respect to the oral health care and treatment of pregnant women.

This may necessitate a re-assessment of the dental curricula in local dental schools and/or the introduction of mandatory training courses into continuing dental education programs.

References

1. World Health Organization (2005) The liverpool declaration: Promoting oral health in the 21st century. A call for action. Geneva: WHO.
2. Azofeifa A, Yeung LF, Alverson CJ, Beltrán-Aguilar E (2014) Oral health conditions and dental visits among pregnant and nonpregnant women of childbearing age in the United States, National Health and Nutrition Examination Survey, 1999-2004. Prev Chronic Dis 11: E163.
3. Healther J, Boggess KA (2008) Periodontal diseases and adverse pregnancy outcomes: A review of the evidence and implications for clinical practice. J Dent Hyg 82: 24.
4. U.S. Department of Health and Human Services (2000) Oral health in America: A report of the surgeon general. Rockville, (MD): U.S. Department of health and human services, National Institute of Dental and Craniofacial Research, National Institutes of Health.
5. Naidu GM, Ram KC, Kopuri RK, Prasad SE, Prasad D, et al. (2013) Is dental treatment safe in pregnancy? A dentist's opinion survey in South India. J Orofac Res 3: 233-239.
6. Turner M, Aziz SR (2002) Management of the pregnant oral and maxillofacial surgery patient. J Oral Maxillofac Surg 60: 1479-1488.
7. Kloetzel MK, Huebner CE, Milgrom P (2011) Referrals for dental care during pregnancy. J Midwifery Womens Health 56: 110-117.
8. Shamsi M, Hidarnia A, Niknami S, Rafiee M, Zareban I, et al. (2014) The effect of educational program on increasing oral health behavior among pregnant women: Applying health belief model. Health Education & Health Promotion 1: 21-36.
9. Silk H, Douglass AB, Douglass JM, Silk L (2008) Oral health during pregnancy. Am Fam Physician 77: 1139-1144.
10. Barak S, Oettinger-Barak O, Oettinger M, Machtei EE, Peled M, et al. (2003) Common oral manifestations during pregnancy: A review. Obstet Gynecol Surv 58: 624-628.
11. Steinberg BJ (1999) Women's oral health issues. J Dent Educ 63: 271-275.
12. Gaffield ML, Gilbert BJ, Malvitz DM, Romaguera R (2001) Oral health during pregnancy: An analysis of information collected by the pregnancy risk assessment monitoring system. J Am Dent Assoc 132: 1009-1016.
13. Laine M (2002) Effect of pregnancy on periodontal and dental health. Acta Odontol Scand 60: 257-264.
14. Rashidi Maybodi F, Haerian-Ardakani A, Vaziri F, Khabbazian A, Mohammadi-Asl S (2015) CPITN changes during pregnancy and maternal demographic factors 'impact on periodontal health. Iran J Reprod Med 13: 107-112.
15. Han YW (2011) Oral health and adverse pregnancy outcomes-what's next? J Dent Res 90: 289-293.
16. Clothier B, Stringer M, Jeffcoat MK (2007) Periodontal disease and pregnancy outcomes: Exposure, risk and intervention. Best Pract Res Clin Obstet Gynaecol 21: 451-466.
17. Xiong X, Buekens P, Fraser WD, Beck J, Offenbacher S (2006) Periodontal disease and adverse pregnancy outcomes: A systematic review. BJOG 113: 135-143.
18. Dasanayake AP, Gennaro S, Hendricks-Muñoz KD, Chhun N (2008) Maternal periodontal disease, pregnancy and neonatal outcomes. MCN Am J Matern Child Nurs 33: 45-49.
19. Hemalatha VT, Manigandan T, Sarumathi T, Nisha VA, Amudhan A (2013) Dental considerations in pregnancy-a critical review on the oral care. J Clin Diagn Res 7: 948-953.
20. Ruma M, Boggess K, Moss K, Jared H, Murtha A, et al. (2008) Maternal periodontal disease, systemic inflammation and risk for preeclampsia. Am J Obstet Gynecol 198: 389.
21. Morgan MA, Crall J, Goldenberg RL, Schulkin J (2009) Oral health during pregnancy. J Matern Fetal Neonatal Med 22: 733-739.
22. Boggess KA, Edelstein BL (2006) Oral health in women during preconception and pregnancy: Implications for birth outcomes and infant oral health. Matern Child Health J 10: S169-174.
23. López NJ, Smith PC, Gutierrez J (2002) Periodontal therapy may reduce the risk of preterm low birth weight in women with periodontal disease: A randomized controlled trial. J Periodontol 73: 911-924.
24. Radha G, Sood P (2013) Oral care during pregnancy: Dentists knowledge, attitude and behaviour in treating pregnant patients at dental clinics of Bengaluru, India. Journal of Pierre Fauchard Academy (India Section) 27:135-141.
25. George A, Shamim S, Johnson M, Dahlen H, Ajwani S, et al. (2012) How do dental and prenatal care practitioners perceive dental care during pregnancy? Current evidence and implications. Birth 39: 238-247.
26. American Academy of Pediatric Dentistry (2011) Guideline on perinatal oral health care. Chicago, Illinois: American Academy of Pediatric Dentistry.
27. Kumar J, Samelson R (2006) Oral health care during pregnancy and early childhood: Practice guidelines. Albany.
28. California Dental Association Foundation (2010) Oral health care during pregnancy and early childhood: Evidence-based guidelines for health professionals. J Calif Dent Assoc 28: 391-403.

29. Achtari MD, Georgakopoulou EA, Afentoulide N (2012) Dental care throughout pregnancy: What a dentist must know. Oral Health Dent Manag 11: 169-176.

30. The american academy of pediatrics and the american college of obstetricians and gynecologists (2007) Guidelines for Perinatal Care 6: 123-124.

31. Lee RS, Milgrom P, Huebner CE, Conrad DA (2010) Dentists' perceptions of barriers to providing dental care to pregnant women. Womens Health Issues 20: 359-365.

32. Pina PM, Douglas J (2011) Practice and opinions of connecticut general dentists regarding dental treatment during pregnancy. Gen Dent 59: e25-e31.

33. Vieira DR, de Oliveira AE, Lopes FF, Lopes e Maia Mde F (2015) Dentists' knowledge of oral health during pregnancy: A review of the last 10 years' publications. Community Dent Health 32: 77-82.

34. National Maternal and Child Oral Health Resource Center (2008) Access to oral health care during the perinatal period: A policy brief. Georgetown University.

35. Gussy MG, Waters EG, Walsh O, Kilpatrick NM (2006) Early childhood caries: Current evidence for aetiology and prevention. J Paediatr Child Health 42: 37-43.

36. Yost J, Li Y (2008) Promoting oral health from birth through childhood: Prevention of early childhood caries. Am J Matern Child Nurs 33: 17-23.

37. Ojeda JC (2013) A literature review on social and economic factors related to access to dental care for pregnant women. The Journal 1: 25.

38. Alves RT, Ribeiro RA, Costa LR, Leles CR, Freire Mdo C, et al. (2012) Oral care during pregnancy: Attitudes of Brazilian public health professionals. Int J Environ Res Public Health 9: 3454-3464.

39. Hwang SS, Smith VC, McCormick MC, Barfield WD (2011) Racial/ethnic disparities in maternal oral health experiences in 10 states, pregnancy risk assessment monitoring system, 2004–2006. J Matern Child Health 15: 722-729.

40. Thomas NJ, Middleton PF, Crowther CA (2008) Oral and dental health care practices in pregnant women in Australia: A postnatal survey. BMC Pregnancy Childbirth 8: 13.

41. George A, Ajwani S, Bhole S (2010) Promoting perinatal oral health in South-Western Sydney: A collaborative approach. J Dent Res 89: 142301.

42. Strafford KE, Shellhaas C, Hade EM (2008) Provider and patient perceptions about dental care during pregnancy. J Matern Fetal Neonatal Med 21: 63-71.

43. Tarannum F, Prasad S, Vivekananda L, Jayanthi D, Faizuddin M (2013) Awareness of the association between periodontal disease and pre-term births among general dentists, general medical practitioners and gynecologists. Indian journal of public health 57: 92.

44. Da Costa EP, Lee JY, Rozier RG, Zeldin L (2010) Dental care for pregnant women: An assessment of North Carolina general dentists. J Am Dent Assoc 141: 986-994.

45. Zanata RL, Fernandes KB, Navarro PS (2008) Prenatal dental care: Evaluation of professional knowledge of obstetricians and dentists in the cities of Londrina/PR and Bauru/SP, Brazil, 2004. J Appl Oral Sci 16: 194-200.

46. Al-Sadhan R, Al-Manee A (2008) Dentist's opinion toward treatment of pregnant patients. Saudi Dent J 20: 24-30.

47. Pertl C, Heinemann A, Pertl B, Lorenzoni M, Pieber D, et al. (2000) Aspects particuliers du traitement dentaire chez la femme enceinte. Rev Men Suisse Odontostomatol 42-46.

48. Luc E, Coulibaly N, Demoersman J, Boutigny H, Soueidan A (2012) Dental care during pregnancy. Schweiz Monatsschr Zahnmed 122: 1047-1063.

49. Navarro PSL, Dezan CC, Melo FJ, Alves-Souza RA, Sturion L, et al. (2008) Prescription medications and local anaesthesia for pregnant women: Practices of dentists in Londrina, PR, Brazil]. Revista da Faculdade de Odontologia de Porto Alegre 49: 22-27.

50. The American academy of pediatrics and the american college of obstetricians and gynecologists (2011) Guidelines for Oral Health Care in Pregnancy.

51. Da Costa EP, Lee JY, Rozier RG, Zeldin L (2010) Dental care for pregnant women: an assessment of North Carolina general dentists. J Am Dent Assoc 141: 986-994.

52. Huebner CE, Milgrom P, Conrad D, Lee RS (2009) Providing dental care to pregnant patients: A survey of Oregon general dentists. J Am Dent Assoc 140: 211-222.

53. Umoh AO, Azodo CC (2013) Nigerian dentists and oral health-care of pregnant women: Knowledge, attitude and belief. Sahel Med J 16: 111.

54. Caneppele TMF, Yamamoto EC, Souza AC, Valera MC, Araújo MAM (2011) Dentists' knowledge of dentists of the care of special patients: Hypertension, diabetes and pregnant women. J Biodentistry Biomaterials 1: 31 41.

55. Enabulele J, Ibhawoh L (2015) Knowledge of Nigerian dentists about drug safety and oral health practices during pregnancy. Indian J Oral Sci 6: 55.

56. Patil S, Thakur R, Madhu K, Paul ST, Gadicherla P (2013) Oral health coalition: Knowledge, attitude, practice behaviours among gynaecologists and dental practitioners. J Int Oral Health 5: 8-15.

Role of Elective Neck Management in Maxillary Sinus Squamous Cell Carcinoma

Pauline Castelnau-Marchand, Eleonor Rivin del Campo and Yungan Tao*

Department of Radiation Oncology, Gustave-Roussy, Paris Sud University, Villejuif, France

***Corresponding author:** Yungan Tao, MD, Ph.D, Department of Radiation Oncology, Institut Gustave Roussy, 114 rue Edouard Vaillant, 94800 Villejuif, France; E-mail: Yungan.TAO@gustaveroussy.fr

Abstract

Maxillary sinus carcinoma is relatively rare. Standard treatment consists in surgery followed by adjuvant radiotherapy or chemoradiotherapy. The rate of neck lymph node metastasis during follow-up is about 5-30% and this event is a poor prognostic factor. It often occurs in large primary tumours (T3-T4). The role of prophylactic neck management, selective neck dissection (SND) or elective neck irradiation (ENI), remains unclear in N0 patients. Few studies specifically discuss the role of SND. A French study suggested SND could be proposed when primary surgery is feasible, especially for high tumour volume (T3-T4). Besides, it can be useful for lymph node staging and determining radiotherapy dose and volume. The role of ENI remains unclear and controversial, although some studies suggest a potential reduction of neck relapse with it. ENI (ipsilateral level II, +/- Ib and III or bilateral neck according to the primary tumour extension) could be proposed in selected patients, especially for T3-4 disease and when SND has not been performed. Intensity-modulated radiotherapy (IMRT) should be considered, whenever feasible, to reduce toxicity.

Keywords: Maxillary sinus; Squamous cell carcinoma; Neck irradiation

Introduction

Paranasal sinus cancers make up less than 3% of head and neck malignancies, of which 80% are located in the maxillary sinus [1]. Squamous cell carcinoma (SCC) represents 60-90% of the histology. They are stage T3-T4 in around 65-70% and are associated with cervical lymph node involvement in around 5-10% [2].

The main issue of this disease is a high local relapse rate [3]. Standard treatment consists in surgery followed by adjuvant radiotherapy or chemoradiotherapy [4]. Positive surgical margins are a significant prognostic factor of local relapse, and adjuvant external-beam radiotherapy (EBRT) is required. When surgery isn't feasible due to high risk of resection morbidity in locally advanced stage (T3-T4) disease, concomitant chemoradiotherapy (CRT) is standard of care [5].

The rate of lymph node metastasis during follow-up is relatively low; it varies between 5% to 30% according to series, but represents a poor prognostic factor [6]. The distinction between isolated regional relapse due to occult nodal involvement causing metastasis, and regional metastatic relapse due to local relapse, remains unclear. Lymphatic drainage of nasal and paranasal cavities occurs in two directions, the anterior facial direction with most frequent sites being levels IIa, Ib and III, and the posterior direction towards retropharyngeal nodes [7,8]. However, the incidence of posterior node invasion is quite low [9]. Controversy remains in the management of the neck when no lymph nodes are involved at diagnosis (clinical N0 disease). The role of selective neck dissection (SND) and elective neck irradiation (ENI) remains unclear. The aim of this short review is to discuss neck management for patients without initial clinical neck node involvement.

Due to the low incidence of this disease, no randomized prospective studies are available on the subject. Table 1 contains the most important retrospective reports that have explored the regional outcome of patients with maxillary sinus cancers.

Neck outcome when no neck management is performed

One of the oldest series by Jiang et al., from 1991, showed 11 neck relapses of 50 patients with N0 maxillary sinus cancer treated exclusively for primary tumour, without prophylactic neck treatment [10]. Of them, 9/11 (81.8%) had isolated neck recurrences. All of the 9 patients received salvage treatment (4/9 underwent definitive EBRT and 5/9 received combined management with EBRT and surgery).

Similarly, Paulino et al. reported 38 N0 diseases of 42 patients with maxillary sinus SCC [11]. None of them received prophylactic neck treatment. They found 11/38 (28.9%) neck metastases during follow-up. Most common sites were levels Ib and II. More recently, Kim et al. and Jang et al. only reported 14/104 (13.5%) and 1/30 (3.33%) neck relapses, respectively, in N0 maxillary sinus cancer patients without any prophylactic management [3,12].

Also, Sakashita et al. reported only 4/48 (8.3%) neck relapses after superelective intra-arterial chemoradiotherapy with Cisplatin, without prophylactic ENI, raising the question of balance between efficiency of elective neck radiotherapy alone and global effect of concomitant chemoradiotherapy [13]. Three out of four patients received salvage neck dissection. Mortality rate from regional disease was 1/48 (2%).

The above results are controversial in regard to the incidence (3.3%-28.9%) of neck relapse, raising the question of which patients should receive prophylactic neck treatment and which modality of treatment should be given to clinically negative neck lymph node maxillary SCC?

Series	Year	n	Maxillary tumour site	Positive Nodal involvement	Neck management	Regional relapse
Jiang et al. [10]	1991	73	73	6	N0: -17/67 ENI - 50/67 NNT N +: Surgery+/-RT	N0: 11/50 NNT N+: 1/6
Paulino et al. [11]	1997	42	42	4	N+: RT+/-surgery N0: NNT	N0: 11/38 (9/11 ipsilateral)
Kim et al. [3]	1999	116	116	12	N0: NNT	14/104 N0
Le et al. [16]	2000	97	97	11 (9/58 SCC)	RT	10
Yagi et al. [26]	2001	118	118	9	RT+surgery	9
Snyers et al. [27]	2006	168		18 (10/55 SCC)	N0: NNT	11% of SCC (19 in maxillary sinus SCC)
Cantù [6]	2008	704	399 (156 SCC)	38 (33/399 maxillary)	N+: ND N0: NNT	66 (16/156 SCC)
Jang et al. [12]	2010	30	30	0	N0: NNT	1
Hinerman et al. [5]	2011	54	54	9	4 neck dissection N0: 23 ENI	10 1/23 (N0 treated with ENI)
Brown et al. [14]	2013	18	18	1	N0: SND+/-RT	4
Homma et al. [28]	2014	128	128	28	N0: 83/100 NNT (0 ENI, 15 SND)	11
Guan et al. [17]	2013	59	19	18	N+: RT N0: 11/41 ENI	7/59 N+:1/48 N0: - 6/4 -0/11 N0 ENI
Sakashita et al. [13]	2014	48	48	0	NN0054	4
Castelnau-Marchand et al. [15]	2016	104	104	17	N0: 9 SND 28 ENI 17 SND +ENI 32 NNT	13

Table 1: Retrospectives series of maxillary sinus squamous cell carcinoma with neck management and regional relapses, NNT=No Neck Treatment, ENI=Elective Neck Irradiation, SND=Selective Neck Dissection, ND=Neck Dissection.

The role of selective neck dissection

Regarding SND, there are very few reports in the literature. Brown et al. presented 18 patients with maxillary sinus SCC treated with this elective treatment [14]. Seventeen out of eighteen had no initial neck involvement. Of them, 13/17 underwent SND in which 1/13 had histologically positive nodes. Four out of eighteen patients presented regional relapse, in which 2/18 (11%) had SND. Regarding the low incidence of neck relapse, affecting only 2 patients with pathologically negative nodes, they concluded that SND did not improve disease control.

A recent French study reported 104 patients with sino-nasal SCC in which 76% were in the maxillary sinus. Eighty-seven of the 104 had N0 disease and only 9 presented regional relapse, principally associated with local relapse as well [15]. A better locoregional control (LRC), but not overall survival (OS), was found according to the management of the neck in favor of SND (94% vs. 47%; p=0.002). However, after excluding patients who had no resection of their primary tumour (n=23), there was no significant difference in LRC of patients with SND (n=27) as compared to others (n=37; p=0.07). None of the 24 patients who were treated with SND and had a pathologically negative neck (pN-) progressed in the neck.

The main risk of failure in these series was still primary site relapse, especially for patients with positive margins. Brown et al. reported 9 local relapses of the 10 patients who had histologically involved margins. No other recent studies exploring exclusive SND in N0 maxillary SCC patients were found. However, from the results of series reporting neck outcome without any prophylactic treatment or with SND only, it appears that regional relapse isn't frequent but associates with a significantly poor prognostic survival. Regional failure occurs more frequently in locally advanced disease, as in a recent report which showed regional failure of 28.4% in 139 patients with hard palate or maxillary SCC, associated with pathologic T classification, from 18.7% in pT1 disease to 37.3% in pT4 [5]. T stage was found to be an independent regional recurrence-free survival factor on multivariate analysis. Thus, SND can be proposed when primitive surgery is feasible, especially for high primary volume (T3-T4). Besides, it can be useful for lymph node staging and for the determination of radiotherapy dose and volume.

The role of elective neck irradiation

The role of ENI, as exclusive neck management or after SND, in patients with N0 disease, remains unclear and controversial. Le et al. reported 5 year neck node relapse of 12% in 97 patients with maxillary cancer (58 with SCC), with higher incidence when histology was SCC. Eleven of the 58 SCC patients presented nodal involvement at initial work-up. None of the patients with N0 neck involvement at diagnosis, treated with ENI, presented neck relapse [16]. They reported a global risk of 28% of neck involvement at diagnosis or during follow-up. As in previous series, most of the regional relapse occurred in T3-T4 disease. Also, 5 year actuarial distant relapse rate was higher when patients presented neck failure, 81% vs 29% for those without neck failure. Significant higher risk of distant metastasis (DM) was estimated in patients with nodal neck failure in multivariate analysis with a hazard Ratio of 4.5 (p=0.006). Only 1/23 patients with N0 initial maxillary sinus SCC treated with prophylactic ENI presented regional relapse in the series of Hinerman et al(5). In the Guan et al. series, none of the 11 patients with N0 paranasal sinus cancer treated with ENI had neck relapse, whereas 6/35 (17.1%) of N0 patients who did not receive any neck prophylactic management did [17].

The recent study of Sakashita et al. showed 4/48 (8.3%) late neck recurrences of 48 patients with N0 maxillary sinus SCC who were treated with superelective intra-arterial chemoradiotherapy without prophylactic neck irradiation, in which 47/48 had stage T3-T4 [13]. Of them, three underwent salvage neck dissection and survived, and one didn't undergo salvage dissection due to DM. They reported a mortality rate of 2% (1/48) from regional disease.

In the Castelnau-Marchand et al. study, of the 87 patients with N0 paranasal sinus SCC, including mostly maxillary sinus SCC primitive sites, neck management consisted in 10/87 (11%) of SND alone, 28/87 (32%) of ENI alone, 17/87 (20%) of an association of SND and ENI, and the 32/87 (37%) left ones did not have any prophylactic neck management(15). Among the 27 patients who underwent SND, 3/27 (11%) had pathologically positive nodes. Eight out of 87 (9%) patients had regional relapses, in which 6/8 were associated with local failure (2 of them with DM). No significant difference of OS neither LRC was found according to the management of the neck.

In a recent meta-analysis with a total of 129 patients with N0 SCC maxillary sinus, including most of the series presented in our review, ENI was considered as a significantly favourable factor of neck nodal recurrence (OR=0.16; 95% CI: 0.04-0.67; p=0.01), compared to management by observation [18]. Considering these results, the prophylactic treatment, SND and/or ENI was recommended in the N0 neck, especially for locally advanced maxillary sinus SCC (T3-T4) where probability of occult lymph node metastasis is >10-20% [19].

Radiation Techniques and Volumes

Between outcome and toxicity: From 3D-CRT to IMRT

Post-operative or exclusive head and neck cancer radiotherapy induced substantial toxicity, especially xerostomia, taste loss and alteration of quality of life, with two-dimensional and even with 3D-conformal radiotherapy (3D-CRT). This morbidity is largely augmented when concomitant chemotherapy and neck irradiation are associated [20]. As a result, neck irradiation was often substituted by neck dissection, without confirmation of any advantages in outcome. In the French series where 90 patients received neck irradiation, 75/90 (83%) were treated with 3D-CRT and only 15/90 (15.7%) with IMRT [15]. For the full population, grade 3 radiomucositis, radiodermatitis and dysphagia were found in 22%, 10% and 21%, respectively. No severe late toxicity was reported.

Intensity-modulated radiotherapy (IMRT) significantly improved dose distribution over 3D-CRT in head and neck cancer, especially when neck irradiation was associated, and reduced acute neck toxicity [21]. As shown in previous series, due to the low incidence of this disease, there is no randomized clinical trial comparing 3D CRT to IMRT in this particular site. However, Suh et al. recently reported, retrospectively, a better 3 year locoregional recurrence-free survival of 89.2% vs 59.5% (p=0.035) with IMRT vs 3D-CRT in 54 patients with maxillary sinus carcinoma, and less toxicity with IMRT [22]. Grade 3 radiomucositis occurred in 31% vs. 0% in 3D-CRT and IMRT, respectively. Grade 2 xerostomia was observed in 9% vs 5%, respectively. These results can be explained by important modification of volume feasible with IMRT, offering higher coverage of primary tumour, which results in better locoregional control. They concluded that IMRT should be privileged over 3D-CRT in maxillary sinus cancer due to proximity of critical organs to the tumour and to improvement of dose distribution, sparing organs at risk.

Doses, levels and side of neck irradiation

Doses: The most widely used prophylactic dose in N0 neck for maxillary sinus SCC is 50-54 Gy. However, as ENI is controversial due to the low incidence of neck relapse, the necessity to reduce post-radiotherapy toxicity is essential. Nevens et al. explored the effect on loco-regional control and toxicity of a reduction of dose of ENI from 50 Gy to 40 Gy with IMRT in 200 patients with head and neck cancer [23]. They reported no significant difference in 2-year disease control and survival between the two groups with a local failure rate of 14.1% vs 14.4% in the 40 Gy and 50 Gy arms, respectively; and regional failure rate of 13.0% and 5.5% (p=0.08), respectively. Significantly less salivary gland toxicity was found in the 40 Gy arm. They suggested that dose de-escalation to the ENI volume in head and neck cancer could be an option to decrease morbidity without compromising disease control or survival.

Levels and sides in N0 disease: In the Le et al. series, they found that 84% of the neck relapses occurred in the ipsilateral side and were mostly limited to levels I, II and then III [16]. Ipsilateral levels Ib and IIa were also the most common sites of nodal recurrence in the Guan et al. series [17]. Suh et al. reported 12 regional recurrences, which occurred in the ipsilateral levels I, II and III in 3, 6 and 2 relapses, respectively, and only one contralateral relapse in the level II [22]. As well, in the French study, neck relapse was ipsilateral for 4 patients, bilateral for 3 and contralateral for one [15]. Most frequent levels were ipsilateral levels II, III (always associated with level II relapse), and Ib. From these retrospective series, most authors suggested that the prophylactic neck volume should include ipsilateral levels Ib, II +/- III for patients without clinical lymph node involvement [24,25].

Conclusion

Neck failure remains an independent poor prognostic factor in maxillary sinus SCC. Prophylactic neck management, whether performed by SND or ENI, seems to improve locoregional control over active monitoring. SND may allow an increase of LRC and a better detection of occult cervical positive LN in order to propose selective post-operative radiotherapy. ENI is still controversial, but considering recent publications, it could be proposed in selected patients, especially with T3-4 stage disease and when SND has not been performed. Volumes of ENI could include ipsilateral level II, +/- Ib and III or bilateral neck, according to the primary tumour extension. IMRT should be considered whenever feasible to reduce toxicity.

References

1. Youlden DR, Cramb SM, Peters S, Porceddu SV, Møller H, et al. (2013) International comparisons of the incidence and mortality of sinonasal cancer. Cancer Epidemiol 37: 770-779.
2. Jégoux F, Métreau A, Louvel G, Bedfert C (2013) Paranasal sinus cancer. Eur Ann Otorhinolaryngol Head Neck Dis 130: 327-335.
3. Kim GE, Chung EJ, Lim JJ, Keum KC, Lee SW, et al. (1999) Clinical significance of neck node metastasis in squamous cell carcinoma of the maxillary antrum. American journal of otolaryngology 20: 383-390.
4. Iyer NG, Tan DSW, Tan VKM, Wang W, Hwang J, et al. (2015) Randomized trial comparing surgery and adjuvant radiotherapy versus concurrent chemoradiotherapy in patients with advanced, nonmetastatic squamous cell carcinoma of the head and neck: 10 year update and subset analysis. Cancer 121: 1599-1607.
5. Hinerman RW, Indelicato DJ, Morris CG, Kirwan JM, Werning JW, et al. (2011) Radiotherapy with or without surgery for maxillary sinus squamous cell carcinoma: Should the clinical N0 neck be treated? Am J Clin Oncol 34: 483-487.
6. Cantù G, Bimbi G, Miceli R, Mariani L, Colombo S, et al. (2008) Lymph node metastases in malignant tumors of the paranasal sinuses: Prognostic value and treatment. Arch Otolaryngol Head Neck Surg 134: 170-177.
7. Day TA, Beas RA, Schlosser RJ, Woodworth BA, Barredo J, et al. (2005) Management of paranasal sinus malignancy. Curr Treat Options Oncol 6: 3-18.
8. Guan X, Wang X, Liu Y, Hu C, Zhu G (2013) Lymph node metastasis in sinonasal squamous cell carcinoma treated with IMRT/3D-CRT. Oral Oncol 49: 60-65.
9. Fernández JMS, Santaolalla F, Del Rey AS, Martínez-Ibargüen A, González A, et al. (2005) Preliminary study of the lymphatic drainage system of the nose and paranasal sinuses and its role in detection of sentinel metastatic nodes. Acta Otolaryngol 125: 566-570.
10. Jiang GL, Ang KK, Peters LJ, Wendt CD, Oswald MJ, et al. (1991) Maxillary sinus carcinomas: Natural history and results of postoperative radiotherapy. Radiother Oncol 21: 193-200.
11. Paulino AC, Fisher SG, Marks JE (1997) Is prophylactic neck irradiation indicated in patients with squamous cell carcinoma of the maxillary sinus? Int J Radiat Oncol Biol Phys 39: 283-289.
12. Jang NY, Wu HG, Park CI, Heo DS, Kim DW, et al. (2010) Definitive radiotherapy with or without chemotherapy for T3-4N0 squamous cell carcinoma of the maxillary sinus and nasal cavity. Jpn J Clin Oncol 40: 542-548.
13. Sakashita T, Homma A, Hatakeyama H, Kano S, Mizumachi T, et al. (2013) The incidence of late neck recurrence in N0 maxillary sinus squamous cell carcinomas after superselective intra-arterial chemoradiotherapy without prophylactic neck irradiation. Eur Arch Otorhinolaryngol.
14. Brown JS, Bekiroglu F, Shaw RJ, Woolgar JA, Triantafyllou A, et al. (2013) First report of elective selective neck dissection in the management of squamous cell carcinoma of the maxillary sinus. Br J Oral Maxillofac Surg 51: 103-107.
15. Castelnau-Marchand P, Levy A, Moya-Plana A, Mirghani H, Nguyen F, et al. (2016) Sinonasal squamous cell carcinoma without clinical lymph node involvement? Which neck management is best? Strahlenther Onkol.
16. Le QT, Fu KK, Kaplan MJ, Terris DJ, Fee WE, et al. (2000) Lymph node metastasis in maxillary sinus carcinoma. International Journal of Radiation Oncology* Biology* Physics 46: 541-549.
17. Guan X, Wang X, Liu Y, Hu C, Zhu G (2013) Lymph node metastasis in sinonasal squamous cell carcinoma treated with IMRT/3D-CRT. Oral Oncol 49: 60-65.
18. Abu-Ghanem S, Horowitz G, Abergel A, Yehuda M, Gutfeld O, et al. (2015) Elective neck irradiation versus observation in squamous cell carcinoma of the maxillary sinus with N0 neck: A meta-analysis and review of the literature. Head Neck 37: 1823-1828.
19. Redaelli de Zinis LO1, Nicolai P, Tomenzoli D, Ghizzardi D, Trimarchi M, et al. (2002) The distribution of lymph node metastases in supraglottic squamous cell carcinoma: therapeutic implications. Head Neck 24: 913-920.
20. McDonald MW, Liu Y, Moore MG, Johnstone PAS (2016) Acute toxicity in comprehensive head and neck radiation for nasopharynx and paranasal sinus cancers: Cohort comparison of 3D conformal proton therapy and intensity modulated radiation therapy. Radiat Oncol 11: 32.
21. Toledano I, Graff P, Serre A, Boisselier P, Bensadoun RJ, et al. (2012) Intensity-modulated radiotherapy in head and neck cancer: Results of the prospective study GORTEC 2004-03. Radiother Oncol 103: 57-62.
22. Suh Y-G, Lee CG, Kim H, Choi EC, Kim SH, et al. (2016) Treatment outcomes of intensity-modulated radiotherapy versus 3D conformal radiotherapy for patients with maxillary sinus cancer in the postoperative setting. Head Neck 1: E207-E213.
23. Nevens D, Duprez F, Daisne JF, Dok R, Belmans A, et al. (2016) Reduction of the dose of radiotherapy to the elective neck in head and neck squamous cell carcinoma; a randomized clinical trial. Effect on late toxicity and tumor control. Radiotherapy and Oncology.
24. Lapeyre M, Miroir J, Biau J (2014) Delineation of the lymph nodes for head neck cancers. Cancer Radiother 18: 572-576.
25. Chao KS, Wippold FJ, Ozyigit G, Tran BN, Dempsey JF (2002) Determination and delineation of nodal target volumes for head-and-neck cancer based on patterns of failure in patients receiving definitive and postoperative IMRT. Int J Radiat Oncol Biol Phys 53: 1174-1184.
26. Yagi K, Fukuda S, Furuta Y, Oridate N, Homma A, et al. (2001) A clinical study on the cervical lymph node metastasis of maxillary sinus carcinoma. Auris Nasus Larynx 28 Suppl: S77-S81.
27. Snyers A, Janssens GORJ, Twickler MB, Hermus AR, Takes RP, et al. (2009) Malignant tumors of the nasal cavity and paranasal sinuses: Long-term outcome and morbidity with emphasis on hypothalamic-pituitary deficiency. International Journal of Radiation Oncology*Biology*Physics 73: 1343-1351.
28. Homma A, Hayashi R, Matsuura K, Kato K, Kawabata K, et al. (2014) Lymph node metastasis in t4 maxillary sinus squamous cell carcinoma: Incidence and treatment outcome. Ann Surg Oncol 21: 1706-1710.

Speech Perception and Subjective Preference with Fine Structure Coding Strategies

Robert Mlynski[1]*, Michael Ziese[2], Thorsten Rahne[3] and Joachim Müller-Deile[4]

[1]*Department of Otorhinolaryngology, Head and Neck Surgery, Otto Körner, Rostock University Medical Center, Germany*
[2]*University Clinic Magdeburg A.ö.R., University Clinic for Otolaryngology, Germany*
[3]*Universitätsklinik und Poliklinik für Hals-Nasen-Ohrenheilkunde, Kopf- und Hals-Chirurgie, Hallesches Hör- und ImplantCentrum (HIC), Deutschland, Germany*
[4]*Universitätsklinikum Schleswig-Holstein, Campus Kiel, Klinik für Hals-, Nasen-, Ohrenheilkunde, Kopf- und Halschirurgie, Deutschland, Germany*

Abstract

This study aimed to determine differences in speech perception and subjective preference after upgrade from the FSP coding strategy to the FS4 or FS4p coding strategies.

Subjects were tested at the point of upgrade (n=10), and again at 1-(n=10), 3-(n=8), 6-(n=8) and 12 months (n=8) after the upgrade to the FS4 or FS4p coding strategy. In between test intervals patients had to use the FS4 or FS4p strategy in everyday life. Primary outcome measures, chosen to best evaluate individual speech understanding, were the Freiburg Monosyllable Test in quiet, the Oldenburg Sentence Test (OLSA) in noise, and the Hochmair-Schulz-Moser (HSM) Sentence Test in noise. To measure subjective sound quality the Hearing Implant Sound Quality Index was used.

Subjects with the FS4/FS4p strategy performed as well as subjects with the FSP coding strategy in the speech tests. The subjective perception of subjects showed that subjects perceived a 'moderate' or 'poor' auditory benefit with the FS4/FS4p coding strategy.

Subjects with the FS4 or FS4p coding strategies perform well in everyday situations. Both coding strategies offer another tool to individualize the fitting of audio processors and grant access to satisfying sound quality and speech perception.

Keywords: Cochlear implant; Fine structure; Coding strategy; Signal; Speech perception

Introduction

Coding strategies are used to process sound signals into deliverable electrical stimuli to the auditory system of cochlear implant (CI) users. The sound signals are decomposed into envelope and fine structure [1,2]. The electrical stimuli are delivered to the auditory nerve through an intra-cochlear electrode array. Most modern CI coding strategies present the signal envelope which, depending on the actual implementation of the coding strategy, includes some fine structure information (e.g. information on pitch). With the commonly used Continuous Interleaved Sampling (CIS) strategy the sound signal is split into a number of frequency bands using band-pass filtering, and the envelope is extracted from each frequency band using rectification and low-pass filtering [1,3,4]. These envelope signals are then used to generate amplitude-modulated biphasic pulses at a constant stimulation rate. Each amplitude-modulated pulse train passes into the cochlea through a contact on the multi-electrode intra-cochlear array to stimulate auditory nerve fibers in a specified region of the cochlea. Cochlear tonotopicity is implemented by sending information from the lowest frequency band envelope to the most apical electrode and information from the highest frequency band envelope to the most basal electrode.

Various forms of the CIS strategy are implemented in all major CI systems (Advanced Bionics Corporation: HiRes, Cochlear Corporation: CIS, MED-EL: CIS, CIS+, HDCIS). In addition to the CIS+ and HDCIS strategy, the MED-EL MAESTRO system currently offers the option to configure low-frequency channels up to 300 Hz by using Channel-Specific Sampling Sequences (CSSS) as described by Zierhofer [5]. Such a strategy with CSSS on low-frequency channels is called the FSP strategy. The FS4 and FS4p strategy are further developments of the FSP strategy and were developed in order to give all users access to refined envelope modulations up to 750-1000 Hz. The fundamental principle as well as the manner of providing refined envelope modulations remains the same in FS4 and FS4p as in FSP. FS4 and FS4p use the same CSSS concept and implementation and the same CSSS-specific default parameter settings as FSP.

Recent publications, comparing FSP to older CIS+ coding strategies, reveal that the FSP coding strategy improves speech perception in noise [6-9]. Thus, a further increase in stimulus variability with FS4 and FS4p might benefit individual speech perception and sound quality even further. The main purpose of this study was to determine the effect of upgrade on the speech perception and subjective perception of sound quality of CI users upgraded from the FSP coding strategy to the FS4 or FS4p coding strategy. Primary outcome measures, chosen to evaluate individual speech understanding, were the Freiburg Monosyllable Test in quiet, the Oldenburg Sentence Test (OLSA) in noise, and the Hochmair-Schulz-Moser (HSM) Sentence Test in noise. Subjective sound quality was determined using the Hearing Implant Sound Quality Index ($HISQUI_{19}$). The Hearing Implant Sound Quality Preference Index was used to determine the subjective differences in sound quality between the two different coding strategies.

***Corresponding author:** Robert Mlynski, Department of Otorhinolaryngology, Head and Neck Surgery, Otto Körner, Rostock University Medical Center, Doberaner Str. 137-139, D-18057 Rostock, Germany; E-mail: robert.mlynski@med.uni-rostock.de

Methods

Subjects

10 adult subjects (9 female, 1 male) with a MED-EL CI were included in this study. Demographic data are presented in Table 1. All subjects had more than 10 active electrodes and used their CI more than 10 h per day.

Speech tests

The test set-up consisted of a computer with an onboard sound card, an audiometer, and an audiometric loudspeaker (calibrated according to DIN 45620 and DIN 45624). All speech tests were performed in a sound-proof room. Software for testing was installed on a PC or laptop. The stimuli were generated by the computer and presented to the subject via loudspeaker. The subject was positioned at a fixed distance of 1 m and 0° from the loudspeaker unable to see any information on the computer screen.

The Freiburg Monosyllable Test in quiet, which consists of 20 lists with 20 words each, was presented at 65 dB sound pressure level (SPL). Each subject was tested with one list (List 1) for training purposes before the start of the actual testing. The results scored in this training session were not analyzed. For the actual test each subject was given 2 lists. These lists were allocated according to a randomization procedure. The outcome was calculated as the number of words repeated in % correct.

Oldenburg Sentence Test (OLSA) in noise was performed with a fixed signal (speech) level and a variable noise level. This test established the speech reception threshold (SRT) in noise. The SRT is defined as 50% speech reception in noise and calculated by counting the number of words understood correctly.

The OLSA, which consists of 40 lists with 30 sentences each was tested first with two lists (List 1 and 2) for training purposes. The training run was conducted as a closed-set test. Subjects were given a print-out of all the possible words used in the test. The results scored in this training session were not analyzed. After the training test was run subjects returned the printed word material. For the actual test each subject was given 2 lists according to a fixed randomization procedure. The actual test was performed as an open-set procedure (no word-material was provided as a print out for the test). The subjects had to repeat the words they understood back to the tester who marked them on the standard OLSA case report form. The outcome evaluates the speech perception in noise at a fixed presentation level (speech was presented at 65 dB SPL. The noise used for this test was the OLSA noise. The test was performed at a starting signal-to-noise ratio of +10 dB.

Hochmair-Schulz-Moser (HSM) Sentence Test in noise is an open-set sentence test, which consists of 30 lists with 20 sentences each. Each subject performed one list (List 1) for training purposes before the start of the actual testing. The results scored in this training session were not analyzed. For the actual test each subject was given 2 lists. These lists were allocated according to a randomization procedure. The outcome evaluates the number of correctly repeated words in % correct at a fixed presentation level. Speech was presented at 65 dB SPL. The test was performed in continuous noise at a signal-to-noise ratio of +10dB.

Audio-processor set-up

The patients' usual fitting with the FSP strategy at the time of the first testing interval was used for initial testing with FSP. After the initial testing with FSP, it was saved on the fitting computer and the FS4 or the FS4p coding strategy was fitted to each subject's individual auditory requirements and also stored on the fitting computer. Following this, only FS4 or FS4p programs were programmed to the audio processor. To ensure reproducibility of the collected data subjects were not able to switch back to the FSP strategy during the study period. Therefore, no FSP program options were uploaded on the audio processor. With the OPUS 1 the FS4 or FS4p strategy was stored in all 3 program options with 9 different volume settings.

The following steps were completed during programming of the FS4 or FS4p strategy:

- For all electrodes the maximum comfortable loudness (MCL level) was measured;
- For all electrodes the threshold level (THR) was measured as standard in clinical practice;
- MCLs and THRs were adjusted in combination with the overall volume (given in percentage of MCL) globally until the speech of the investigator was perceived as comfortably loud;
- MCLs and THRs were adjusted until the sound quality was satisfying (test the loudness with spoken voice e.g. 's', 'sh', 'f', 'bub' and environmental sounds e.g. rattling a key, scrunching paper, etc.);
- Optional: The overall volume was adjusted using recorded speech in quiet using an OLSA sentence test at 65 dB SPL.
- The investigator informed the subject about the process in the case of necessary reprogramming of the strategy or any other complications with the study equipment.

Subjective Assessment

The Hearing Implant Sound Quality Index ($HISQUI_{19}$) is a questionnaire used in this study to gain overall information about the

Subject	Gender	Age at time of assessment (years)	Implant Type	Type of Speech Processor	Age at implantation Right Ear (years)	Age at implantation Left Ear (years)	Coding Strategy
1	Female	60.6	PULSAR	OPUS 2	55.7		FS4p
2	Female	67.4	SONATA	OPUS 2		65.0	FS4p
3	Female	72.6	PULSAR	OPUS 2	65.9		FS4p
4	Female	53.4	PULSAR	OPUS 2	47.4		FS4p
5	Female	68.4	PULSAR	OPUS 2		64.6	FS4p
6	Female	54	PULSAR	OPUS 2	49.9		FS4p
7	Female	80.9	SONATA	OPUS 2		78.7	FS4
8	Female	40.9	SONATA	OPUS 2	38.2		FS4
9	Female	56.6	CONCERTO	OPUS 2		55.3	FS4
10	Male	65.8	SONATA	OPUS 2	63.7		FS4

Table 1: Demographic data.

sound quality in personal, everyday listening situations of a hearing implant user. It consists of 19 items on a seven-point Likert scale, with possible answers ranging from 'Always' (7) to 'Never' (1) [10]. A total score is obtained by adding the numerical values of all 19 questions, ranging between 19 and 133 points. A score <30 indicates 'very poor sound quality', a score between 30 and 60 indicates 'poor sound quality', a score between 60 and 90 indicates 'moderate sound quality', a score between 90 and 110 indicates 'good sound quality' and a score between 110 and 133 indicates 'very good sound quality'.

The investigator explained the procedure for filling out the HISQUI questionnaires to the subject. The questionnaires were filled out at each test interval directly after speech testing at the study site.

Test intervals

The study was of an ABAB design. Every uneven patient number was first tested with the familiar FSP fitting strategy, whereas every even patient number was initially tested with the new fitting strategy (FS4 or FS4p).

Test Interval 1: At switch-over

Speech testing with the FSP or FS4/FS4p (if necessary fit FS4/FS4p before), switch over to other speech coding strategy and do speech testing with this second speech coding strategy, subject to fill out the Hearing Implant Sound Quality Index ($HISQUI_{19}$); send subject home with FS4/FS4p only.

Test Interval 2: One month after switch-over

Speech testing with FSP or FS4/FS4p (use "old" FSP program), switch over to other speech coding strategy and do speech testing with this second coding strategy; subject to fill out the Hearing Implant Sound Quality Index ($HISQUI_{19}$); send subject home with FS4/FS4p only.

Test Interval 3: Three months after switch-over

speech testing with FSP or FS4/FS4p (use "old" FSP program), switch over to other speech coding strategy and do speech testing with the second speech coding strategy; subject to fill out the Hearing Implant Sound Quality Index ($HISQUI_{19}$); send subject home with FS4/FS4p only.

Test Interval 4: Six months after switch over

speech testing with FSP or FS4/FS4p, (use "old" FSP program), switch over to other speech coding strategy and do speech testing with the second speech coding strategy; send subject home with FS4/FS4p only.

Test Interval 5: Twelve months after switch over

speech testing with FSP or FS4/FS4p (use "old" FSP program), switch over to other speech coding strategy and do speech testing with the second speech coding strategy; subject to fill out the Hearing Implant Sound Quality Index ($HISQUI_{19}$); send subject home with FS4/FS4p only.

Statistical Analysis

Group outcome variables were tested for Gaussian distribution and are described by mean values plus standard deviation. In a first step speech performance (Monosyllables in quiet, OLSA in noise and HSM in noise) over time (Interval 1-5) was examined for each coding strategy (FSP and FS4/FS4p), applying repeated measure ANOVAs. Wilcoxon signed-rank test was used to test for a significant difference between the two coding strategies at each tested interval. Additionally, multivariate ANOVAs were conducted to look for a statistically significant effect of coding strategy. Wilcoxon signed-rank test was performed for the $HISQUI_{19}$ to test for a significant difference between the tested intervals.

All p-values are results of two-sided tests, and generally p-values ≤ 0.05 were considered to indicate statistical significance. In cases of multiple comparisons, a p-value of ≤ 0.01 was considered statistically significant. For multiple pairwise comparisons such as analyses between the two coding strategies on speech performance, p-values were adjusted with the Bonferroni correction method. In this case, a p-value ≤ 0.01 indicates statistical significance.

The software tool IBM SPSS Statistics 22 (IBM, Armonik, New York) was used for the statistical analyses.

Results

Speech tests

Freiburg monosyllables in quiet: Over time (Interval 1-5) there were no significant differences in the mean percentage on the Freiburg monosyllables in quiet with the FSP coding strategy ($F(4; 24)=1.989$; $p=0.128$) or with the FS4/FS4p coding strategy ($F(4; 24)=1.343$; $p=0.283$) (Figure 1 and Table 2a).

Overall (across all tested intervals) subjects did not perform significantly better on the Monosyllables in quiet with the FS4/FS4p coding strategy than with the FSP coding strategy (Table 2b).

Oldenburg sentence test (OLSA) in noise: Over time (Interval 1-5) there were no significant differences in the mean score on the OLSA in noise with the FSP coding strategy ($F(4; 24)=1.659$; $p=0.192$) or with the FS4/FS4p coding strategy (Figure 2). However, over time there was a tendency towards an improvement on the OLSA in noise with the FSP/FS4p coding strategy ($F(4; 24)=2.667$; $p=0.057$) (Figure 2 and Table 3a).

Overall (across all tested intervals) subjects did not perform significantly better on the OLSA in noise with the FS4/FS4p coding strategy than with the FSP coding strategy. There was a tendency towards an improvement on the OLSA in noise with the FSP/FS4p coding strategy at test Interval 2 ($p=0.066$) (Table 3b).

Hochmair-Schulz-Moser (HSM) sentence test in noise: Over

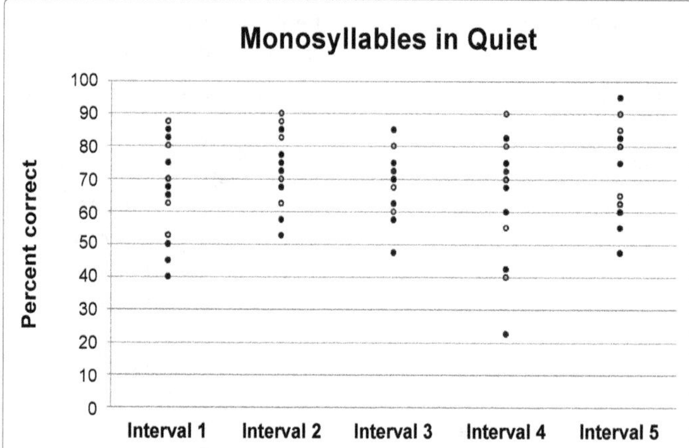

Figure 1: Individual results of monosyllables in quiet (%). Black dots represent results of the FSP coding strategy; black circles represent results of the FS4/FS4p coding strategy.

	Interval 1		Interval 2		Interval 3		Interval 4		Interval 5			
ID	FSP	FS4/FS4p	FSP	FS4/FS4p	FSP	FS4/FS4p	FSP	FS4/FS4p	FSP	FS4/FS4p	Mean FSP	Mean FS4/ FS4p
1	65	65	75	82,5	72,5	80	75	90	60	62,5	69,5	76,0
2	75	70	77,5	85					95	90	82,5	81,7
3	67,5	52,5	72,5	72,5			67,5	70			69,2	65,0
4	82,5	80	85	87,5	85	85	82,5	82,5	82,5	85	83,5	84,0
5	45	50	72,5	67,5	62,5	67,5	60	70	60	62,5	60,0	63,5
6	65	70	67,5	67,5	72,5	60	72,5	80	75	80	70,5	71,5
7	50	50	52,5	62,5	57,5	57,5	22,5	40	55	47,5	47,5	51,5
8	40	52,5	57,5	62,5	47,5	62,5	42,5	55	47,5	65	47,0	59,5
9	85	87,5	85	90	75	70	75	82,5	82,5	80	80,5	82,0
10	67,5	62,5	67,5	70	70	70					68,3	67,5

Bold font shows better value

Table 2A: Individual results on Freiburger Monosyllables in Quiet plus mean over all test intervals.

	FSP	FS4/FS4p	p-value*
Interval 1 (n=10)	64.2 ± 15.14	64.0 ± 13.08	0.943
Interval 2 (n=10)	71.2 ± 10.55	74.7 ± 10.50	.048**
Interval 3 (n=8)	67.8 ± 11.60	69.1 ± 9.53	0.588
Interval 4 (n=8)	62.2 ± 20.15	71.2 ± 16.58	.018**
Interval 5 (n=8)	69.7 ± 16.44	71.6 ± 14.39	0.67

*Results of Wilcoxon signed-rank test

**Because of multiple comparisons, a p-value ≤ 0.01 indicates statistical significance

Table 2B: Freiburger monosyllables in quiet as mean percent ± standard deviation.

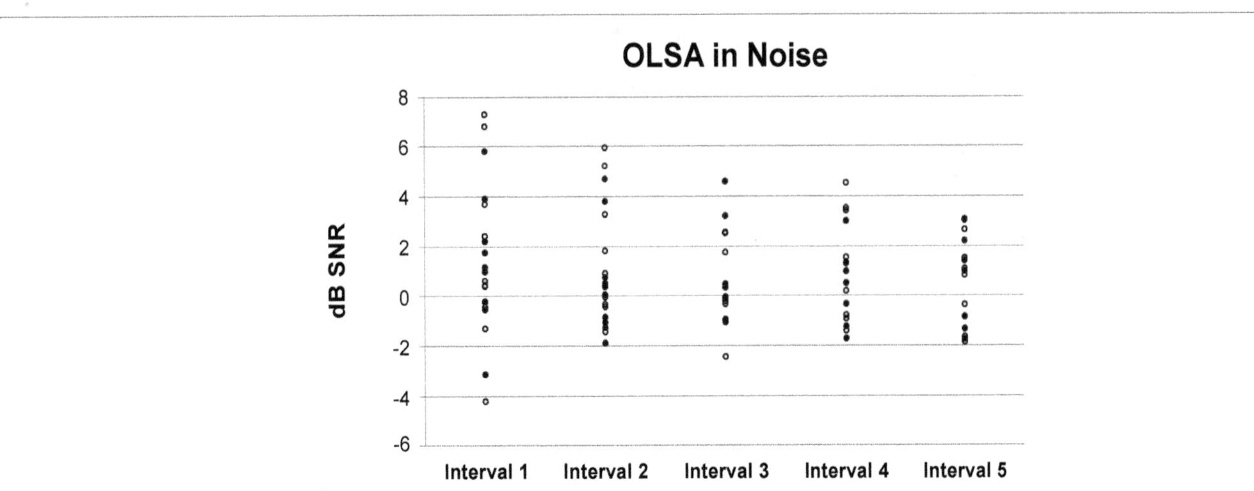

Figure 2: Individual results of OLSA in noise (dB SNR). Black dots represent results of the FSP coding strategy; black circles represent results of the FS4/FS4p coding strategy.

time (Interval 1-5) there were no significant differences in the mean percentage on the HSM in noise with the FSP coding strategy (F(4; 24)=0.234; p=0.917) or with the FS4/FS4p coding strategy F(4; 24)=0.660; p=0.626) (Figure 3 and Table 4a).

Overall (across all tested intervals) subjects there were no significant differences between the mean percentage with the FS4/FS4p coding strategy and the mean percentage with FSP coding strategy on the HSM in noise (Table 4b).

Subjective assessment

Hearing implant sound quality index (HISQUI$_{19}$): The mean average score on the HISQUI$_{19}$ was 78.5 (± SD=21.9) at Interval 1, 41.7 (± SD=24.4) at Interval 2, 47.7 (± SD=30.3) at Interval 3 and 77.9 (± SD=20.2) at Interval 5. Subjects reported 'moderate' self-perceived sound quality at Interval 1 and 5 and 'poor' self-perceived sound quality at Interval 2 and at Interval 3. The results show a significant deterioration at Interval 2 and 3 compared to Interval 1 (p=0.005 and

	Interval 1		Interval 2		Interval 3		Interval 4		Interval 5			
ID	**FSP**	**FS4/FS4p**	**FSP**	**FS4/FS4p**	**FSP**	**FS4/FS4p**	**FSP**	**FS4/FS4p**	**FSP**	**FS4/FS4p**	**Mean FSP**	**Mean FS4/ FS4p**
1	1,745	0,6	0,365	-0,05	-0,135	-0,23	-1,725	-0,785	3,045	1,515	0,659	0,21
2	-0,215	0,425	-1,91	-0,33					-1,765	-1,865	-1,297	-0,59
3	1,155	6,8	-0,86	3,29			-0,33	4,52			-0,012	4,87
4	-0,235	-0,445	-1,285	0,405	-0,95	-0,33	-1,25	-0,92	-1,35	-0,375	-1,014	-0,333
5	0,995	2,395	0,49	1,8	-0,105	1,745	0,5	0,19	1,385	1,085	0,653	1,443
6	5,8	3,7	4,7	5,2	3,2	2,5	1,3	3,4	2,2	1,5	3,44	3,26
7	3,9	7,3	3,8	5,95	4,6	2,55	3	3,5	3,05	2,65	3,67	4,39
8	-0,55	-1,3	-1,05	-1,45	-1,05	-2,45	1	-1,4	-0,85	-1,65	-0,5	-1,65
9	2,21	0,395	0,75	0,925	0,32	-0,075	1,345	1,525	1	0,8	1,125	0,714
10	-3,14	-4,21	0,05	-0,45	0,475	-0,975					-0,872	-1,878

Bold font shows better value

Table 3A: Individual results on OLSA in noise plus mean over all test intervals.

	FSP	**FS4/FS4p**	**p-value***
Interval 1 (n=10)	1.17 ± 2.49	1.57 ± 3.57	0.959
Interval 2 (n=10)	0.50 ± 2.16	1.53 ± 2.51	0.066
Interval 3 (n=8)	0.79 ± 2.02	0.34 ± 1.77	0.263
Interval 4 (n=8)	0.48 ± 1.54	1.25 ± 2.31	0.208
Interval 5 (n=8)	0.84 ± 1.94	0.46 ± 1.61	0.123

*Results of Wilcoxon signed-rank test

Table 3B: OLSA in noise as dB SNR ± standard deviation.

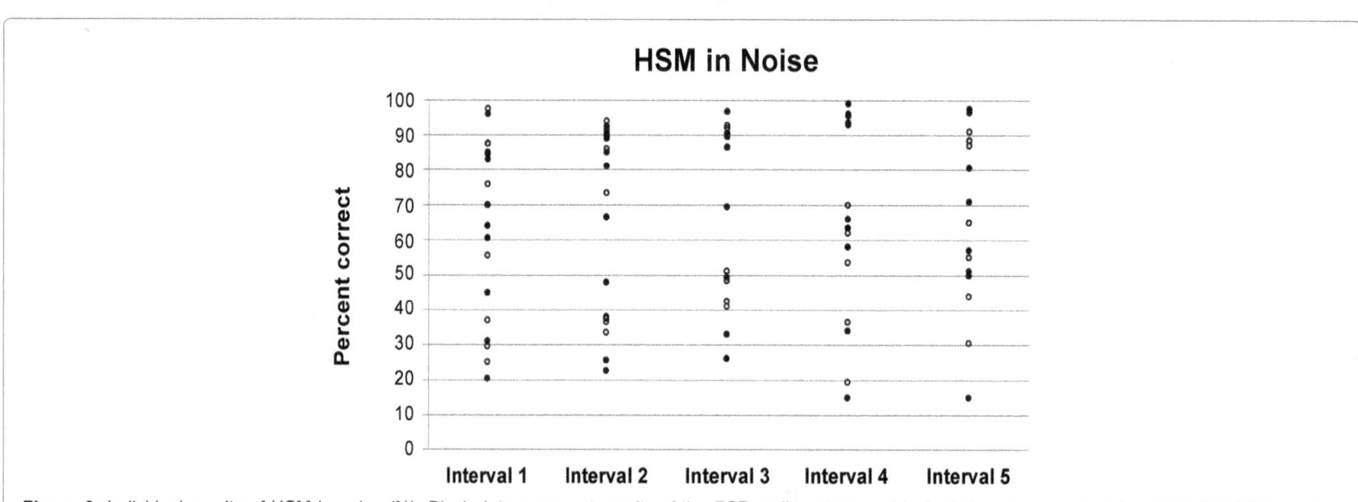

Figure 3: Individual results of HSM in noise (%). Black dots represent results of the FSP coding strategy; black circles represent results of the FS4/FS4p coding strategy.

p=0.012), but in turn a significant improvement from Interval 2 and 3 to Interval 5 (p=0.018 and p=0.028).

Discussion

This study compared subjects with the FSP coding strategy after upgrade to the FS4 and the FS4p (FS4/FS4p) coding strategies, over 12 months. Subjects with the FS4/FS4p strategy performed as well as subjects with the FSP coding strategy. The primary outcomes measures: the Freiburg monosyllables in quiet, OLSA and HSM test, determined that the performance with both coding strategies were similar. The subjective assessment of subjects showed that half of the time they perceived a moderate improvement in auditory benefit or a poorer sound quality with the FS4/FS4p than with the FSP coding strategy.

The subjects tested herein did not perform significantly differently on the Freiburg monosyllables in quiet test with the FS4/FS4p coding strategy than with the FSP coding strategy. In contrast, Riss et al. [11] had shown that subjects tested on the Freiburg monosyllables in quiet with FS4 had a small, but significant difference in favour of the FSP strategy. A possible explanation for the difference between the Riss et

	Interval 1		Interval 2		Interval 3		Interval 4		Interval 5			
ID	FSP	FS4/FS4p	FSP	FS4/FS4p	FSP	FS4/FS4p	FSP	FS4/FS4p	FSP	FS4/FS4p	Mean FSP	Mean FS4/ FS4p
1	85	87,5	85	86	90	92	99	96	71	65	86	85,3
2	64	76	92,5	91,5					97,5	88,5	84,7	85,3
3	70	70	90	90			63,5	70			74,5	76,7
4	83	87,5	89	94	86,5	90,5	93	93,5	96,5	91	89,6	91,3
5	45	37	66,5	38	69,5	51	58	53,5	57	55	59,2	46,9
6	20,5	25	22,5	36,5	49,5	41	66	19,5	15	30,5	34,7	30,5
7	31	29,5	25,5	33,5	33	48,5	15	36,5	51	44	31,1	38,4
8	60,5	55,5	48	37,5	26	42,5	34	62	50	87	43,7	56,9
9	96	97,5	90,5	89	86,5	92,75	96	95,5	80,5	88,5	89,9	92,7
10	84,5	84,5	81	73,5	96,7	89,62					87,4	82,5

Bold font shows better value

Table 4A: Individual results on HSM in Noise plus mean over all test intervals.

	FSP	FS4/FS4p	p-value*
Interval 1 (n=10)	63.9 ± 25.02	65.0 ± 26.51	0.623
Interval 2 (n=10)	69.0 ± 27.40	66.9 ± 26.89	0.722
Interval 3 (n=8)	67.2 ± 27.57	68.5 ± 24.52	0.889
Interval 4 (n=8)	65.6 ± 30.26	65.8 ± 28.65	0.833
Interval 5 (n=8)	64.8 ± 27.54	68.7 ± 23.56	0.779

*Results of Wilcoxon signed-rank test

Table 4B: HSM in Noise as mean percent ± standard deviation.

al. study and the present data may be the difference in follow-up period [11]. The Riss et al. study followed-up patients over 4 months; whereas the present study looked at the patients over 12 months [11]. Punte et al. and Vermiere [6,12] have both shown that subjects tend to need some experience (12-24 months) before fine structure becomes useful to them [6-9]. The subjects included herein had at least 12 months, of more than 10 h per day FSP use, before upgrade to the FS4/FS4p coding strategy. However, upon upgrade the subjects may have needed even more time to appreciate the differences or were already well adjusted to fine structure conditions in quiet.

Comparing FSP to older CIS+ coding strategies has shown that the provision of fine structure via an audio processor improves speech perception in noise [13-16]. As the subjects in the present study are already so used to their CI with fine structure coding from the FSP strategy, it could be that the differences were not obvious. Similarly, some published literature indicates that with other approaches to better code the temporal structure, by enhancing the channel envelope modulations, changes in speech perception scores are relatively small (as mainly areas of low frequencies are stimulated) [13-16]. Thus, on the speech tests subjects did not perform significantly better than with the FSP coding strategy. Nonetheless, the hearing performance of the subjects was no worse with the new FS4/FS4p coding strategy than with FSP.

However, the outcomes of the $HISQUI_{19}$ showed that at 2 out of 4 intervals (Interval 1 and 5) subjects perceived the level of auditory benefit as 'moderate'. It is difficult to compare different subjective measures between studies. The $HISQUI_{19}$ is a newly validated and reliable questionnaire designed to be used across all studies to determine the subjectively perceived sound quality of hearing implant users [10]. Introduced in 2014, there are to date few studies available with the $HISQUI_{19}$. However, the aforementioned studies, by Punte et al. and Vermeire et al., performed over a longer follow-up period, used the Speech; Spatial and Qualities of Hearing Scale (SSQ) to determine subjective perception [6,12]. $HISQUI_{19}$ outcomes correlate strongly with the SSQ [17]. Comparing, FSP to traditional CIS+ coding strategies showed that subjects benefitted significantly from the provision of fine structure on the SSQ questionnaire in both studies. In the Riss et al. study, one of the few studies to compare FSP and FS4/FS4p very little difference in the subjective perception of sound quality between coding strategies was described [12]. With two subjects detecting 'very little difference' in sound quality between the FSP and FS4 coding strategies, and another two subjects stating that they experienced 'less recognized differences'. Similarly, in the present study, at Interval 2 and 3, the perception of auditory benefit was perceived as 'poor'. Although, we suspect that because subjects were already used to the fine structure coding from the FSP strategy the perceived differences were less obvious but subjects generally appreciated the new coding strategy.

To establish a complete picture of the rehabilitation of CI users, quantification of sound quality is of increasing importance [17,18]. Therefore, given the preference of some individuals to particular coding strategies and that satisfaction cannot be predicted from speech testing; the subjective preference of a certain speech coding strategy should be recognized as an outcome of growing importance. Identification of an individual's subjective preference for a given coding strategy gives audiologists and clinicians greater opportunities to meet the individual needs of the implant recipient.

Conclusion

The FS4/FS4p coding strategy works well in experienced CI recipients and represents a further tool to individualize the fitting of audio processors. This grants access to more satisfying sound quality and speech perception. The subjective perception of individual's experiences indicates that in a real life situation many subjects benefit from the use of the FS4/FS4p coding strategy.

References

1. Hilbert D (1912) Grundzüge Einer AllgemeinenTheorie Der Linearen Integralgleichungen, Leipzig und Berlin.
2. Smith ZM, Delgutte B, Oxenham AJ (2002) Chimaeric sounds reveal dichotomies in auditory perception. Nature 416: 87-90.
3. Zeng FG, Nie K, Stickney G, Kong YY (2004) Auditory perception with slowly-varying amplitude and frequency modulations. New York.
4. Wilson BS, Lawson DT, Finley CC, Wolford RD (1991) Coding strategies for multichannel cochlear prostheses. Am J Otol 12 Suppl: 56-61.
5. Zierhofer CM (2001) Analysis of a linear model for electrical stimulation of axons--critical remarks on the "activating function concept". IEEE Trans Biomed Eng 48: 173-184.
6. Kleine Punte A, De Bodt M, Van De Heyning P (2014) Long-term improvement of speech perception with the fine structure processing coding strategy in cochlear implants. ORL J Otorhinolaryngol Relat Spec 76: 36-43.
7. Chen X, Liu B, Liu S, Mo L, Li Y, et al. (2013) Cochlear implants with fine structure processing improve speech and tone perception in Mandarin-speaking adults. Acta Otolaryngol 133: 733-738.
8. Galindo J, Lassaletta L, Mora RP, Castro A, Bastarrica M, et al. (2013) Fine structure processing improves telephone speech perception in cochlear implant users. Eur Arch Otorhinolaryngol 270: 1223-1229.
9. Müller J, Brill S, Hagen R, Moeltner A, Brockmeier SJ, et al. (2012) Clinical trial results with the MED-EL fine structure processing coding strategy in experienced cochlear implant users. ORL J Otorhinolaryngol Relat Spec 74: 185-198.
10. Amann E, Anderson I (2014) Development and validation of a questionnaire for hearing implant users to self-assess their auditory abilities in everyday communication situations: the hearing implant sound quality index (HISQUI19). Acta Otolaryngol 134: 915-923.
11. Riss D, Hamzavi JS, Blineder M, Honeder C, Ehrenreich I, et al. (2014) FS4, FS4-p, and FSP: A 4-month crossover study of 3 fine structure sound-coding strategies. Ear Hear 35: e272-281.
12. Vermeire K, Punte AK, Van de Heyning P (2010) Better speech recognition in noise with the fine structure processing coding strategy. ORL J Otorhinolaryngol Relat Spec 72: 305-311.
13. Geurts L, Wouters J (2001) Coding of the fundamental frequency in continuous interleaved sampling processors for cochlear implants. J Acoust Soc Am 109: 713-726.
14. Green T, Faulkner A, Rosen S (2004) Enhancing temporal cues to voice pitches in continuous interleaved sampling cochlear implants. J Acoust Soc Am 116: 2298-2310.
15. Green T, Faulkner A, Rosen S, Macherey O (2005) Enhancement of temporal periodicity cues in cochlear implants: effects on prosodic perception and vowel identification. J Acoust Soc Am 118: 375-385.
16. Vandali AE, Sucher C, Tsang DJ, Mckay CM, Chew JW, et al. (2005) Pitch ranking ability of cochlear implant recipients: A comparison of sound-processing strategies. J Acoust Soc Am 117: 3126-3138.
17. Mertens G, Kleine Punte A, De Bodt M (2015) Sound quality in adult cochlear implant recipients using the HISQUI19. Acta Otolaryngol 135: 1138-1145.
18. Humes LE (1999) Dimensions of hearing aid outcome. J Am Acad Audiol 10: 26-39.

Sphenoid Aspergilloma: Diagnosed as a Malignancy

Gray MR[1], Thrasher JD[2*], Dennis Hooper[3], Dumanov MJ[4], Cravens R[5] and Jones T[6]

[1]*Progressive Healthcare Group, Benson, Arizona, USA*
[2]*Retired, Consultant to Progressive Healthcare Group, Benson Arizona, USA*
[3]*RealTime: Laboratories, Carrollton, Texas, USA*
[4]*Mycological Institute Subclinical Research Group, USA*
[5]*Tucson Ear, Nose and Throat, Tucson, USA*
[6]*Husband of the Affected Woman, USA*

Abstract

Purpose: This case study was undertaken to demonstrate the important aspects of the differentiation between a fungal infections of the sphenoid sinus vs a diagnosis of cancer. It is important to consider fungal disease in the differential diagnosis when treating masses in the sinuses. A 55 year old female employee was exposed to a water-damaged office that had fungal and bacterial growth. She developed a sphenoid mass that was first diagnosed as cancer. After surgery, radiation, chemotherapy and a second biopsy she discharged fungal hyphae from the opened sphenoid sinus.

Methods: In 2005 her workplace was noted to have water intrusion and was inspected and tested for the presence of fungi and Gram negative bacteria. Wipe samples of dust were collected for culturing and identification of mold and bacteria. Biopsy specimens were tested by PCR DNA analysis for species of mold. The biopsy specimens were reviewed by a Medical Mycologist. The histology slides were stained with Giemsa. Sphenoid discharged materials were stained with fungalase.

Results: The sphenoid mass was shown to be an aspergilloma, *Aspergillus terreus*. Mycotoxins detected in urine were macrocyclic trichothecenes, aflatoxins and ochratoxin. The sphenoid aspergilloma completely resolved following oral and intranasal administration of antifungals. Multiple organ symptoms resulting from her exposure and chronic inflammation abated following detoxification and supportive antioxidant therapy. Clinical observations and diagnostic testing ruled out other causes, revealing chronic inflammation and an infection resulting from exposure to fungi and bacteria in the work environment.

Conclusions: Sphenoid aspergilloma can be medically treated with a combination of voriconazole and cyclosporine when they are administered intranasally. The required duration antifungal therapy can be determined by DNA PCR in combination with MRI and appropriate follow up. The findings are discussed and the rational for accepting the aspergilloma rather than a sphenoid malignancy is presented. It is imperative that fungal origins be considered in cases of suspected sinus neoplasms.

Introduction

Fungal Rhinosinusitis (FRS) is a relatively common, often misdiagnosed disease process of the paranasal sinuses [1-3]. The incidence of the disease is 37 million cases that encompass a wide spectrum of immune and pathological responses, including invasive, chronic granulomatous and allergic conditions. A recent attempt was made to classify the various types of fungal sinusitis [4]. The current schema still includes 1) invasive diseases (acute invasive, granulomatous invasive and chronic) FRS and 2) noninvasive disease (saprophytic fungal infections, fungal ball and fungus related eosinophilic FRS that includes AFRS (allergic fungal rhinosinusitis). Thus, FRS results from multiple of fungal genera, including *Aspergillus* species [1-8]. *Aspergillus* species are involved in invasive FRS in immunocompetent individuals [9-12]. In all cases the condition is refractory to antibiotic regimens and is improved with intranasal antifungals [2,13,14]. The use of corticosteroids should be limited because of the potential for suppression of the neutrophil migration and killing action on fungal spores and hyphae by both neutrophils and macrophages [15-17]. In addition, *Aspergillus* sinusitis can mimic malignant disease and even appear as pituitary tumor [18-20]. Presented herein is a case of a 55 year old woman who developed a sphenoid sinus infection by *Aspergillus terreus*. The infection was initially diagnosed and treated as a neuroblastoma and a pituitary adenoma. She had endoscopic surgery followed with radiation and chemotherapy based upon misdiagnosis. Of interest, *A. terreus* produces mycotoxins citreoviridin, citrinin, and territrems [21]. The bio-complexity of water-damaged indoor environments has been reviewed by two independent sources [22,23].

Methods and Results

The building

The patient worked as a book keeper in an old building that had water intrusion, musty odors, dead animals in the attic and visible mold growth. The building was inspected, tested for mold and partially remediated. Technicians removed bat and bird dropping, nesting material and insulation from the attic area in August, 2005. However visible mold and musty odors were still present. The testing and identification of mold in the office was conducted by Richard L.

***Corresponding author:** Jack Dwayne Thrasher, Retired, Consultant to Progressive Healthcare Group, Benson Arizona, USA; E-mail: toxicologist1@msn.com

Lipsey. Ph.D. and Associates, Jacksonville, FL. Swab samples of dust and visible growth were obtained in July 2009. They were sent under chain of custody to EMLab P and K, Cherry Hill, NJ for culturing and identification of molds (MEA medium) and bacteria (TSA medium), wall cavity contamination and ERMI-36. The results are summarized in Table 1. The results showed typical mold and bacteria present that have been identified in water damaged buildings [24-29]. The potential pathogens found in the Gram negative rods are the following genera: *Acinetobacter, Klebsiella, Aeromonas, Campylobacter, Pseudomonas,* and *Legionella*. However, bacterial cultures for infections were not performed in this case.

Nonviable spores present in the two wall check samples of *Aspergillus/Penicillium Stachybotrys* and *Cladosporium*. MEA cultures from various areas revealed several species of mold, except *Aspergillus terreus*. Similarly, the Q-PCR (ERMI Tests) did not reveal *A. terreus*. However, the data did demonstrate the presence of *Aspergillus fumigatus, penicillioides, niger, unguis* and *ustus* along with *Eurotium amstelodami*, three species of *Penicillium* and *Wallemia*. Almost all are known producers of mycotoxins of which several have been identified in water-damaged buildings [23-29]. In addition, it is also recognized that analysis or air and bulk samples may not identify all molds and bacterial toxins present in an indoor environment [27-29]. Thus, absence of *A. terreus* in the limited sampling conducted in the office of this case is not surprising.

The patient

The past medical history of this 55 year old female included: childhood illnesses (measles, mumps, ear infections and Chicken pox). Adult conditions: surgical excision of let lower leg of melanoma with no recurrence, smokes 10 cigarettes per day, hypertension, and hyperlipidemia. No history of asthma or atopic dermatitis. She had a 15 year history of mild rhino-conjunctivitis using OTC self-medication to control symptoms. She had an episode of pneumonia in 1986, successfully treated. At this time tests for TB and Valley Fever were negative. Shortly after beginning employment she began experiencing persistent health conditions that included but were not limited to the following: Headaches, nasal congestion, chronic sinusitis, tearing of eyes, fullness of ears, sneezing, chronic fatigue, decreased sense of smell, and decreased vision of the left eye. Her treating physician sent her to an allergist to determine the nature of her condition (see below).

Following the allergy workup, she continued to have severe health problems that included but not limited to the following: series of upper respiratory infections, continued decline of vision in the left eye, headaches, and congestion from sinusitis. The loss of vision precipitated a cardiovascular work up for stroke, which was negative.

Allergy testing and medications

Prick/Puncture and intradermal testing for inhalant allergens revealed positive reactions to tree pollens; dust mites and mold groups (*A. fumigatus, Fusarium, Penicillium*, minor reactions to weed pollens, cat, dog, feather and cockroach allergens and negative to grass, and ragweed. Her medications were Nasonex (2 puffs per nostril per day), Prednisone (40 mg/day for a 4 week tapering), Prevacid, Crestor, Premarin, Atenolol, Triamterene/HCTZ, Ecotrin, folic acid, CoQ_{10}, omega-3 fish oil and flaxseed oil. Her condition continued to deteriorate with eventual loss of vision. She was then subjected to a series of MRIs, PET and CT scans to determine the nature of her condition (CT and PET scans and MRIs below).

Initial MRI, CT, PET scans, endoscope, diagnoses and treatment

The initial PET scan performed in January, 2006 was negative for involvement of other areas of the body (data not shown). The MRI scans revealed the following: A skull base tumor that occupied the bilateral sphenoid sinuses extending into the clivus and sella, encroaching into the posterior maxillary sinuses. In addition, involvement of the left lenticular nucleus, left basal ganglia and cerebellum was noted. The tumor had an axial measurement 3.3×4.2 cm and 8.7 cm in the cranial-caudal length. Erosion of the bone included temporal, posterior maxillary sinuses with abutment of the carotid canals bilaterally.

Endoscopic examination revealed a peduncle with a bulbous mass extending from the sphenoid Ostia into the Nasopharynx. The peduncle and mass were surgically removed and sent for pathological examination. The initial diagnosis was esthesionneuroblastoma. However, additional pathology reports did not agree, naming it a neuroblastoma and/or non-secretory adeno-pituitary tumor (see initial pathology below). She was given two courses of Cisplatin Etoposide chemotherapy in October and November, 2005 with minimal tumor response (reduction in size of 20-25%). In January of 2006 she underwent a sphenoid surgery to remove the mass; this also failed to alleviate the condition. Following the surgery and opening of the sphenoid sinuses, she began and continued to discharge material from her nasal cavity. In February and March of 2006 she was given 36 radiation treatments for the suspected malignancy, again with minimal tumor response. At this time fungal sinusitis, which had been rejected by the pathologists, was suspected. The lack of response to radiation and chemotherapy it was decided to seek assistance for possible samples fungal involvement. Nasal discharge material, tissue samples and pathology slides were sent to Dumanov, Mycological Institute for further evaluation (see mycology below). This material was identified by fungalase staining to contain hyphal fragments

Sample Location	Culture Medium	Fungi CFU/ Swab	Culture Medium	Bacteria CFU/ Swab
Vent – Top	MEA	840,000	TSA	3,000,000
Vent - Bottom	MEA	1,100,000	TSA	60,000
AHU – Bottom Front	MEA	310,000	TSA	110,000
AHU- Bottom Center	MEA	490,000	TSA	3,100,000
AHU- Bottom Back	MEA	130,000	TSA	100,000
AHU – Floor on Left	MEA	2,500,000	TSA	3,00,000
Blackened Paper – Floor	MEA	1,200,000	TSA	31,000,000

AHU = Air Handling Unit
Most Common Fungi: *Aspergillus niger, Aureobasidium pullulans, Mucor plumbeus, Rhizopus stolonifer, Rhodotorula mucilagenous, Cladosporium, Penicillium spp, Trichoderma hazarianumm, Cunningham elegans*, yeast.
Most Common Bacteria: *Bacillus* spp, Gram negative rods, Gram positive cocci.
Non-Viable Spores: Non-viable spore samples were taken from a wall cavity with a telephone jack: *Penicillium/Aspergillus; Cladosporium and Stachybotrys chartarum*.
Q-PCR: ERMI tests: ERMI tests were performed on two samples. Identified fungi were: following: *Acremonium strictum, Aspergillus fumigatus, penicillioides, niger, unguis, and ustus, Aureobasidium pullulans, Cladosporium herbarium, Eurotium amstelodami, Mucor/Rhizopus, Paecilomyces variotii, Penicillium chrysogenum, purpurogenum, spinulosum and variable, Rhizopus stolonifer and Wallemia sebi*
Wall Cavities: Wall check samples at two outlets (electrical and phone jack) collected by Air-0-Cell cassettes (14 L/min for 5 minutes) detected *Aspergillus/ Penicillium* at 95 and 87.5 % of the total spore counts of 390 and 1,600, respectively. Stachybotrys spores were detected in the phone jack outlet at 0.008 % if the total spore counts.

Table 1: This table summarizes the Fungi and bacteria identified in the building from cultures of swab samples obtained from patient's office. All areas were contaminated with fungi and bacteria.

Initial pathology

The results of the pathology of the original peduncle and bulbous mass are summarized in Table 2. The original diagnosis was esthesio-neuroblastoma based upon positive immuno-histochemical staining for synaptophysin, cytokeratin 903, chromogranin and inconclusive GMC staining. The potential cross-reactivity with of synaptophysin with Leukophysin, chromogranins and other hematopoietic markers were not considered in the final diagnosis [20,30-34]. In addition, fungi are known to disrupt, utilize and disrupt the actin-cytoskeleton matrix during infection [33-36]. Additional biopsies and histological staining were not done to determine if fungal elements were present. The pathology description on the same biopsy specimen also varied from one laboratory to another, resulting in diagnoses of Esthesionneuroblastoma neuroblastoma, olfactory neuroblastoma and pituitary adenoma.

MRI

The results of MRI scans are summarized in Table 3 and Figure 1. The MRIs and other scans (data not shown) revealed chronic inflammatory changes in the sphenoid, ethmoid and maxillary sinuses, nasal and paranasal sinus inflammation and chronic inflammatory changes in the left mastoid air cells. In addition, the optic chiasm was displaced by the mass in the sella, along with thinning of adjacent bony cortex. In addition, areas of enhancement were observed bilaterally in

Column1	Column2	Column3	Column4	Column5	Column6	Column7	Column8	Column9
Place		FMH	UMMC	UMMC3	Hopkins	AFIP	Pitts	RTL
Date			10/10/2005	1/3/2006	Aug 30,2006	28-Jul-06	11/11/2008	5/1/2009
SX Number		05-sp-9599	01-SC-05-00439	01-S-06-00041 Nasal Neoplasm			PHS08-37373	
DX		Favor OFN#	NE Neoplasm*	Esrhesioneuroblastoma	Pitutary Adenoma	Pit. Adenoma A	NE Neoplasm	
			PV Pseudo ros	perivascular pseudorosettes				
	IPX							
	synaptophysin	POS	POS	POS	POS		POS	WK+
	NSE			POS			POS	POS
	CD56			POS				
	Cam 5.2			POS				
	CD99			NEG				
	Cytokeratin 903	POS		NEG				
	S-100	NEG		NEG	NEG		NEG	NEG
	HMB-45			NEG				
	prolactin			NEG				
	GH	SCATTERED +		NEG	WK+	POS	NEG	NEG
	LH			NEG		NEG		
	FSH			NEG		NEG		
	TSH			MINIMAL		NEG		
	ACTH			NEG	POS	NEG		
	Chromagranin	POS	POS		NEG		NEG	NEG
	Keratin		POS					
	Melan A	NEG						NEG
	Silver Stain	NEG						
	AE1: AE3				NEG		NEG	NEG
	EMA				NEG			
	GMS					NEG		
		#Olfactory	*can't exclude			^inconsistent	Difficult see	Agree with
		Neuroblast	a non-secreting			with Olf Neuro	dx form	Pitts.
		cannot r/O	pituitary adenoma					
		pit adenoma						

Table 2: Summary of the Initial Pathology: This table summarizes the 7 different pathology reports done on the original biopsy taken from the nasopharyngeal area described as a peduncle with a bulbous growth arriving from the sphenoid Ostia. Note that the diagnoses were esthesioneuroblastoma, NE neoplasm, and pituitary adenoma.

Jones MRI Summaries

MRI Date	Summary of MRI Findings
09/20/05 (A)	Near complete opacification of the sphenoid sinuses with associated thinning of adjacent bony cortex. Destructive changes from either sinusitis or soft tissue mass.
06 2006 (B)	This MRI and the one in Figure C show minimal response of the sphenoid mass to radiation and chemotherapy.
10/26/06 (C)	large mass replacing the clivus and filling the sella extending into the cavernous sinuses. The mass abuts the undersurface of the optic chiasm. Diffuse inflammatory and post-surgical changes involving the nasal cavity and paranasal sinuses. Diffuse small high signal intensity lesions scattered throughout the cerebral white matter bilaterally, unchanged from prior studies.
June/July, 2007 (D)	Post esthesionneuroblastoma. Persistent mass lesion within the clivus. Appears much more cystic. Near optic chiasm with mild mass effect against the chiasm. Left sphenoid more involved than right. Mild maxillary sinus disease.
02/08/07	There continues to be a large mass replacing the clivus, filling the sella, extending into both cavernous sinuses. Mucosal thickening throughout the sphenoid sinuses bilaterally. Also mild chronic appearing inflammatory changes in the left mastoid. Other paranasal sinuses and right mastoid sinus cells are clear. Very mild diffuse white matter disease, which appears stable when compared to the previous study. Multiple new areas of chronic lacuna infarction within the right corona radiate, head of right caudate nucleus, anterior limb of the right internal capsule and right lentiform nucleus (MRI not shown)
07/26/07 (D)	The mass in the clivus and sella decreased to 2×3.4×2.9 from 3.7×2.8×4.1 cm. Mild mucosal thickening in the sphenoid and ethmoid sinuses that has not resolved. Appearance of small cystic area in the right head of caudate nucleus
02/15/08	Small region of encephalomalacia changes involving the right caudate nucleus. Moderate mucosal thickening of left maxillary sinus as well as ethmoid air cells. Minimal mucosal thickening of sphenoid sinuses. Increased severity of the left maxillary sinus. 8 mm enhancing nodule in the putamen (MRI not shown).
06/30/08	Pituitary follow-up. Abnormal signal involving the clivus with diffuse enhancement. Pituitary bland measures 1.8×0.9×2.1 cm with heterogeneous enhancement. Abnormal enhancement in the left putamen, 6.4×5.2 mm, stable since previous exam. There are no abnormal signals seen within the brain. – DR. Gray.
09/10/08 (G)	Dr Gray: Follow up of fungus infection in sinuses. There is mucosal thickening in left maxillary sinus with mucous retention cyst, new since previous exam. Mucosal thickening in sphenoid sinus, stable since last exam. Increased signal in the clivus, stable since last exam. Right caudate nucleus without enhancement. Enhancement in left posterior aspect of the putamen (6.9×5.2 mm). No other abnormal signals in the brain.
03/30/09	Dr. Gray: Mild encephalomalacia, has been stable. Abnormal signal in clivus and mild enhancement of the in the region of cavernous sinus bilaterally. There are no new sites of disease seen. (MRI not shown).

Table 3: This table summarizes the findings of the MRIs done on the plaintiff's sinuses from September 09, 2005 to March 30, 2009.

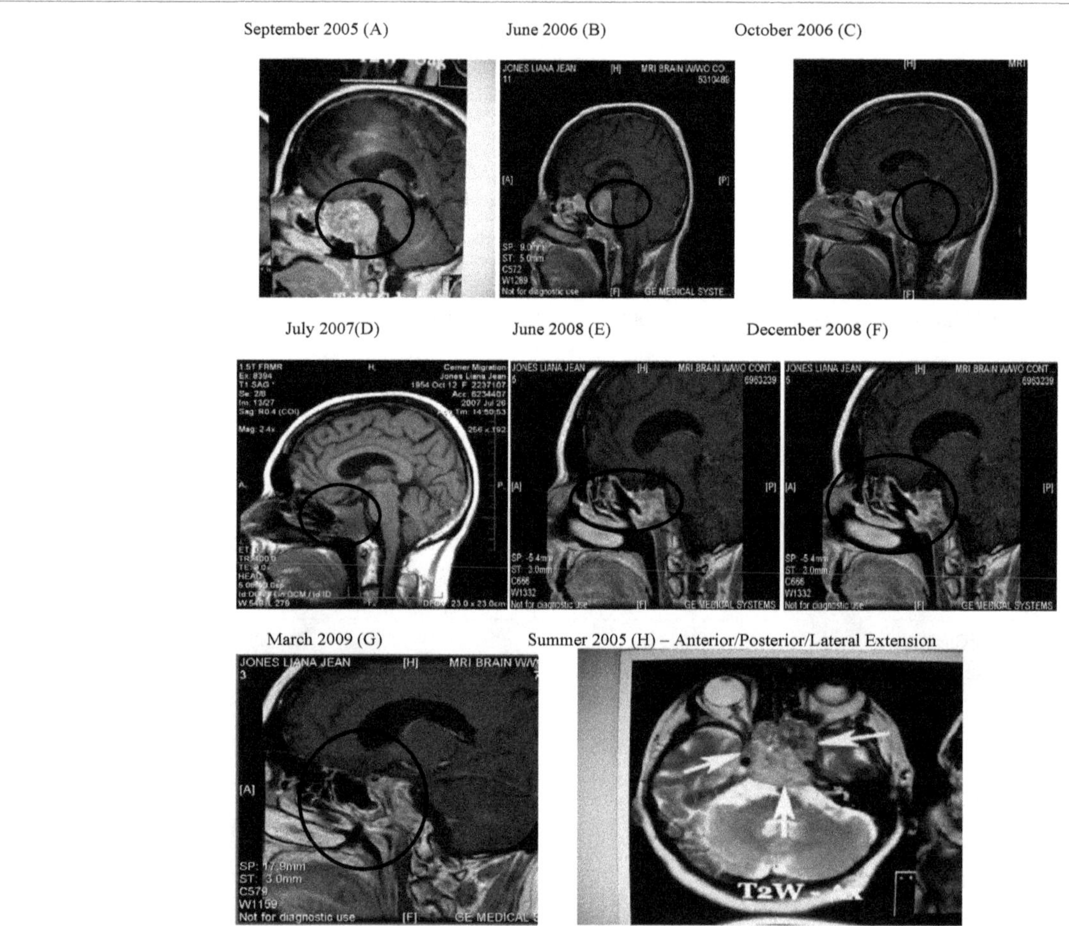

Figure 1: This figure shows the series of MRI images from September 2005 through March 2009 demonstrating the sphenoid Aspergilloma and its successful treatment with antifungals. The bottom right figure shows the Posterior/Anterior lateral dimensions of the Aspergilloma.

the cerebral white matter, the left putamen encephalomalacia changes involving the right caudate nucleus. These observations were apparent even after surgical removal the sphenoid mass (see MRIs, 02/08/07 and 07/26/07). Figure 1 summarizes the results of the MRIs from initial diagnosis if 09/20/05 through 03/30/09. Following radiation treatment (32 in 2006) chemo-therapy (cisplatin/etoposide and surgery the mass was still present in the sphenoid sinuses (Figure 1A-1E). The mass cleared following intranasal antifungal treatments (Figure 1F-1H and Table 4).

Mycology and mycotoxins

Pathology materials were sent to RealTime Laboratories, Carrollton, Texas for differential staining for fungi and RT-PCR-DNA testing for *Aspergillus* species. In addition, urine specimens were evaluated for the presence of macrocyclic trichothecenes, aflatoxins and ochratoxin as previously reported [37,38]. The differentially stained microscope slides were sent to Joseph Dumanov, Mycological Institute of the Study of Fungal Mold in Human Habitation, Sparta, for pathology evaluation [39].

The results of these evaluations were as follows: (1) Fungalase staining revealed septate hyphae and conidia in nasal discharge following sphenoid surgery [39] (Figure 2).

(2) the pathology (Giemsa Stain) evaluation revealed discernable septate hyphae, phialides and conidia characteristic of the genus, *Aspergillus* (Figure 2).

(3) PCR DNA testing identified *Aspergillus terreus* in the pathology specimens [39]

(4) The urine was positive for macrocyclic trichothecenes and aflatoxins as listed in Table 5.

Antifungals

The regime of antifungal treatments is summarized in Table 4. Upon Identification of the sphenoid aspergilloma, a regimen of antifungals was initiated. The initial treatment was orally and followed by intranasal sprays. The antifungal regimen eliminated the sphenoid mass. The MRI (March 2009) showed residual sphenoid sinus disease with abnormal signal in the clivus and mild enhancement in the region of the cavernous sinus bilaterally described above. It could be related to mycotic fungus infection versus mucocele. The findings in this area have been stable since previous exam. There were no new sites of disease seen (Figure 1E-G).

Date	Antifungal	Route – Dose
6/3/2007	Fluconazole	Oral -150 mg/day
14-Jun-07	Fluconazole Itraconazole	Oral – 150 mg/day Oral – 250 mg/day
10-Jul-07	Itraconazole Fluconazole	Oral - 200 mg/day x 4 days Oral – 150 mg/day
13-Aug-07	Fluconazole Fluconazole	Oral – 600 mg/day Oral – 150 mg/day
21-Aug-07	Ketoconazole Cyclosporine	Intranasal - 4 times/day/per nostril (2%)
9-Sep-07	Amphotericin + Ketoconazole Nasal Spray	Intranasal – 5 mg/ml Ketoconazole (2%). 2X /day, once per nostril
11-Apr-08	Voriconazole and Cyclosporine Itraconazole	Intranasal – Dosage Not Available

Table 4: This table summarizes the administration of antifungals beginning in June 2007 through April 2008.

Discussion

The role of mold in chronic rhinosinusitis was introduced by Ponikau et al., [1]. Since then numerous reports have appeared demonstrating that mold are associated with Fungal Rhinosinusitis (FRS) [1-5,8-14,40]. An attempt to classify the disease led to the following classification of FRS: 1) Invasive disease (acute, granulomatous and chronic); 2) Noninvasive: (saprophytic fungal infestations, fungal ball, and fungus eosinophilic FRS that includes AFRS – Allergic AFR [4]. FRS results from multiple fungal genera, including *Aspergillus* species [1-8] *Aspergillus* species are often involved in invasive FRS [10-12]. The invasive FRS requires surgical intervention and favorably responds to oral as well as intranasal antifungals [1-4,11,14,40]. Invasive FRS is associated with erosion of surrounding bone, intracerebral extension and vascular invasion [4,9,11,14]. The use of corticosteroids should be limited because of the potential suppression of neutrophil migration and oxidative burst of neutrophils and macrophages [15-17]. Finally, Aspergillus sinusitis can mimic malignant disease and even appear as a pituitary adenoma [18-20]. With respect to *A. terreus* it has been identified as the causative fungus in bronchitis, Onchymycosis, pulmonary Aspergillosis, and sphenoid sinusitis with orbitocranial extension [41-45].

The patient presented herein had a 15 year history of mild-rhino-conjunctivitis that was symptomatically treated with OTC medications. Commensurate and shortly after employment in a water-damaged building she developed multiple symptoms that included: headaches, nasal congestion, chronic sinusitis, fullness of ears, sneezing, fatigue, tearing of eyes, decreased sense of smell, and loss of vision in the left eye. Allergy workup demonstrated positive reactions to tree pollens, dust mites, and mold (*A. fumigatus, Fusarium, and Penicillium*). The symptoms and sinus involvement are consistent with microbial growth in water-damaged buildings and FRS [4,46,47]. However, because of the loss of vision she underwent diagnostic MRIs, CT scan and PET studies that can detect invasive fungal infections and determine the cause of lost vision [48-51]. The results these of diagnostics demonstrated maxillary, ethmoid and mastoid sinuses involvement was well as a large mass in the sphenoid that appeared to be pressing on the optic nerves. The sphenoid mass appeared to cause loss of bony structures in the area (Figure 1). Unfortunately, the initial diagnostics were interpreted as a malignancy treated with chemotherapy, radiation and surgical intervention. None of the cancer treatments were successful in alleviating the mass. Because of the persistence of the mass, nasal discharge and sphenoid tissue samples were examined for evidence of fungal growth. *Aspergillus* was detected in the biopsy and RT-QPCR identified *Aspergillus terreus* (Figure 1). In addition, hyphae fragments and conidia were identified in nasal discharges by fungalase staining (Figure 1). As a result oral and intranasal antifungals were initiated in June, 2007. MRIs images from studies in June 2009 through March 2009 showed resolution of the sphenoid mass (Figure 2E-2G). The enhancements seen the MRIs in the caudate nucleus, putamen, white matter, lentiform nucleus and other areas of brain may be indicative of intracerebral extension. The detection of mycotoxins in the urine samples (Table 1) are consistent with previous findings that exposure to molds in water-damaged homes and buildings results in the presence of these toxins in autopsy and biopsy specimens from various organs, sinuses, canine sebaceous tumors and urine [37,40,50,51].

In this case the issue of whether or not the presence of Aspergillus terreus in the sphenoid sinus resulted from the initial diagnosis of a malignancy, rather than being a primary infection that was misdiagnosed. We have several reasons to state that the fungal infection of the sinus was primary [52-54]. These are as follows:

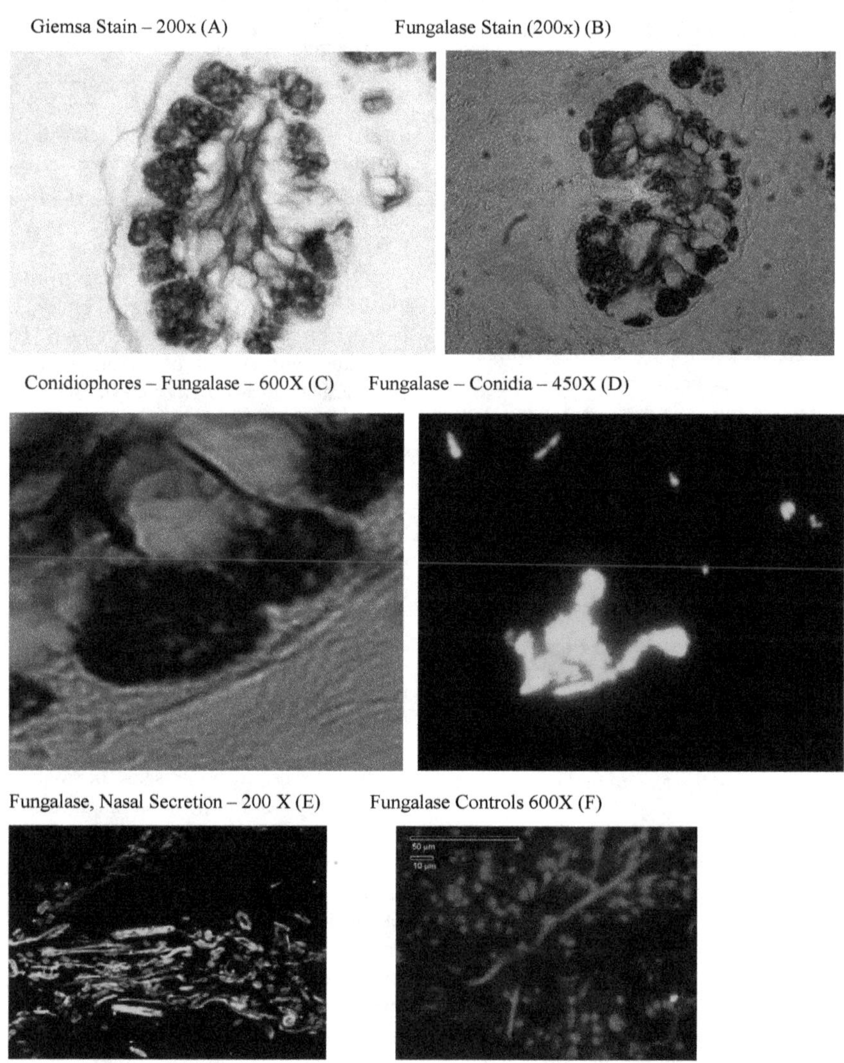

Figure 2: Giemsa stains of *Aspergillus terreus* identified in the biopsy from the sphenoid sinus (Figures A-C). Fungalase staining of nasal drainage following sphenoidotomy (Figures D and E) and Fungalase control(F).

Date	Aflatoxins (ppb)[1]	Trichothecenes (ppb)[2]
3/27/2007	21	1.51
4/11/2007	5	0.53
6/3/2007	4	1.38
7/10/2007	12	3.44
7/14/2007	9	0.73
8/21/2007	5	21.3
12/12/2007	20	1.9

[1,2]Limit Detection for Aflatoxins - <1.8 ppb (negative); 1.8-2.0 ppb (equiv0cal); ≥ 2.0 ppb (positive)

Table 5: Urine Mycotoxins. This table summarizes the concentrations of Aflatoxins and Macrocyclic Trichothecenes detected in urine specimens. Mycotoxins continue to be released from intracellular storage and appear in the urine during detoxification.

(1) At least three different cancers were diagnosed by different pathologist (NE neoplasm, Esthesionneuroblastoma, and Pituitary adenoma (Table 2)

(2)The immunochemistry used markers that are known to cross react with other cellular constituents of normal cells [30-34,48-51] leading to a possible misdiagnosis

(3) The sphenoid tumor did not favorably respond to either radiation or chemotherapy

(4) The opening of the sphenoid sinus lead to the nasal discharge of fungalase positive mycelial fragments (Figure 2).

(5) Treatment with antifungals successfully removed the sphenoid mass without a recurrence of the mass (Figure 1G and 1H)

(6) Fungal infections are difficult to identify histological material; without appropriate staining appropriate staining procedures [54]. In this case Giemsa and fungalase staining identified the fungal hyphae as well as *Aspergillus* (Figure 2) and finally

(7) *Aspergillus* species are involved in fungal sinusitis, rhinosinusitis, and pituitary masses [1-4,13-14,17,18].

Conclusion

The patient in this case study was initially misdiagnosed as a malignancy associated with the sphenoid mass. The initial sphenoid sinus biopsy the lesion was diagnosed as an Esthesionneuroblastoma. Subsequent diagnoses included NE neoplasm and pituitary adenoma. The lesion did not respond to surgical biopsies, radiation treatment and chemotherapy. Subsequent follow up for potential fungal involvement demonstrated the presence of *Aspergillus terreus* DNA in the sphenoid sinus along with fungalase positive hyphal fragments and conidia in nasal discharged fluids. Mycetoma should be included in the differential diagnosis of masses in the sinuses. Finally it is currently recognized that molds and bacteria present in water-damaged indoor environments leads to multiple health problems of the occupants [52-54].

References

1. Ponikau JU, Sherris DA, Kern EB, Homburger HA, Frigas E, et al. (1999) The diagnosis and incidence of allergic fungal sinusitis. Mayo Clin Proc 74: 877-884.
2. Ponikau JU, Sherris DA, Kita H, Kern EB (2002) Intranasal antifungal treatment in 51 patients with chronic rhinosinusitis. J Allergy Clin Immunol 110: 862-866.
3. Ponikau JU, Sherris DA, Kephart GM, Kern EB, Congdon DJ, et al. (2005) Striking deposition of toxic eosinophil major basic protein in mucus: implications for chronic rhinosinusitis. J Allergy Clin Immunol 116: 362-369.
4. Chakrabarti A, Denning DW, Ferguson BJ, Ponikau J, Buzina W, et al. (2009) Fungal rhinosinusitis: a categorization and definitional schema addressing current controversies. Laryngoscope 119: 1809-1818.
5. Braun H, Buzina W, Freudenschuss K, Beham A, Stammberger H (2003) 'Eosinophilic fungal rhinosinusitis': a common disorder in Europe? Laryngoscope 113: 264-269.
6. Katzenstein AL, Sale SR, Greenberger PA (1983) Allergic Aspergillus sinusitis: a newly recognized form of sinusitis. J Allergy Clin Immunol 72: 89-93.
7. Schubert MS (2009) Allergic fungal sinusitis: pathophysiology, diagnosis and management. Med Mycol 47 Suppl 1: S324-330.
8. Shin SH, Ponikau JU, Sherris DA, Congdon D, Frigas E, et al. (2004) Chronic rhinosinusitis: an enhanced immune response to ubiquitous airborne fungi. J Allergy Clin Immunol 114: 1369-1375.
9. Reddy CE, Gupta AK, Singh P, Mann SB (2010) Imaging of granulomatous and chronic invasive fungal sinusitis: comparison with allergic fungal sinusitis. Otolaryngol Head Neck Surg 143: 294-300.
10. Milroy CM, Blanshard JD, Lucas S, Michaels L (1989) Aspergillosis of the nose and paranasal sinuses. J Clin Pathol 42: 123-127.
11. Siddiqui AA, Shah AA, Bashir SH (2004) Craniocerebral aspergillosis of sinonasal origin in immunocompetent patients: clinical spectrum and outcome in 25 cases. Neurosurgery 55: 602-611.
12. Sivak-Callcott JA, Livesley N, Nugent RA, Rasmussen SL, Saeed P, et al. (2004) Localised invasive sino-orbital aspergillosis: characteristic features. Br J Ophthalmol 88: 681-687.
13. Dennis DP (2003) Chronic sinusitis: defective T-cells responding to superantigens, treated by reduction of fungi in the nose and air. Arch Environ Health 58: 433-441.
14. Dennis DP, Robertson D, Curtis L, Black J (2009) Fungal exposure endocrinopathy in sinusitis with growth hormone deficiency: Dennis-Robertson syndrome. Toxicol Indust Health 25: 669-680.
15. Gan WQ, Man SF, Sin DD (2005) Effects of inhaled corticosteroids on sputum cell counts in stable chronic obstructive pulmonary disease: a systematic review and a meta-analysis. BMC Pulm Med 5: 3.
16. Palmer LB, Greenberg HE, Schiff MJ (1991) Corticosteroid treatment as a risk factor for invasive aspergillosis in patients with lung disease. Thorax 46: 15-20.
17. Philippe B, Ibrahim-Granet O, Prévost MC, Gougerot-Pocidalo MA, Sanchez Perez M, et al. (2003) Killing of Aspergillus fumigatus by alveolar macrophages is mediated by reactive oxidant intermediates. Infect Immun 71: 3034-3042.
18. Larranaga J, Fandiño J, Gomez-Bueno J, Rodriguez D, Gonzalez-Carrero J, et al. (1989) Aspergillosis of the sphenoid sinus simulating a pituitary tumor. Neuroradiology 31: 362-363.
19. Lee JH, Park YS, Kim KM, Kim KJ, Ahn CH, et al. (2000) Pituitary aspergillosis mimicking pituitary tumor. AJR Am J Roentgenol 175: 1570-1572.
20. Daghistani KJ, Jamal TS, Zaher S, Nassif OI (1992) Allergic aspergillus sinusitis with proptosis. J Laryngol Otol 106: 799-803.
21. Samson RA, Peterson SW, Frisvad JC, Varga J (2011) New species in Aspergillus section Terrei. Stud Mycol 69: 39-55.
22. WHO (2009) Dampness and Mould: Who Guidelines for indoor air quality, Euro non serial publications.
23. Thrasher JD, Crawley S (2009) The biocontaminants and complexity of damp indoor spaces: more than what meets the eyes. Toxicol Ind Health 25: 583-615.
24. Thrasher JD, Gray MR, Kilburn KH, Dennis DP, Yu A (2012) A water-damaged home and health of occupants: a case study. J Environ Public Health 2012: 312836.
25. Bloom E, Nyman E, MustA, Pehrson C, Larsson L (2009) Molds and mycotoxins in indoor environments--a survey in water-damaged buildings. J Occup Environ Hyg 6: 671-678.
26. Polizzi V, Delmulle B, Adams A, Moretti A (2009) JEM spotlight: Fungi, mycotoxins and microbial volatile organic compounds in mouldy interiors from water-damaged buildings. J Environ Monit 11: 1949-1958.
27. Taubel M, Sulyok M, Vishwanath V, Bloom E, Turunen M, et al. (2011) Co-occurrence of toxic bacterial and fungal secondary metabolites in moisture-damaged indoor environments. Indoor Air 21: 368-375.
28. Smoragiewicz W, Cossette B, Boutard A, Krzystyniak K (1993) Trichothecene mycotoxins in the dust of ventilation systems in office buildings. Int Arch Occup Environ Health 65: 113-117.
29. Tuomi T, Reijula K, Johnsson T, Hemminki K, Hintikka EL, et al. (2000) Mycotoxins in crude building materials from water-damaged buildings. Appl Environ Microbiol 66: 1899-1904.
30. Ebener U, Wehner S, Cinatl J, Gussetis ES, Kornhuber B (1990) Expression of markers shared between human haematopoietic cells and neuroblastoma cells. Anticancer Res 10: 887-890.
31. Abdelhaleem MM, Hatskelzon L, Dalal BI, Gerrard JM, Greenberg AH (1991) Leukophysin: a 28-kDa granule membrane protein of leukocytes. J Immunol 147: 3053-3059.
32. Abdelhaleem MM, Hameed S, Klassen D, Greenberg AH (1996) Leukophysin: an RNA helicase A-related molecule identified in cytotoxic T cell granules and vesicles. J Immunol 156: 2026-2035.
33. Mendes-Giannini MJ, Taylor ML, Bouchara JB, Burger E, Calich VL, et al. (2000) Pathogenesis II: fungal responses to host responses: interaction of host cells with fungi. Med Mycol 38 Suppl 1: 113-123.
34. Kogan TV, Jadoun J, Mittelman L, Hirschberg K, Osherov N (2004) Involvement of secreted Aspergillus fumigatus proteases in disruption of the actin fiber cytoskeleton and loss of focal adhesion sites in infected A549 lung pneumocytes. J Infect Dis 189: 1965-1973.
35. Baker RD (1956) Pulmonary mucormycosis. Am J Pathol 32: 287-313.
36. Taylor MJ, Ponikau JU, Sherris DA, Kern EB, Gaffey TA, et al. (2002) Detection of fungal organisms in eosinophilic mucin using a fluorescein-labeled chitin-specific binding protein. Otolaryngol Head Neck Surg 127: 377-383.
37. Hooper DG, Bolton VE, Guilford FT, Straus DC (2009) Mycotoxin detection in human samples from patients exposed to environmental molds. Int J Mol Sci 10: 1465-1475.
38. Hooper DG, Bolton VE, Sutton JS, Guilford T (2012) Assessment of Aspergillus

fumigatus in Guinea pig bronchoalveolar lavages and pulmonary tissues by culture and realtime polymerase chain reaction studies. Int J Mol Sci 13:726-36.

39. Dumanov J (2008) Pathology report by Dr. Dumanov. Mycological Institute for the Study of Fungal Mold in Human Habitations, Sparta, NJ.

40. Thrasher JD, Gray MR, Kilburn KH, Dennis DP, Yu A (2012) A water-damaged home and health of occupants: a case study. J Environ Public Health 2012: 312836.

41. Chrdle A, Mustakim S, Bright-Thomas RJ, Baxter CG, Felton T, et al. (2012) Aspergillus bronchitis without significant immunocompromise. Ann N Y Acad Sci 1272: 73-85.

42. Fernandez MS, Rojas FD, Cattana ME, Sosa Mde L, Mangiaterra ML, et al. (2013) Aspergillus terreus complex: an emergent opportunistic agent of Onychomycosis. Mycoses 56: 477-481.

43. Guinea J, Padilla C, Escribano P, Muñoz P, Padilla B, et al. (2013) Evaluation of MycAssayâ„¢ Aspergillus for diagnosis of invasive pulmonary aspergillosis in patients without hematological cancer. PLoS One 8: e61545.

44. Akhaddar A, Gazzaz M, Albouzidi A, Lmimouni B, Elmostarchid B, et al. (2008) Invasive Aspergillus terreus sinusitis with orbitocranial extension: case report. Surg Neurol 69: 490-495.

45. Schubert MS (2009) Allergic fungal sinusitis: pathophysiology, diagnosis and management. Med Mycol 47 Suppl 1: S324-330.

46. Takahashi H, Hinohira Y, Hato N, Wakisaka H, Hyodo J, et al. (2011) Clinical features and outcomes of four patients with invasive fungal sinusitis. Auris Nasus Larynx 38: 289-294.

47. Brewer JH, Thrasher JD, Straus DC, Madison RA, Hooper D (2013) Detection of mycotoxins in patients with chronic fatigue syndrome. Toxins (Basel) 5: 605-617.

48. Brewer JH, Thrasher JD, Hooper D (2013) Chronic illness associated with mold and mycotoxins: is naso-sinus fungal biofilm the culprit? Toxins (Basel) 6: 66-80.

49. Gray MR, Thrasher JD, Crago R, Madison RA, Arnold L, et al. (2003) Mixed mold mycotoxicosis: immunological changes in humans following exposure in water-damaged buildings. Arch Environ Health 58: 410-420.

50. Fisk WJ, Eliseeva EA, Mendell MJ (2010) Association of residential dampness and mold with respiratory tract infections and bronchitis: a meta-analysis. Environ Health 9: 72.

51. NIOSH Mold Alert, 2013

52. Alrajhi AA, Enani M, Mahasin Z, Al-Omran K (2001) Chronic invasive aspergillosis of the paranasal sinuses in immunocompetent hosts from Saudi Arabia. Am J Trop Med Hyg 65: 83-86.

53. Aribandi M, McCoy VA, Bazan C 3rd (2007) Imaging features of invasive and noninvasive fungal sinusitis: a review. Radiographics 27: 1283-1296.

54. Gorovoy IR, Kazanjian M, Kersten RC, Kim HJ, Vagefi MR (2012) Fungal rhinosinusitis and imaging modalities. Saudi J Ophthalmol 26: 419-426.

Sudden Sensorineural Hearing Loss After Total Thyroidectomy Surgery Under General Anesthesia

Mitat Arıcıgil[1*], Abitter Yucel[2], Mehmet Akif Alan[1], Fuat Aydemir[1] and Suayp Kuria Aziz[1]

[1]*Department of Otorhinolaryngology, Meram Faculty of Medicine, Necmettin Erbakan University, Turkey*

[2]*Department of Otorhinolaryngology, Horasan State Hospital, Erzurum, Turkey*

[*]**Corresponding author:** Mitat Arıcıgil, Associate Professor, Department of Otorhinolaryngology, Meram Faculty of Medicine, Necmettin Erbakan University, Turkey; E-mail: maricigil79@gmail.com

Abstract

Introduction: Sudden sensorineural hearing loss that developes after surgery which has been done under general anesthesia is quite rare and mostly occurs after otologic and coronary artery bypass surgery.

Case-report: A 43 year old female patient who developed right sided hearing loss 6-7 h after a total thyroidectomy operation was diagnosed as sudden sensorineural hearing loss and treated succesfully at our clinic.

Discussion: Sudden sensorineural hearing loss that develops after surgical operations under general anesthesia are quite rare and frequently occur after otologic and coronary artery bypass surgeries. patients should be informed before the operation and awareness should be created by educating anesthesiologist, surgeons and assisting health personels.

Keywords: Sudden sensorineural hearing loss; Total thyroidectomy; General anesthesia

Introduction

Sudden sensorineural hearing loss is defined as sensorineural hearing loss of 30 dB or greater in at least three contiguous frequencies as recorded in audiometry developing within a period of three days or less. Even though many etiologic factors have been brought forward, only 10-15% of cases have had their etiologies shedlight on [1]. In most patients the sudden sensorineural hearing loss is regarded idiopathic. The approximate incidence of sudden sensorineural hearing loss is 5-20/100.000 and its potential causes that can be brought forward are infectious, autoimmune, traumatic, vascular, neoplastic, metabolic and neurologic cases. In a meta-analysis consisting of 23 idiopathic sudden sensorineural hearing loss case studies, infectious agents were reported to be the most common cause [2].

Excluding otologic interventions, sudden hearing loss is a condition that rarely occurs after surgical operations done under general anesthesia. Most of these develop after cardiopulmonary bypass surgery where extracorporeal circulation is used. In addition to this, sudden sensorineural hearing loss has been reported to develop after surgical operations with the exclusion of otologic and cardiopulmonary interventions [3].

In this case report, the clinical case of a patient diagnosed with multinodular goiter who developed unilateral sudden sensorineural hearing loss at an early postoperative stage after total thyroidectomy under general anesthesia together with a review of the literature wil be discussed.

Case Report

Our department was consulted on the case of a 43 year old female patient who developed right sided hearing loss 6-7 h after a total thyroidectomy operation. The patient affirmed to having no ear complaint and that her hearing was normal prior to the operation. Together with hearing loss the patient also complained of ear fullness without tinnitus and dizziness. The patient had no history of chronic disease or use of ototoxic drugs. The patient's intraoperative blood pressure level, heart rate and oxygen saturation were within normal limits.

The patient's otologic examination was unremarkable. There was no spontaneous nystagmus and fistula test was negative. The routine blood tests and electrocardiography done before the operation were normal. According to the American Society of Anesthesiologists (ASA) classification, the patient was taken to operation with a status of ASA 1 and was administered with midazolam 1-2 mg/kg, lidocaine 1 mg/kg, propofol 2 mg/kg, rocuronium 0.6 mg/kg, sevoflurane and remifentanil 0.2 mcg/kg/min. Nitrous oxide was not used during anesthesia.

In the patient's pure tone audiometry test a sensorineural hearing loss of 53 dB was confirmed (Figure 1) at the bone conduction thresholds. The patient was diagnosed with sudden sensorineural hearing loss and decreasing doses of systemic steroid (Metilprednizolon sodyum süksinat 1 mg/kg, terminated within three weeks with decreasing doses) and plasma volume expansion solution (dextran 40) was started. At the same time hypocalcemia was confirmed in the blood test and calcitriol medication started . The right ear audiometry test was done on the 4th day of treatment and the hearing level was found to be at 43 dB (Figure 2) at the bone conduction thresholds. However the audiometry test of both ears done on the 10th day of treatment showed the hearing levels to be within normal limits (Figure 3). The patient's calcium level normalized 3 days after resolution of the hearing loss. The patient did not have any synthetic thyroid hormone replacement treatment between the time hearing loss developed to the time it resolved. With resolution of the hearing loss the patient was discharged and is still under follow up.

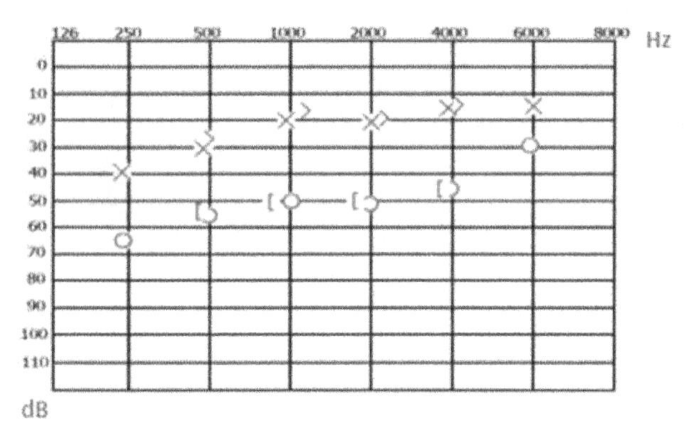

Figure 1: Audiometry of the patient at the time of diagnosis.

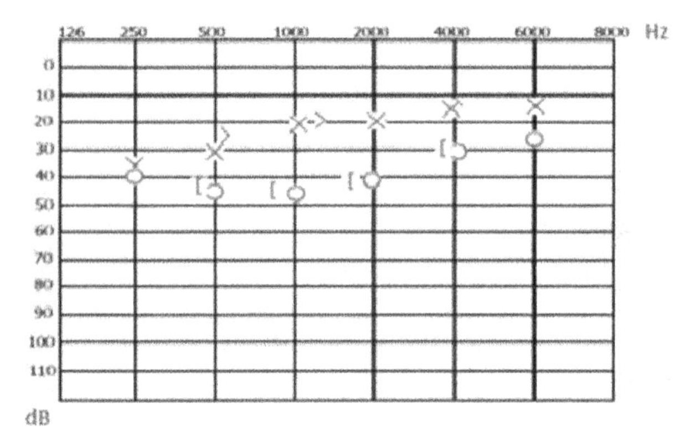

Figure 2: Audiometry of the patient at 4th treatment day.

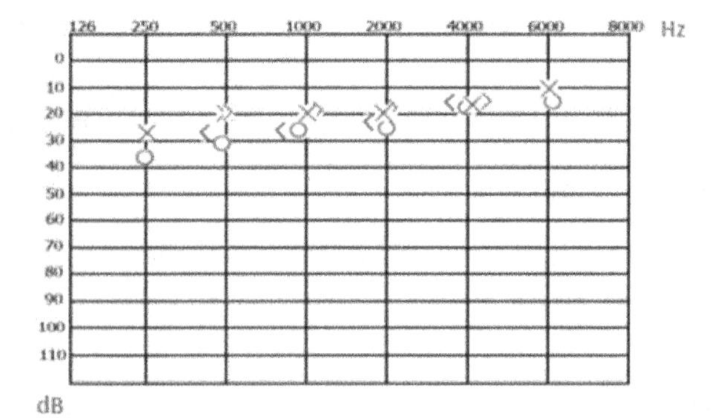

Figure 3: Audiometry of the patient at 10th treatment day.

Discussion

Sudden sensorineural hearing loss is frequently encountered in ear nose and throat practice and up to date it is a well-recognized otological emergency. Even though it is a pathology that has been recognized for a long time, its etiopathogenesis and treatment is still debatable. As much as many etiologic factors have been put forward, most of the cases are idiopathic. Sudden sensorineural hearing loss that develops after surgical operations under general anesthesia are quite rare and frequently occur after otologic and coronary artery bypass surgeries. However sudden sensorineural hearing loss has also been reported to occur after other surgical interventions. Consequently not only does this condition occur under general anesthesia but also in interventions where spinal anesthesia is used.

Arenberg [4] repoted a case of sudden sensorineural hearing loss after cardiopulmonary bypass surgery in 1972. Even though the etiologic factors of sudden sensorineural hearing loss that develops under general anesthesia have been put forward, determining the exact cause is quite difficult. The potential causes include ototoxic drug use, nitrous oxide, variations in middle ear pressure, vascular pathologies, perioperative hypoperfusion, variations in cerebrospinal fluid pressure, valsalva maneuver, perilymphatic fistula, microemboli and viral infections [5,6].

Sudden sensorineural hearing loss that develops after spinal anesthesia was first reported in 1914. As sudden sensorineural hearing loss can be unilateral or bilateral, it can also occur at an early or late stage. Hearing loss that occurs during spinal anesthesia is thought to develop due to changes in cerebral spinal fluid pressure. Decrease in pressure and leakage of cerebral spinal fluid after dural puncture results in a quick decrease in perilymphatic pressure. Sudden decrease in cerebral spinal fluid can cause unmeasurable changes in endolymphatic pressure and consequently can result in reissner membrane and basilar membrane damage. As a result, changes in the position of the hair cells causes hearing loss. Moreover acute increase in cerebral spinal fluid pressure and conduction to the perilymph causing damage to the basilar membrane has been thought to result in hearing loss [6].

Microembolism is one of the most culpable factors of sudden sensorineural hearing loss that is seen after general anesthesia. Increased platelet count and platelet aggregability is thought to be a source of microembolism during the postoperative period [4]. Especially, sensorineural hearing loss that develops after cardiovascular surgery is mostly as a result of emboli particles created during cardiopulmonary bypass. The number of arterial microembolism significantly increases during extracorporeal perfusion and hearing loss is believed to be as a result of microemboli that occurs between the basilar artery and its branches to the inner ear [6].

Hearing loss that develops during anesthesia for cardiopulmonary bypass procedures has a generally bad prognosis. In most patients full recovery never occurs. This is believed to be as a result of an emboli that blocks microcirculation of the inner ear causing ischemic injury to stria vascularis and hairy cells. Sudden sensorineural hearing loss that develops after general anesthesia for procedures other than bypass surgery have relatively good prognosis. It has been reported that approximately 50% of patients have at least partial recovery. From these facts microembolism plays a very small role than expected as an etiologic factor of sudden sensorineural hearing loss after general anesthesia for interventions other than cardiopulmonary bypass surgery. For this reason, the other etiologic factors are more prominent in these patients.

The type of anesthesia used during the operation can also cause hearing loss. Nitrous oxide is one of the well-recognized agents in this field. Nitrous oxide has a dissolution of 30 folds compared to nitrogen and can therefore quickly penetrate into the middle ear and increase the pressure in the middle ear . This high pressure is directed towards the inner ear and by means of the oval and round window, can cause perilymphatic fistula resulting in sensorineural hearing loss [3,4]. For this reason, vestibular symptoms should be checked and fistula test done during the postoperative period. In our case nitrous oxide was not used during any stage of the anesthesia.

In this case sudden sensorineural hearing loss developed after total thyroidectomy operation. The total excision of thyroid gland was thought to be able to cause sudden hearing loss as it produces thyroid hormone which affects general metabolism. The effects of serum thyroid hormone levels on hearing function has been known for a long time. Both hyperfunction and hypofunction of thyroid gland can cause dynamic changes on hearing. In a cross sectional study, Oiticica et al. [7] studied the metabolic defects of 166 patients who presented with sudden hearing loss within a period of 10 years. They found that thyroid hormone levels was normal in 116 patients (78.4%) whereas in 32 patients (21.6%) it was not normal. Long periods of thyroid hormone deficiencies has been shown to cause hearing function variations in both humans and experimental animal studies. Psaltakos et al. [8] determined the hearing levels of 52 patients who had undergone total thyroidectomy using pure tone audiometry and transient evoked otoacoustic emission before and 6-8 weeks after the operation. The patients were not given levothyroxine and Thyroid Stimulating Hormone(TSH) was monitored during the postoperative period. An increase in all of the hearing levels was noted in the postoperative audiometry and the S/N ratio on otoacoustic emission was seen to be lower in the postoperative period compared to the preoperative period. On the contrary, Mra and Wax [9] did not find any changes on audiogram and otoacoustic emission during the 6 week period of acute thyroxin depletion after total thyroidectomy. Whereas in our case hearing loss developed at an early postoperative period (~ 6 h) after total thyroidectomy and taking into account the half life of thyroid hormone we came to the conclusion that hypothyroidism could not be an etiologic factor in this case.

Hypocalcemia whether symptomatic or asymptomatic is frequently seen after thyroid surgery and even though most cases resolve spontaneously it can be permanent in conditions where parathyroid gland is damaged. Sensorineural hearing loss is a less known sign of hypoparathyroidism. In a study on 20 idiopathic hypoparathyroidsm patients, pure tone audiometry was done and bilateral sensorineural hearing loss found in 15% of the patients and this hearing loss was thought to be as a result of long periods of low calcium levels in the inner ear fluids [10]. In our case while the preoperative calcium levels were normal, hypocalcemia developed at the same postoperative period as hearing loss.

Even though there were no signs of hypocalcemia on physical examination of the patient, calcitriol treatment was started and on approximately the 10th postoperative day calcium levels normalized. Hearing loss and hypocalcemia developed at the same period whereas hearing loss resolved 3 days before calcium levels normalized. For this reason this patient's hearing loss most probably did not occur as a result of sudden changes in calcium level.

We have presented a rare case of sudden sensorineural hearing loss in this case report. Sudden sensorineural hearing loss has been reported to occur after many different operations under general anesthesia. Even though many etiologic factors have been put forward in these patients, generally a definite factor is not clear. In this study occurance of metabolic changes that can cause hearing loss in the postoperative period is seen in patients undergoing endocrine surgery under general anesthesia however it was found that the patient's hearing loss was not in a correlated progression with these factors. The patient's TSH levels gradually increased in the postoperative period but the hearing levels resolved to normal limits. Similarly hearing resolved before calcium levels came within normal limits. In the period when hearing had normalized hypocalcemia was still present.

Conclusion

Sudden sensorineural hearing loss is a rare condition that develops after surgical interventions under general and spinal anesthesia. For this reason patients should be informed before the operation and awareness should be created by educating anesthesiologist, surgeons and assisting health personnels.

References

1. Oiticica J, Bittar RS (2010) Metabolic disorders prevalence in sudden deafness. Clinics (Sao Paulo) 65: 1149-1553.
2. Kuhn M, Heman-Ackah SE, Shaikh JA, Roehm PC (2011) Sudden sensorineural hearing loss: a review of diagnosis, treatment and prognosis. Trends Amplif 15: 91-105.
3. Pau H, Selvadurai D, Murty GE (2000) Reversible sensorineural hearing loss after non-otological surgery under general anaesthetic. Postgrad Med J 76: 304-306.
4. Evan KE, Tavill MA, Goldberg AN, Silverstein H (1997) Sudden sensorineural hearing loss after general anesthesia for nonotologic surgery. Laryngoscope 107: 747-752.
5. Girardi FP, Cammisa FP Jr, Sangani PK, Parvataneni HK, Khan SN, et al. (2001) Sudden sensorineural hearing loss after spinal surgery under general anesthesia. J Spinal Disord 14: 180-183.
6. Sprung J, Bourke DL, Contreras MG, Warner ME, Findlay J (2003) Perioperative hearing impairment. Anesthesiology 98: 241-257.
7. Narozny W, Kuczkowski J, Mikaszewski B (2006) Thyroid dysfunction-underestimated but important prognostic factor in sudden sensorineural hearing loss. Otolaryngol Head Neck Surg 135: 995-996.
8. Psaltakos V, Balatsouras DG, Sengas I, Ferekidis E, Riga M, et al. (2013) Cochlear dysfunction in patients with acute hypothyroidism. Eur Arch Otorhinolaryngol 270: 2839-2848.
9. Mra Z, Wax MK (1999) Effects of acute thyroxin depletion on hearing in humans. Laryngoscope 109: 343-350.
10. Garty BZ, Daliot D, Kauli R, Arie R, Grosman J, et al. (1994) Hearing impairment in idiopathic hypoparathyroidism and pseudohypoparathyroidism. Isr J Med Sci 30: 587-591.

Supraglottic Obstruction in an Adult with Inspiratory Arytenoid Cartilage Prolapse

Amy L Rutt*, **James P Dworkin and Noah Stern**

Department of Otolaryngology Head and Neck Surgery, Detroit Medical Center/Michigan State University, USA

Abstract

Laryngomalacia (LM) has become the default diagnostic term for any patient who might struggle with stridor and dyspnea secondary to floppy, insufficient, hypotonic, or passively collapsing supraglottal tissue characteristics. Despite the increasing incidence of this diagnosis, the etiology, work-up, and pathophysiology of LM remain poorly understood and controversial to date.

Objectives: The purpose of this paper is to illustrate the history, unique physical examination findings, and multi-varied and creative treatments rendered to an adult patient of ours who struggled with profound signs and symptoms of Type 1 LM.

Methods: This is a case study of idiopathic aerodynamic supraglottic collapse that occurred in an otherwise healthy individual who had no prior history of connective tissue disorder, neurodegenerative disorder, or trauma. The patient's history, examination, treatment, and review of the literature are discussed.

Results: Laryngoscopy is the definitive test to evaluate supraglottic airway collapse. Supraglottoplasty is a safe and effective treatment for adult LM.

Conclusions: The diagnosis of adult aerodynamic supraglottic collapse is an important entity to consider in patients presenting with dyspnea, stridor, or other breathing complaints. This case description illustrates the importance of laryngoscopy when evaluating patients with such signs and symptoms.

Keywords: Laryngomalacia; Supraglottic collapse; Supraglottic obstruction; Stridor

Introduction

The most common cause of stridor and dyspnea in infants is LM. The nominal derivation of this congenital condition arises from the Greek word "malakia", which refers to morbid softening of an organ part. It has been sub-classified into 3 primary variants: Type 1 is characterized by antero-medial prolapse or collapse of the bodies of the arytenoid cartilages over the laryngeal inlet. In Type 2, the antero-posterior dimension of the airway is significantly reduced by abnormally short aryepiglottic folds. The Type 3 form involves abnormal degrees of posterior deflection of the epiglottis during inspiratory aerodynamics, which results in pronounced narrowing of the laryngeal lumen [1]. In the vast majority of these cases, watchful surveillance is indicated as the treatment of choice, owing to the probability of gradual spontaneous resolution of signs and symptoms without medical-surgical management. For those children with intractable LM several surgical approaches have been successfully employed, including lengthening the aryepiglottic folds and de-bulking or anchoring redundant supraglottic mucosa and/or cartilage [2-4].

Acquired airway obstruction in adults caused by excessive, hypotense, hyperactive, or floppy supraglottic tissue has also been described and classified as LM [4,5]. Irritable larynx syndrome and paradoxical vocal fold motion disorders can also result in intermittent occurrences of breathing difficulties. The etiologies in these cases may include vigorous exercise, chronic use of inhaled steroids, and asthmatic bronchospasms with upstream laryngeal sequelae, neurodegenerative illnesses, traumatic brain injury, cerebral vascular accident, connective tissue diseases, laryngeal trauma, and idiopathic laryngeal synkinesis [6-8]. None of these alternative explanations was considered applicable to the diagnosis of airway collapse in the current patient presentation, inasmuch as her symptoms and signs of dyspnea and stridor were clinically significant during restful breathing as well as exertional activities.

The purpose of this paper is to illustrate the history, unique physical examination findings, and multi-varied and creative treatments rendered to an adult patient of ours who struggled with profound signs and symptoms of Type 1 LM.

Case Report

A 61 year old African American female presented to Detroit Receiving Hospital with chief complaints of dyspnea and stridor on exertion, at rest, and during sleep. These symptoms had persisted for several months prior to her visit to our Otolaryngology clinic. She had a past medical history of hypertension, hypercholesterolemia, gastro esophageal reflux disease, diabetes mellitus, and asthma. At the time of our initial examination she was 6 weeks status post C4-C5 and C5-C6 anterior cervical discectomy with fusion for severe neural foraminal stenosis. It should be noted that her breathing difficulties were first diagnosed approximately one year ago prior to this surgical experience. At that time, she was using a CPCP apparatus to improve sleep apnea symptoms. This device was titrated to the minimum

***Corresponding author:** Amy L Rutt, Department of Otolaryngology Head and Neck Surgery, Detroit Medical Center/Michigan State University, USA; E-mail: scse9000@aol.com

level required to eliminate sleep breathing difficulty and snoring. At a pressure of 9 cm H_20, disordered breathing ceased, and the tight-fitting mask was well tolerated. Additionally, within the same time frame, the patient underwent pulmonary function testing to evaluate symptoms of suspected exercise induced asthma. At baseline, FVC, FVC1, and FEV1/FVC results were all within normal limits, with excellent efforts given by the patient throughout testing. Methacholine challenge result was next performed, followed by post-bronchodilator response testing via a small-volume nebulizer, with 0.083% albuterol solution over 10 minutes. At first dose of methacholine there was a 23% decrease in FEV1. This finding was interpreted by the attending pulmonologist as suggestive underlying asthma. It should be noted that significant improvement in FVC or FEV1 occurred immediately after administration of the bronchodilator, and flow volume loops had normal configuration. Based on all these pulmonary function test results, the patient's primary care physician concluded that her breathing disturbances during exercise and sleep were likely casually related to moderately severe asthma.

The patient's immediate post-operative history was uncomplicated and she was discharged home successfully, without the need for supplemental oxygen therapy. Soon after discharge she developed oropharyngeal dysphagia to solids and liquid, in addition to more severe dyspnea, snoring, and sleep apneic symptoms than were evident before such surgery. These exacerbations lead to multiple ER visits over the course of two months for profound dyspnea and intermittent Globus sensations. On each occasion, she was discharged without hospital admission or prescription medication, with the diagnosis of idiopathic breathing complaints likely secondary to asthmatic bronchospasms. As an outpatient, she underwent a polysomnogram. Results revealed mild sleep disordered breathing, with an apnea-hyponea index of 7.8; she was fitted subsequently for a CPAP unit. She was referred to our clinic and pulmonary medicine for follow-up evaluations of her dysphagia and breathing complaints. The pulmonologist reinforced her daily inhaler regimen and recommended that she avoid strenuous physical exercise activities. No other treatments were rendered.

During our examination in the Voice and Swallowing Laboratory the patient appeared well nourished and her speech, voice, and language behaviors were all within normal limits. Stridor was not evident at rest, but deep inspiratory-expiratory exchanges evoked mild-to-moderate bi-phasic noisy breathing sounds. She reported that she had voluntarily altered her food intake to a mechanically soft diet with all liquid preferences. This resulted in a marked improvement in swallowing ability. Anterior rhinoscopy demonstrated a severely deviated left nasal septum. Oral examination results were within normal limits. Videostroboscopy of laryngeal anatomy and physiology revealed an elongated uvula as well as marked inflammation of the arytenoid and corniculate cartilages bilaterally, which aerodynamically prolapsed antero-medially during inspiration. This resulted in near complete obstruction of the laryngeal lumen (Figure 1). The true vocal folds were fully mobile, without identifiable growths or lesions. The false vocal folds, ventricles, epiglottis, and peri-laryngeal boundaries were similarly unremarkable anatomically and physiologically. We elected to refer the patient to the pulmonary service, concurrent with her admission to hospital for airway monitoring and anticipated surgical intervention, Vis a vis a partial uvulectomy and excisional debulking of the left redundant corniculate cartilage and ipsilateral arytenoid body apex. Such surgery was accomplished using the CO_2 OmniGuide laser apparatus. On her postoperative visit, the surgical site was healing well and the airway dimensions improved by approximately 50% over the preoperative status (Figure 2). The patient reported significantly

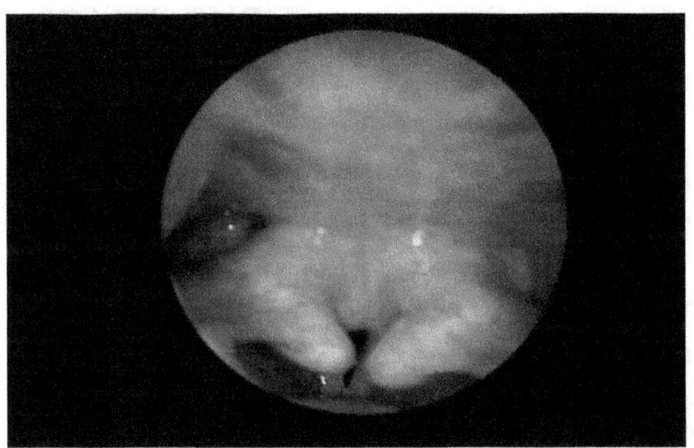

Figure 1: Marked inflammation of the arytenoid and corniculate cartilages, which aerodynamically prolapsed antero-medially during inspiration.

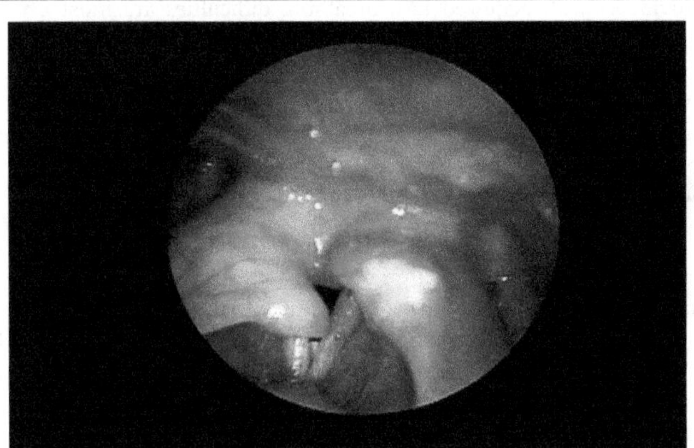

Figure 2: Post-operative picture from the first surgery. The surgical site healed well and the airway dimensions improved by approximately 50 % over the preoperative picture.

less sleep difficulties, dyspnea at rest and upon exertion, and noisy breathing. The prolapsing arytenoid and corniculate cartilages was eliminated on the operated side, accounting for these symptomatic gains. Six weeks later the patient was taken to the operating room for the same surgical procedure on the contralateral side of the larynx. Figure 3 illustrates the successful anatomical and physiological treatment outcome. The patient shortly thereafter experienced near complete resolution of her sleep apnea symptoms and dyspnea at rest and with exercise; there was no perceptible degree of stridor at the 1 week post-operative examination. To date, more than 18 months following these staged surgical procedures, the patient continues to maintain her improvements.

Discussion

LM has become the default diagnostic term for any patient who might struggle with stridor and dyspnea secondary to floppy, insufficient, hypotonic, or passively collapsing supraglottal tissue characteristics. Despite the increasing incidence of this diagnosis, the etiology, work-up, and pathophysiology of LM remain poorly understood and controversial to date. It is a rare diagnosis in older children and adults because in the vast majority of cases the condition is congenital and it either spontaneously improves or is treated surgically early in life. A subset of adolescents and adults occasionally present to ER, pulmonary, and ENT physicians with signs and symptoms

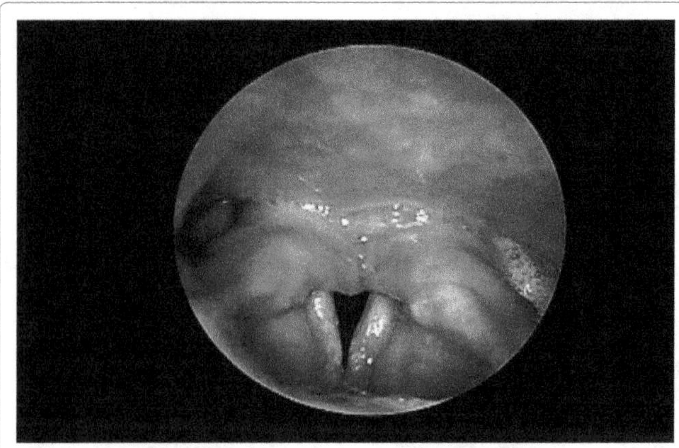

Figure 3: Post-operative picture from second surgery.

that closely mimic those observed in children with congenital LM. In individuals with acquired LM, breathing difficulties are most often experience during exertional activities and delta sleep stages 3 and 4. In cases like this, flexible nasolaryngoscopy during sleep has demonstrated invagination or obstructive prolapse of the arytenoid bodies toward the laryngeal lumen during inspiration [2]. When these signs are observed, they may be considered causally related to associated stridor, intermittent hypoxia, hypercapnia, and hypopnea.

Two alternative LM etiologic theories have been postulated by clinical researchers: neuromuscular and structural. The former explanation suggests the principle feature of supraglottic narrowing or collapse results from underlying muscular incoordination and hypotonia of the components of the unified airway; that ill-coordinated respiratory drive, pulmonary load, and airflow dynamics cause hyper-reflexive supraglottal resistance, motion, and medial prolapse of these tissues into the lumen of the larynx [9-12]. Those individuals who possess unusually tall and prominent arytenoid and cuneiform cartilages are considered to be most susceptible to developing LM, whether congenital or acquired. Proponents of this theory believe that the brisk air velocities and negative pressure associated with labored respirations and the Bernoulli Effect induce supraglottic collapse and airway obstruction in this population.

Those who support the structural theory of origin propose that congenital or acquired supraglottal tissue anatomic insufficiency or redundancy produces intermittent or persistent laryngeal inlet narrowing [3,13,14]. Factors such as laryngo-pharyngeal reflux, post-nasal drainage, and smoking may exacerbate baseline supraglottic edema and airway compromise, especially during exertional breathing and delta sleep.

Laryngoscopy is the definitive test to appreciate supraglottic airway collapse. This collapse may result as redundant mucosa of the arytenoids cartilages, ventricular folds, or aryepiglottic folds are drawn into the laryngeal lumen during deep inspiration. Patients usually experience stridor during sleep and/or exertion. Supraglottic airway collapse must be differentiated from paradoxical vocal fold movement and vocal fold paralysis, both of which may cause similar airway compromising signs and symptoms.

Our patient was seen by her pulmonary physician for breathing difficulty and pulmonary function tests. She had demonstrated a positive methacholine test challenge result, which led to the presumed diagnosis of asthma, to which her dyspnea and obstructive sleep apnea were attributed. Unfortunately, at that time of testing she did not undergo bronchoscopy or laryngoscopy to rule out other possible etiologies for these conditions. In retrospect, had the pulmonologist placed a stethoscope on the larynx as the patient took deep breaths, evidence of bi-phasic stridor would have been detected as a competing challenge to the sole diagnosis of asthma. In retrospect, the patient's pulmonologist and primary care physician concluded that in her case of coexisting asthma and LM these two conditions likely acted synergistically to compound her exercise induced dyspnea and sleep apnea; akin to a respiratory mechanical double whammy.

We would suggest that possible upstream airway compromise should always be a component of the differential diagnostic algorithm in patients with clinically significant dyspnea, stridor, and/or sleep apnea. Laryngeal stridor, in particular, requires further work-up via endoscopic examination, preferably with the aid of videostroboscopy for detailed imaging and analysis of the anatomy and bio-mechanics of the glottal and supraglottal tissues. Such examination is often beneficial in the post-treatment period as well, for comparative purposes. Had video endoscopy been performed on outpatient early in her course, accurate diagnosis of LM would have been reached, and appropriate treatments would have been rendered sooner?

The origin of our patient's LM remains a mystery to us. We have asked ourselves whether her condition was congenital. Was LPR a factor in her presenting signs? Could the condition have been a result of aging hypotonia? Perhaps a combination of anatomical and physiological factors? In cases like ours, treating physicians would be wise to examine the status of all components of the unified airway before concluding the diagnostic process and prescribing treatments. In our clinical experiences, numerous patients have been erroneously treated for asthma with undiagnosed laryngeal pathologies, such as vocal fold paralysis, obstructive tumors, or LM.

Our case study of idiopathic aerodynamic supraglottic collapse occurred in an otherwise healthy individual who had no prior history of connective tissue disorder, neurodegenerative disorder, or history of airway trauma. Referral to our service was made only after several failed treatments for asthma, an otherwise negative cardiopulmonary workup, and following the onset of transient dysphagia. Videostroboscopy revealed the likely cause of her external dyspnea, sleep apnea, and stridor. She suffered from collapse of the redundant arytenoid body mucosa and corniculate cartilages into the airway lumen during inspiration. Her glottis dimension was markedly compromised as a result, with associated noticeable stridor and dyspnea. The impending diagnosis was LM of an acquired form. Surgical management was recommended for definitive airway improvement.

A causal link between supraglottic collapse and obstructive sleep apnea may be more common than we may believe. Comprehensive evaluation is of paramount importance to the differential diagnosis. Surprisingly supraglottic mucosal redundancy in conjunction with adult obstructive sleep apnea/hyponea syndrome has only been described sporadically over the past 15 years [3,4]. Rodriquez et al. [15] reported a case of a 48-year-old female whose obstructive sleep apnea and CPAP/Bi-PAP failure was attributable to severe arytenoid mucosal hyperplasia, her airway symptoms resolved after endoscopic laser excision of the excessive mucosa. Similarly, our patient‘s degree of supraglottic collapse negatively impacted her sleep activity. After supraglottic surgery, she experienced markedly improved sleep patterns and airway relief, as demonstrated by her post-treatment AHI of 5.2.

In cases of adult LM, surgical management may prove necessary for long-term airway improvement, especially during exertional activities and deep sleep. For many years, CO_2 laser supraglottoplasty has been shown to be the treatment of choice for infants and children with LM [5]. Supraglottoplasty is a well-established method to relieve the airway obstruction without the need for concurrent tracheostomy. Several surgical approaches have been proposed, including 1) excision of the redundant arytenoid mucosa on the arytenoids, 2) division of the aryepiglottic folds to lengthen the laryngeal inlet in the anteroposterior axis, and 3) resection of the aryepiglottic folds followed by glossoepiglottopexy [6-8]. In order to prevent the complication of postoperative interarytenoid scarring, a mucosal bridge between the resected areas must be preserved. These procedures may be carried out with microscissors and microforceps, or using CO_2 laser [16,17]. Our patient's positive response to surgery was consistent with the outcomes of other clinical researchers who employed the supraglottoplasty technique for their adult patients with LM [18-20]. Use of laser technology during such surgery offers the advantage of hemostasis, blood vessel coagulation with little bleeding, and precision repair [21,22].

Conclusion

Acquired adult LM is very rare. The diagnosis of adult aerodynamic supraglottic collapse is an important entity to consider in anyone presenting with dyspnea, stridor, or other breathing complaints. The importance of conducting laryngoscopy to appraise the upper airway in these patients must be considered. In most cases, supraglottoplasty is a safe and effective treatment for long-term symptomatic relief.

References

1. Olney DR, Greinwald JH Jr, Smith RJ, Bauman NM (1999) Laryngomalacia and its treatment. Laryngoscope 109: 1770-1775.
2. Richter GT, Thompson DM (2008) The surgical management of laryngomalacia. Otolaryngol Clin North Am 41: 837-864, vii.
3. Beaty MM, Wilson JS, Smith RJ (1999) Laryngeal motion during exercise. Laryngoscope 109: 136-139.
4. Siou GS, Jeannon JP, Stafford FW (2002) Acquired idiopathic laryngomalacia treated by laser aryepiglottoplasty. J Laryngol Otol 116: 733-735.
5. Gessler EM, Simko EJ, Greinwald JH Jr (2002) Adult laryngomalacia: an uncommon clinical entity. Am J Otolaryngol 23: 386-389.
6. Wiggs WJ Jr, DiNardo LJ (1995) Acquired laryngomalacia: resolution after neurologic recovery. Otolaryngol Head Neck Surg 112: 773-776.
7. Murry T, Tabaee A, Owczarzak V, Aviv JE (2006) Respiratory retraining therapy and management of laryngopharyngeal reflux in the treatment of patients with cough and paradoxical vocal fold movement disorder. Ann Otol Rhinol Laryngol 115: 754-758.
8. Fahey JT, Bryant NJ, Karas D, Goldberg B, Destefano R, et al. (2005) Exercise-induced stridor due to abnormal movement of the arytenoid area: videoendoscopic diagnosis and characterization of the "at risk" group. Pediatr Pulmonol 39: 51-55.
9. Belmont JR, Grundfast K (1984) Congenital laryngeal stridor (laryngomalacia): etiologic factors and associated disorders. Ann Otol Rhinol Laryngol 93: 430-437.
10. Purser S, Irving L, Marty D (1994) Redundant supraglottic mucosa in association with obstructive sleep apnea. Laryngoscope 104: 114-116.
11. Sataloff RT, Chowdhury F, Joglekar S, Hawkshaw M [2011] Atlas of Endoscopic Laryngeal Surgery. Jaypee Brothers Medical Publishers; New Delhi, India.
12. Hui Y, Gaffney R, Crysdale WS (1995) Laser aryepiglottoplasty for the treatment of neurasthenic laryngomalacia in cerebral palsy. Ann Otol Rhinol Laryngol 104: 432-436.
13. Giannoni C, Sulek M, Friedman EM, Duncan NO 3rd (1998) Gastroesophageal reflux association with laryngomalacia: a prospective study. Int J Pediatr Otorhinolaryngol 43: 11-20.
14. Solomons NB, Prescott CA (1987) Laryngomalacia. A review and the surgical management for severe cases. Int J Pediatr Otorhinolaryngol 13: 31-39.
15. Rodriguez Adrados F, Esteban Ortega F, Peña Griñán N (1999) [Massive hyperplasia of the arytenoid mucosa with sleep apnea and stridor. Endoscopic resection by CO2 laser]. Acta Otorrinolaringol Esp 50: 664-666.
16. Archer SM (1992) Acquired flaccid larynx. A case report supporting the neurologic theory of laryngomalacia. Arch Otolaryngol Head Neck Surg 118: 654-657.
17. Thompson DM (2007) Abnormal sensorimotor integrative function of the larynx in congenital laryngomalacia: a new theory of etiology. Laryngoscope 117: 1-33.
18. Woo P (1992) Acquired laryngomalacia: epiglottis prolapse as a cause of airway obstruction. Ann Otol Rhinol Laryngol 101: 314-320.
19. Matthews BL, Little JP, Mcguirt WF Jr, Koufman JA (1999) Reflux in infants with laryngomalacia: results of 24-hour double-probe pH monitoring. Otolaryngol Head Neck Surg 120: 860-864.
20. Lane RW, Weider DJ, Steinem C, Marin-Padilla M (1984) Laryngomalacia. A review and case report of surgical treatment with resolution of pectus excavatum. Arch Otolaryngol 110: 546-551.
21. Seid AB, Park SM, Kearns MJ, Gugenheim S (1985) Laser division of the aryepiglottic folds for severe laryngomalacia. Int J Pediatr Otorhinolaryngol 10: 153-158.
22. Jani P, Koltai P, Ochi JW, Bailey CM (1991) Surgical treatment of laryngomalacia. J Laryngol Otol 105: 1040-1045.

Evaluation of TSH And T4 Levels in Idiopathic Sudden Sensorineural Hearing Loss Patients

Arıcıgil M*

Department of Otorhinolaryngology, Necmettin Erbakan University, Turkey

***Corresponding author:** Arıcıgil M, Meram Faculty of Medicine, Department of Otorhinolaryngology, Necmettin Erbakan University, Turkey; E-mail: maricigil79@gmail.com

Abstract

Objectives: to research on TSH, T4 levels and audiologic values of unilateral ISSNHL patients.

Methods: The files of patients who treated with sudden sensorineural hearing loss diagnosis were retrospectively reviewed. Hematologic and biochemical parameters, vitamin B-12, free T4 (tetraiodothyronine), TSH (thyroid stimulating hormone), the initial and last audiologic report after treatment were recorded.

Results: The study group consist of 60 patients (32 patients responder, 28 patient nonresponder) and the control group had 30 healthy persons. There was no significant difference in TSH and free T4 between the responder group and the control group. Serum free T4 was significantly lower in the nonresponder group comparing to the control group. There was no significant difference in TSH and T4 levels between subgroups of sudden hearing loss.

Conclusion: Small variations in T4 levels can be a risk factor for ISSNHL even if the patient has euthyroidism and these changes can be either acute or chronic.

Keywords: Sudden; Hearing loss; Thyroid

Introduction

Sudden sensorineural hearing loss (SSNHL) is defined as hearing loss of at least 30 dB at 3 consecutive frequencies in less than 3 days. A number of agents are responsible for its etiology but they have only been determined in 10-15% of cases [1]. Viral infections, vascular reasons, intracochlear membrane rapture, perilymphatic fistula, metabolic diseases, inner ear autoimmune disease, acoustic tumors, psychogenic diseases are at the forefront of its etiology [2]. 95% of the cases are unilateral and appoximately 90% of cases with unknown etiology are defined as idiopathic sudden sensorineural hearing loss [3] (ISSNHL).

Metabolic diseases are a risk factor for sudden hearing loss and one of these diseases is thyroid hormone disorders. Thyroid hormone levels are quite important for normal functioning of the cochlear and it has been reported that hearing functions have dynamic changes in hyper-hypothyroidism states [4]. Thyroid hormones are crucial for complete normal development of cochlear. Thyroid hormones are also necessary for normal development of middle ear and ossicular chain [5]. It is a well known fact that children born with congenital hypothyroidism can develope sensorineural hearing loss if thyroid hormone replacement is not done [6].

The etiology of ISSNHL has not been completely shed light on. It has been reported in a study that the rate of partial and total recovery of ISSNHL patients is 57% and the average recovery is 15 Db [7]. The etiology of one case in these patients was found to be history of thyroid gland disease and in the other cases cigarette was found to be responsible. Studies that research on the relationship between idiopathic sudden sensorineural hearing loss and thyroid hormones are limited in the literature. In this study we aimed to research on TSH, T4 levels and audiologic values of unilateral ISSNHL patients who were treated and either recovered or didn't recover by comparing them to a healthy control group.

Materials and Method

The files of patients who presented with sudden sensorineural hearing loss and were treated in Necmettin Erbakan University Meram Medical Faculty Ear Nose and Throat department between the years 2007 and 2016 were retrospectively reviewed. A total of 352 patient files were collected. Hematologic (leukocyte, hemoglobin, hematocrit, platelet values) and biochemical results, vitamin B-12, free T4 (tetraiodothyronine), TSH (thyroid stimulating hormone), temporal bone MRI, the initial and last audiologic report after treatment, history and physical examination were recorded from the patient files. Cigarette smokers, those with blood disorders, coronary artery disease, hypertension, lipid and cholesterol metabolic disorders, endocrine disorder, diabetes melitus, peadiatric patients, those with audiovestibular tumors, those with a history of drug use that is ototoxic and that affects thyroid function, those who have had a viral infection in the last 1 month, and those with abnormal hematologic and biochemical blood parameters were excluded from the study. After this exclusion sudden hearing loss with unkown etiologic risk factor was termed ISSNHL.

A total of 32 patients who met the criteria for recovery of more than 10 dB (the group that responded to treatment) and a total of 28 patients with a recovery of less than 10 dB (the group that didn't respond to treatment) in the audiologic tests were included into the study therefore forming two groups. Healthy individuals without any documented disease in the hospital's data base were chosen to form the control group. TSH, free T4, initial and last audiologic values after treatment of the 60 patient group and 2 subgroups accepted to have ISSNHL were evaluated by comparing to healthy individuals. Calculation of the average audiologic values was done by dividing the total of 250 Hz, 500 Hz, 1000 Hz, 2000 Hz, 4000 Hz and 8000 Hz by six. Treatment of ISSNHL was done by administration of 1 mg/kg/day prednizolon (I,V.), pirasetam (nootropil) ampul 8 mg/day (I.V.) (UCB Pharma, Turkey), and Dextran RMI (Rheomacrodex) 1000 ml/day (I.V.) (Eczacıbaşı,Turkey). ADVIA Centaur™ Siemens Healthcare (NY, USA) equipment was used for measurement of TSH and T4 values. Audiometric measurements were done with Clinical Audiometer AC33 (Denmark) in a sound proof cabin. This study was approved by the Local Ethics Committee of Necmettin Erbakan University Meram Medical Faculty.

Statistical analysis

Data was analyzed using SPSS 23.0 (USA) program. Comparison between those that showed recovery, those that didn't show recovery and the control group was done by Kruscal Wallis analysis of variance whereas post-hoc comparison was done by Mann Whitney U test with Bonferroni correction. Pearson correlation test was done to investigate whether or not there was any correlation between T4, TSH and the initial and last audiologic value in the groups. $P<0,05$ was accepted to be significant.

Results

There were 18 females and 14 males in the 32 patient group that responded to treatment (responders) and their average age was 42,75 (18-72) years. There were 16 females and 12 males in the 28 patient group that did not respond to treatment (non-responders) and their average age was 44,50 (19-68) years. The control group had 30 healthy persons, 16 females and 14 males with an average age of 47,21 (19-68) years. There was no significant difference in age and sex between the groups ($p>0,05$). There was no significant difference in TSH and free T4 between the responder group and the control group ($p>0,05$). Comparing the nonresponder group to the control group, there was no significant difference in TSH ($p>0,05$), whereas T4 was significantly lower in the nonresponder group ($p<0,05$). Comparing the subgroups of sudden hearing loss, there was no significant difference in TSH and T4 ($p<0,05$). Comparing the sudden hearing loss groups to the control group, the initial and last audiologic values were significantly higher in the sudden hearing loss groups ($p<0,05$). Comparing the sudden hearing loss groups, the last audiometric values were significantly higher in the nonresponder group ($p<0,05$). TSH and T4 values in all the patients that were diagnosed with ISSNHL without discriminating between the groups were compared to those in the control group and only T4 levels were found to be significantly lower in the sudden hearing loss group ($p<0,05$). TSH and free T4 values in the sudden hearing loss groups had no significant correlation with the initial and last audiometric values (average values ± standard deviation have been given in Tables 1 and 2).

	Responder group ISSNHL (n=32)	Nonresponder group ISSNHL (n=28)	Control (n=30)	p value
Age	42,75 ± 18,73	44,50 ± 21,820	47,21 ± 14,62	0,098
Gender (female/ male)	18/14	16-12-2016	16/14	0,883
TSH µIU/mL	1,617 ± 1,131	1,987 ± 1,032	1,691 ± 0,69	0.753
Free T4 ng/dL	1,240 ± 0,208	1,106 ± 0,127	1,30 ± 0,62	0,007
Initial air conduction (dB)	65,63 ± 26,107	80,57 ± 24,77	12,21 ± 3,42	0,001
Initial bone conduction (dB)	57,93 ± 57,50	61,93 ± 17,77	11,36 ± 3,53	0,001
Lasta air conduction (dB)	20,31 ± 18,147	76,00 ± 25,997		
Last bone conduction (dB)	16,94 ± 15,178	58,29 ± 15,993		

Table 1: Demographic features, Laboratory and audiometeric results of the study groups ISSNHL: idiopatic sensorineural sudden hearing loss, TSH: thyroid stimulating hormone. T4: tetraiodothyronine, dB: desibel, Initial air-bone conduction: Initial values at the time of diagnosis, Last air-bone conduction: values after medical treatment.

Comparison of Group	Control - Responders	Control - Nonresponders	Responders - Nonresponders	Control - ISSNHL* group
	p value	p value	p value	p value
Age	0,098	0,088	0,076	0,337
Gender	0,083	0,094	0,079	0,445
TSH	0,753	0,784	0,682	0,148
Free T4	0,382	0,003	0,412	0,007
Initial air conduction	0,001	0,001	0,06	0,001
Initial bone conduction	0,001	0,001	0,06	0,001
Last air conduction	0,208	0,001	0,017	0,001
Last bone conduction	0,704	0,001	0,024	0,001

Table 2: P values are showing comparison between the groups.

Discussion

In this study free T4 levels in sudden hearing loss patients who did not respond to treatment was found to be lower than in the control group. Furthermore evaluation of ISSNHL patients without dividing into subgroups , free T4 levels was also found to be lower than in the control group. From this it can be hypothesized that even with small variations of T4 levels hearing function can be affected.

The relationship between hearing and thyroid function has been identified in various studies. It has been reported that hearing function can be impaired in congenital and acquired hypothyroidism, endemic cretinism, pendred syndrome, and in patients resistant to thyroid hormone [8–11].

The relationship between thyroid hormone and hearing function dates back to the prenatal period. Thyroid hormone is necessary for the development of hearing function [9]. In the prenatal period organ of corti is quite sensitive to thyroid hormone at the maturation stage and lack of it can cause permanent hearing loss. Thyroid hormone increases the expression of genes that encode for thyroid hormone receptor [8]. Even though important proteins coded by these genes are present for the physiologic process and structural development of the inner ear [12] , the molecular mechanism behind permanent hearing loss due to hypothyroidism is still unknown (Figure 1).

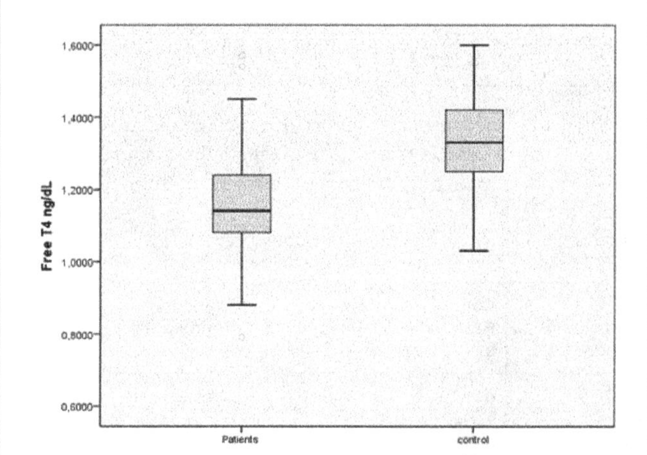

Figure 1: Mean free T4 values of ISSNHL patients and control groups.

Hearing function can be affected by both hyperfunction and hypofunction states of the thyroid gland. Oiticica et al. [13] did a cross sectional study where they studied for a period of 10 years the metabolic disorders of 166 patients diagnosed with sudden hearing loss. They reported that thyroid hormone levels were normal in 116 (78.4%) patients and abnormal in 32 (21.6%) patients. It is indicated in this study that abnormal thyroid hormone levels can be a risk factor for sudden hearing loss. Whereas in our study the effects of thyroid hormine levels on hearing and its prognosis in patients without any known risk factor including hyper-hypothyroidism was investigated and it was found that free T4 levels were lower in the group that did not respond to treatment than in the control group. Moreover even though free T4 levels were between the normally accepted reference range from the results in our study, the hypothesis that small variations in the level of this hormone can cause sudden hearing loss or can affect its prognosis comes to mind.

Through human and animal studies acute thyroid hormone deficiency states have been shown to result in changes in hearing function. Psaltakos et al. [14] used pure tone audiometry and transient evoked otoacoustic emission to record the hearing levels of 52 patients who had thyroidectomy operation before and 6-8 weeks after the operation. Levothyroxine was not administered to the patients and a follow up of thyroid stimulating hormone was done after the operation. Hearing levels increased in all the postoperative audiometric measurements and when otoacoustic measurements were compared before and after surgery, S/N ratio was found to be lower after surgery. Changes in the levels of thyroid hormone and its effects on hearing function in this study coincided with our thesis. However changes in free T4 levels of the groups in our study were neither determined to be acute nor chronic. This is because in our study even though thyroid hormone levels were within the normal reference range, hearing function can be affected by small variations in the level of free T4 and this should not be ignored. Contrary to this Mra and Wax [15] did not identify any changes on either audiogram or otoacoustic emission for a period of 6 weeks of acute decrease in thyroxin after total thryroidectomy operation. As for this study it was suggested that acute changes in thyroid hormone levels did not affect hearing function and therefore it was thought that chronic changes might be more effective.

Thyroid hormone level is an important prognostic factor as an etiology for sudden hearing loss. In a study done by Narozny et al. [16] high dose steroid treatment for 10 days, normal thyroid function tests, preserved labyrinth function and disease being diagnosed during spring season were taken to be positive progenostic factors. This study is supported by the fact that that there is a positive correlation between free T4 levels and response to treatment in our study. In a case-control study done by Nakashima et al. [17] 109 ISSNHL patients were evaluated and it was reported that sensitivity to cold, hypertension and history of thyroid disease were risk factors for sudden hearing loss. Just like in the last study even though patients in our study had euthyroidism it should be kept in mind that history of thyroid gland disease can be a risk factor for hearing loss. This is supported by the fact that 6 of the patients in our study had a history of thyroid disease.

At a glance the limitations of our study is it being a retrospective study and the number of patients being relatively small. Patients were not questioned on the possible risk factors and data was only obtained from evaluation of the patient files. A meaningful free T4 cut off value that can be used to predict the risks and prognosis of sudden hearing loss was not calculated.

Conclusion

Thyroid hormone level is an important factor for normal hearing function. Small variations in T4 levels can be a risk factor for ISSNHL even if the patient has euthyroidism and these changes can be either acute or chronic. To clear these uncertainties controlled prospective studies with wider patient population is required.

References

1. Hughes GB, Freedman MA, Haberkamp TJ, Guay ME (1996) Sudden sensorineural hearing loss. Otolaryngol Clin North Am 29: 393-405.
2. Wang Y, Zhang L, Zhang J, Zhang X, Zhang W, et al. (2016) The clinical analysis of bilateral successive sudden sensorineural hearing loss. Eur Arch Otorhinolaryngol .

3. Stachler RJ, Chandrasekhar SS, Archer SM, Rosenfeld RM, Schwartz SR, et al. (2012) Clinical practice guideline: Sudden hearing loss. Otolaryngol Head Neck Surg 146: S1-35.

4. Himelfarb MZ, Lakretz T, Gold S, Shanon E (1981) Auditory brain stem responses in thyroid dysfunction. J Laryngol Otol 95: 679-686.

5. Cordas EA, Ng L, Hernandez A, Kaneshige M, Cheng SY, et al. (2012) Thyroid hormone receptors control developmental maturation of the middle ear and the size of the ossicular bones. Endocrinology 153: 1548-1560.

6. Geptner EN (2014) [The hearing function in the patients presenting with congenital primary hypothyroidism]. Vestn Otorinolaringol 3: 32-34.

7. Brors D, Eickelmann AK, Gäckler A, Sudhoff H, Lautermann J, et al. (2008) [Clinical characterization of patients with idiopathic sudden sensorineural hearing loss]. Laryngorhinootologie 87: 400-405.

8. Wasniewska M, De Luca F, Siclari S, Salzano G, Messina MF, et al. Hearing loss in congenital hypothalamic hypothyroidism: A wide therapeutic window. Hear Res 172: 87-91.

9. Debruyne F, Vanderschueren-Lodeweyckx M, Bastijns P (1983) Hearing in congenital hypothyroidism. Audiology 22: 404-409.

10. Bhatia PL, Gupta OP, Agrawal MK, Mishr SK (1977) Audiological and vestibular function tests in hypothyroidism. Laryngoscope 87: 2082-2089.

11. Anand VT, Mann SB, Dash RJ, Mehra YN. Auditory investigations in hypothyroidism. Acta Otolaryngol 108: 83-87.

12. Karolyi IJ, Dootz GA, Halsey K, Beyer L, Probst FJ, et al. (2007) Dietary thyroid hormone replacement ameliorates hearing deficits in hypothyroid mice. Mamm Genome 18: 596-608.

13. Narozny W, Kuczkowski J, Mikaszewski B (2006) Thyroid dysfunction--underestimated but important prognostic factor in sudden sensorineural hearing loss. Otolaryngol Head Neck Surg 135: 995-996.

14. Psaltakos V, Balatsouras DG, Sengas I, Ferekidis E, Riga M, et al. (2013) Cochlear dysfunction in patients with acute hypothyroidism. Eur Arch Otorhinolaryngol 270: 2839-2848.

15. Mra Z, Wax MK (1999) Effects of acute thyroxin depletion on hearing in humans. Laryngoscope 109: 343-350.

16. Narozny W, Kuczkowski J, Kot J, Stankiewicz C, Sicko Z, et al. (2006) Prognostic factors in sudden sensorineural hearing loss: Our experience and a review of the literature 115: 553-558.

17. Nakashima T, Tanabe T, Yanagita N, Wakai K, Ohno Y (1997) Risk factors for sudden deafness: A case-control study. Auris Nasus Larynx 24: 265-270.

The Silent Sinus Syndrome: A Collaborative Approach between Rhinologists and Oculoplastics

Yaser Najaf[1*], **Abdulmohsen AlTerki**[2] **and Adel Al-Buluoshi**[3]

[1]*Zain & Al-Sabah Hospital, Al-Jabriyah, Kuwait*

[2]*Chairman of ENT College, Postgraduate Training, Kuwait Institute of Medical Specialization, Head of Unit &Consultant, ENT Department, Zain & Al-Sabah Hospitals, Kuwait*

[3]*Consultant Ophthalmologist and Oculoplastic and Reconstructive Surgery, Al-Bahar Eye Center, Kuwait*

[*]**Corresponding author:** Yaser Najaf, Zain & Al-Sabah Hospital, Al-Jabriyah, Kuwait; Email: yaser.najaf@gmail.com

Abstract

The Silent Sinus Syndrome (SSS) is a rare phenomenon originally described in 1964 by Montgomery, which often occurs unilaterally in the maxillary sinus with opacification and collapse. It is characterized by ipsilateral enophthalmos and hypoglobus or mistakenly as an exophthalmos of the contralateral eye. The pathophysiology is caused by obstruction of the ostiomeatal complex with subsequent maxillary sinus hypoventilation and development of negative intra-sinus pressure resulting in bony changes and sinus collapse. Radiographic evaluation by the mean of CT scan orbits and paranasal sinuses as well as nasal endoscopic examination are mandatory in diagnosing such cases. Treating such cases require a collaborative multidisciplinary approach to ensure the best possible results. In this case report, we discuss this rare phenomenon in terms of clinical presentation, clinical and radiological evaluation and conclude with the optimal treatment approach.

Keywords: Silent sinus syndrome; Enophthalmos; Hypoglobus; Ostiomeatal complex; Maxillary sinus

Introduction

Silent Sinus Syndrome (SSS) is a rare clinical disorder that is typically characterized as spontaneous, painless, progressive enopthalmos and hypoglobus. It results from downward bowing of the orbital floor secondary to maxillary sinus collapse, in the absence of any symptoms of sinonasal disease [1]. In 1964, Montgomery was the first to present and publish two cases of unilateral enopthalmos and hypoglobus associated with ipsilateral maxillary sinus collapse; however, SSS term was only used 30 years later by Soparkar and colleagues [1,2]. Interestingly, the term imploding antrum is another term used for silent sinus syndrome in literatures review [3]. Recent to this in 2008, Brandt and wright suggested SSS to be included under the general term of chronic maxillary atelectasis [4]. It has been noticed that increasing numbers of case reports were published on SSS recently, which could be explained by the widespread use of Computed Tomography (CT) and endoscopic interventions in diagnosing such cases. This case report will illustrate the clinical and the imaging features of this rare phenomenon. Our aim from this report is to emphasize in the collaborative approach required to manage such patients with this syndrome. Additionally, this report will highlight the significance of rare but not to be missed differential diagnosis in any unexplained enophthalmos, hypoglobus or even exphthalmos.

Case Report

A 47-year-old, previously healthy, Caucasian presented to the orbital and oculoplastic clinic complaining of 2 weeks duration of occasional binocular vertical diplopia associated with right eye exophthalmos. On further questioning the patient, he denied having pain, loss of vision, rhinorrhea or any history of facial trauma. Moreover, he denied any past ophthalmic or sino-nasal surgeries. Careful ophthalmic examination revealed his Best -Corrected Visual Acuity (BCVA) to be 20/25 of the Right Eye (RE) and 20/30 of the Left Eye (LE). Exophthalmometer measurement of the RE was 17 mm compared to 14 mm for the LE (3 mm difference) and facial asymmetry was noticed. Full ocular movements were intact with normal findings on anterior and posterior segments' examination. Initial diagnosis was RE exophthalmos; hence, thyroid function test was ordered with 3 weeks follow-up appointment given. The patient was seen in the follow-up visit but this time with new symptoms and complaints (Figure 1) as follow:

- More diplopia in primary gaze.
- Worse proptosis (4 mm) of the RE
- More pronounced facial asymmetry.
- Deep upper lid sulcus of the LE
- LE hypoglobus.

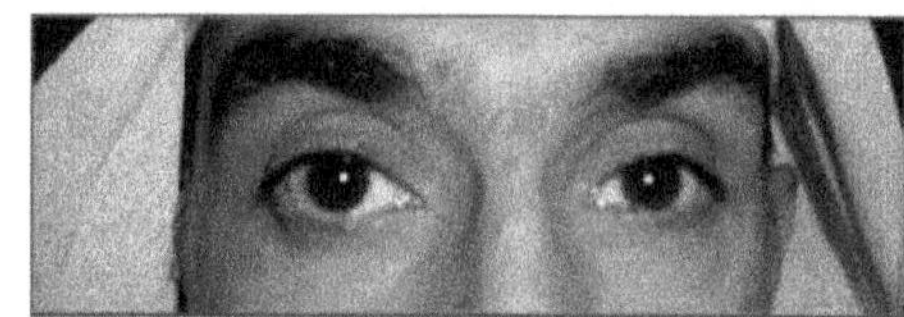

Figure 1: Follow-up visit symptoms and complaints

Consequently, axial and coronal CT scan images of the orbits and paranasal sinuses (Figures 2 and 3) were ordered. Radiological findings showed partial opacification of the left maxillary sinus with reduced maxillary sinus volume and ipsilateral globe prolapse associated with almost complete bony resorption of the left orbital floor. All of these findings were consistent with the diagnosis of Silent Sinus Syndrome.

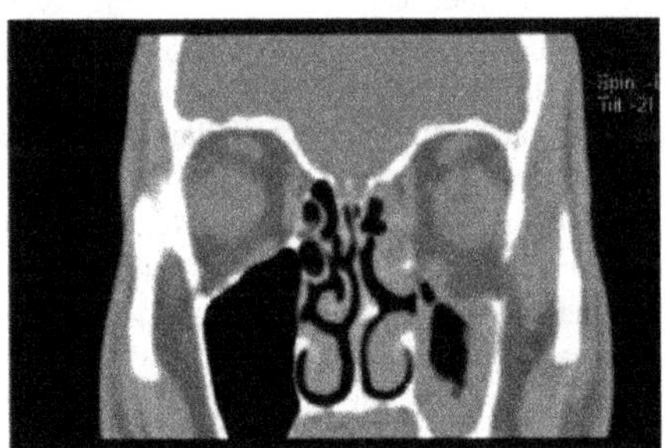

Figure 2: Axial and Coronal CT scan images of the orbits.

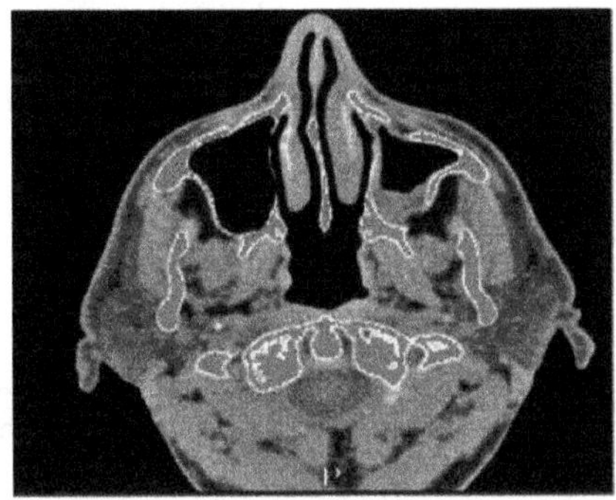

Figure 3: Axial and Coronal CT scan images of the paranasal sinuses

To ensure the best possible outcomes, the decision was made to do Combined Functional Endoscopic Sinus Surgery (FESS) with orbital floor reconstruction under the same anaesthesia and the same surgical table in a teamwork approach. FESS, in the form of uncinectomy and middle meatal antrostomy was performed. The left maxillary sinus was filled with secretions and polypoidal mucosa. Following the rhinologist's intervention, oculoplastic took over performing anterior orbitotomy via transconjuctival approach with lateral canthatomy-cantholysis. Due to significant orbital floor loss, a Synpor titanium mesh 43 mm (radius) X 15 mm was fashioned and implanted to support the globe inferiorly. The histopathological examination showed non-specific chronic inflammation within the sinus mucosa. Bacterial and fungal cultures were negative. The patient was followed up for 12 months and showed dramatic improvement of the initially reported symptoms and signs. The patient reported no diplopia and thorough ophthalmic examination revealed good restoration of the upper lid sulcus with no signs of enopthalmos or hypoglobus (Figures 4 and 5) show almost normal maxillary sinus volume with restored orbital architecture supported by the titanium mesh implant in the left orbital floor.

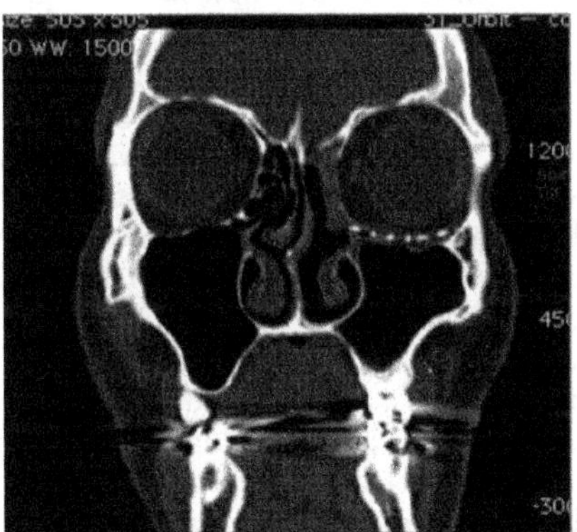

Figure 4: Maxillary sinus volume with restored orbital architecture

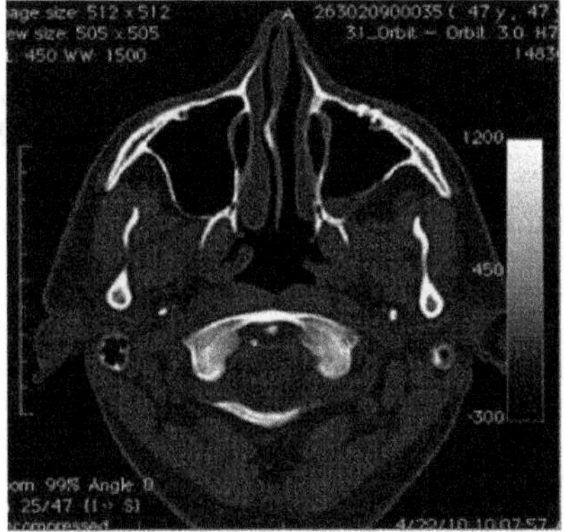

Figure 5: Maxillary sinus volume with restored orbital architecture supported by the titanium mesh implant in the left orbital floor

Discussion

Upon reviewing literatures, several case reports have explained different presentations of this phenomenon; however, they all shared the combination of enophthalmos and hypoglobus in the presenting complaint. Due to its insidious course of presentation with no linked past history; SSS poses diagnostic challenge to otolaryngologists, ophthalmologists as well as general practitioners. When Soparkar et al. published his observations of SSS; only 30% of the cases had past history of sinus disease in childhood [5]. SSS is found to affect adults between the third and the fifth decades of life with no gender variation [4]. Additionally, experts of this phenomenon have found no association between smoking, alcohol consumption and genetics with the development of this rare syndrome [6]. The most common reported complaint to an ophthalmologist is changes to the facial appearance experienced by the patient or noticed by friends or family members [7]. It presents typically as unilateral asymmetry and can be sometimes misinterpreted as exophthalmos of the contralateral eye. According to Stevens et al. [3], approximately 50% of patients with enophthalmos are initially referred to ophthalmologists for investigations of contralateral exophthalmos or ptosis. Other presenting symptoms include lid lag, lagophthalmos, oscillopsia and transient vertical diplopia [8]. While enophthalmos is present in all cases, diplopia occurs in about one - quarter and it is typically vertical and painless [7,9]. These orbital symptoms can suggest a possible neuro-opthalmic disorder; however, the presence of enophthalmos with hypoglobus in previously healthy patients will narrow the differential diagnosis towards Silent sinus syndrome. In order to diagnose SSS; other causes that might present with similar symptoms must be ruled out first such as Horner's syndrome, facial hemiatrophy, developmental anomalies or any past history of facial trauma [10]. In our case, the history was negative for the mentioned above disorders and his endocrine and autoimmune markers were negative too. Many theories have explained the pathophysiological process of this disease with varying degrees of evidence in literature. Gillman et al. in 1999 described the most acceptable theory behind the disease process [11]. Gillman et al. suggested that in SSS patients, obstruction of the Ostio Meatal Complex (OMC) leads into hypoventilation of the maxillary sinus with the subsequent development of intra-sinus negative pressure and thinning of the sinus wall. This chronically causes remodeling and bone resorption of the orbital floor causing malposition of the ipsilateral eye. Although this theory is widely accepted among observers of this phenomenon; however, no one yet knows the reason behind OMC obstruction [4]. Radiographic evaluation by the mean of CT scan orbits and paranasal sinuses is crucial to assess the anatomy of orbito-maxillary sinus structure and is mandatory upon labeling patients with such a disease.

Diagnosis	Value
Enopthalmos	ranging from 1-6mm
Hypoglobus	ranging from 0 -6mm
Lid retraction Deeping of superior sulcus Exophthalmos	mistakenly diagnosed

Table 1: Shows most clinical manifestations of SSS.

CT scan findings show opacification (complete or partial) of the maxillary sinus and collapse with inferior bowing of the orbital floor towards affected maxillary sinus [12]. Cobb et al. further explains CT scan findings by linking the pathophysiological process to the radiological findings, 'the maxillary sinus roof loses its normal upward convexity and the orbital floor is bowed downwards giving the appearance of reduced sinus volume with increased orbital volume'. This orbital volume expansion causes horizontal displacement of the eye level appearing as hypoglobus. Treating such cases require a collaborative multidisciplinary approach to ensure the best possible results. It involves the input of rhinology, oculoplastics as well as anesthesia with the availability of good nursing team in the operating theatre. Treatment from the otolaryngology points of view is aimed in restoring drainage and maintaining good aeration of the occluded maxillary sinus. Traditionally, the Caldwell-Luc procedure used to be the gold standard in treating such cases; however, this has been complicated by adhesions that cause stagnation of mucus clearance with re-obstruction of the maxillary sinus outlet [13]. Nowadays this approach was replaced by performing endoscopic maxillary antrostomy and uncinectomy with the aim of enlarging the maxillary ostium [10]. In many cases where the bony orbital floor is intact, the ENT intervention will be sufficient in restoring the sinus obstruction as well as orbital misalignment associated with ipsilaterally. Some publishers argue that it is advised to do Functional Endoscopic Sinus Surgery (FESS), then use the approach of 'wait and see' for few months to assess the need for oculoplastic intervention [14]. However, in our case, due to the extensive bony resportion of the left orbital floor with the poor inferior support of the orbital globe seen in the CT scan (Figures 2 and 3), the decision was made to do combined FESS with orbital floor repair. According to Cobb et al. reconstruction can be simultaneous or delayed to reduce the risk of visual loss or infection. Nevertheless, our combined approach yielded in rapid alleviation of symptoms as well as symmetrical cosmetic outcomes reported by our patient. When surgical intervention is required, otolaryngologists take over firstly to perform FESS then oculoplastic surgeons involve in intervening with orbital floor. The use of titanium mesh fixed with Leibinger screws is the preferred material in reconstructing and maintaining the normal orbital architecture, classically through transconjunctival or external lower lid approaches [4,15]. Again, it is important to emphasis that the decision to perform both combined procedures should take the teamwork approach with the patient's view took in great consideration while weighing up the risks and benefits of such a decision.

Conclusion

Silent sinus syndrome is rare and often misdiagnosed pathology with a unilateral progressive and asymptomatic collapse of the maxillary sinus. The pathogenesis is not completely understood but appears to result from maxillary sinus collapse due to acquired obstruction of the maxillary sinus drainage. CT scan is usually required for a definite diagnosis. Treatment of such a disease consists of restoration of maxillary sinus aeration and reconstruction of the orbital floor in case needed. Any unexplained enophthalmos especially if associated with hypoglobus should hint for silent sinus syndrome as a differential diagnosis.

References

1. Soparkar CN, Patrinely JR, Cuaycong MJ, Dailey RA, Kersten RC, et al. (1994) The silent sinus syndrome. A cause of spontaneous enophthalmos. Ophthalmology 101: 772-778.
2. Montgomery Ww (1964) Mucocele of the Maxillary Sinus Causing Enophthalmos. Eye Ear Nose Throat Mon 43: 41-44.
3. Stevens K, Omer S, Toocaram B, Rich P, Almemar A (2010) The imploding antrum syndrome: an unusual cause of double vision. Pract Neurol 10: 101-104.
4. Cobb AR, Murthy R, Cousin GC, El-Rasheed A, Toma A, et al. (2012) Silent sinus syndrome. Br J Oral Maxillofac Surg 50: e81-85.
5. Hobbs CG, Saunders MW, Potts MJ (2004) Spontaneous enophthalmos: silent sinus syndrome. J Laryngol Otol 118: 310-312.
6. Wang XR, Zhao XD (2004) Secondary silent sinus syndrome: case report. Chin Med J (Engl) 117: 785-786.
7. Numa WA, Desai U, Gold DR, Heher KL, Annino DJ (2005) Silent sinus syndrome: a case presentation and comprehensive review of all 84 reported cases. Ann Otol Rhinol Laryngol 114: 688-694.
8. Borruat FX, Jaques B, Durig J (1999) Transient vertical diplopia and silent sinus disorder. J Neuroophthalmol 19: 173-175.
9. Rose GE, Sandy C, Hallberg L, Moseley I (2003) Clinical and radiologic characteristics of the imploding antrum, or "silent sinus," syndrome. Ophthalmology 110: 811-818.
10. Bossolesi P, Autelitano L, Brusati R, Castelnuovo P (2008) The silent sinus syndrome: diagnosis and surgical treatment. Rhinology 46: 308-316.
11. Gillman GS, Schaitkin BM, May M (1999) Asymptomatic enophthalmos: the silent sinus syndrome. Am J Rhinol 13: 459-462.
12. Bahgat M, Bahgat Y, Bahgat A (2012) Silent sinus syndrome. BMJ Case Rep 2012.
13. Blackwell KE, Goldberg RA, Calcaterra TC (1993) Atelectasis of the maxillary sinus with enophthalmos and midface depression. Ann Otol Rhinol Laryngol 102: 429-432.

The Effect of Novel Combination Therapy with Azelastine Hydrochloride and Fluticasone Propionate in Allergic Rhinitis

Amtul Salam Sami[1*], **Nida Ahmed**[2] **and Sabahat Ahmed**[3]

[1]*ENT and Allergy department, Royal National Throat, Nose and Ear Hospital, UK*

[2]*Acute Medicine, Ealing Hospital, UK*

[3]*Guys, Kings College and St Thomas's School of Medical Education, King's College, UK*

[*]**Corresponding author:** Amtul Salam Sami, MBBS, BSc, ODTC, MCPS, MA, M.Sc., ENT and Allergy department, Royal National Throat, Nose and Ear Hospital, UK; E-mail: amtul_salam@hotmail.com

Abstract

Background: Allergic rhinitis is a prevalent condition in the community and impairs quality of life. Treatment often requires combination of different topical treatment. We wanted to assess the effect of combination steroid and antihistamine nasal spray in patients who have failed primary therapy. Secondary aims were to analyse the multi-domain impact of rhinitis, financial costs incurred and impact on quality of life.

Method: We analysed fifty-three patients who were referred to the specialist hospital having failed primary care treatment for nasal and sinus disease. The MSNOT-20 is a disease specific validated questionnaire to identify rhinitis and its response to treatment. Patients were re-assessed following one month of treatment use. Skin prick testing and nasal inspiratory peak flow were also used.

Results: All subjects had improvement in their symptoms following treatment (31.6 (10.69) vs. 11 (4.18)-mean and standard deviation before and after treatment respectively, $p<0.05$). There was improvement in each subgroup, statistically significant in all except the emotional subgroup. Common allergens identified in sufferers were grass, house dust mite and tree pollen. The majority of patients were in the working age bracket and 90% had to take time off work due to their symptoms.

Conclusion: There is significant impact on quality of life and education/work-based complications of rhinitis. Combination intranasal steroid with intranasal antihistamine is effective at improving symptomatology of allergic rhinitis, this was also demonstrated through patient comments. MSNOT-20 is once again proven as a useful tool in detecting rhinitis, its impact and disease response to treatment.

Keywords: Allergic rhinitis; Questionnaire; Nasal sprays; Intranasal; Fluticasone propionate; Azelastine hydrochloride

Background

Seasonal allergic rhinitis, or hay fever as it is also known, is a prevalent condition effecting 1 in 4 persons in the UK [1,2], in fact it is becoming increasingly common especially in developed countries [3-5]. Rhinitis itself means inflammation of the nasal mucous membrane and often precedes sinusitis (inflammation of the lining of the paranasal sinuses), it is rare for sinusitis to occur without coexisting rhinitis and as such the most appropriate term for both is rhinosinusitis [6,7].

Allergic rhinitis has been found to be one of the commonest causes of presentation to primary care [8], causing nasal congestion, rhinorrhea, itching and/or sneezing. Allergic rhinoconjucntivitis is the associated watery eyes, itching, burning/irritability, redness and injection of the conjunctiva which has been documented in 71% of European patients who concurrently had nasal symptoms [9].

Skin prick testing (SPT) has been shown to be superior to patient-reported allergen identification or allergens as identified on allergy history take [10]. One meta-analysis reported that on SPT the top three allergens identified in 15 developed countries (covering Europe including the UK, USA and Australia) were house dust mite, grass pollen and cat (median prevalence across all centres 21.7%, 16.9% and 8.8%, respectively) [11].

Allergic rhinitis has been shown to be a risk factor for developing asthma, often preceding it, in fact it has been shown that optimal management of allergic rhinitis may improve coexisting asthma control [12-14]. Rhinitis has also been shown to affect quality of life as well as impacting on education and productivity. The British Society of Allergy and Clinical Immunology (BSACI) have developed a pathway for the treatment of Rhinitis, adapted in Figure 1 [15,16].

One meta-analysis looked into the role of intranasal corticosteroids in patients with allergic rhinitis (n=2,267) and showed that it provides significantly greater relief of nasal congestion than oral antihistamines [17]. It is, however, combination therapy which has proven to not only improve symptomatology but also be found to be more convenient and effective when used by patients [18-20].

The MSNOT-20 is a validated, disease specific questionnaire (Appendix 1) which can identify rhinitis and rhinosinusitis, its associated impact on quality of life and disease response to treatment in the adult population, its modified version has proven similar qualities in the paediatric/young person's population of 11-16 year old [1].

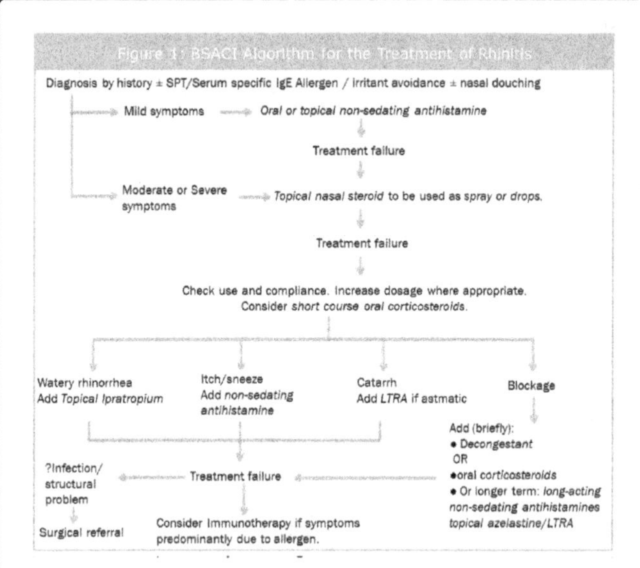

Figure 1: BSACI algorithm for the treatment of rhinitis.

The primary aim of this study is to assess the effect of combination nasal spray (azelastine hydrochloride and fluticasone propionate) on disease in patients who have failed primary therapy in the GP setting. Secondary aims include evaluation of the cost of disease to patients and impact on quality of life, relationship between the different subgroups defined by MSNOT-20 questionnaire and comparison between allergic and non-allergic rhinitis.

Methods

Inclusion criteria- patients being referred from their GP to the ENT and Allergy department at Royal National Throat, Nose and Ear hospital, London due to nasal and sinus symptoms. These patients showed no response to optimal primary care treatment along the Figure 1 algorithm or practice-specific guidelines. Participants were enrolled in a four-month period, February-May 2016.

Exclusion criteria- patients with nasal polyposis

The tool used was the MSNOT-20 questionnaire which has been proven to be diagnostic for rhinitis [1]. It consists of three sections; section one comprises of demographic details, section two is the disease specific section and section three is the quality of life section. Its disease specific section is split into subgroups each of which is composed of the following questions from this section:

Nasal: questions 1, 2, 3, 19

Paranasal: 5, 6, 7, 8, 9, 10-can be further split into the below for further analysis

Sinus: 5, 6, 10

Ear: 7, 8, 9

Sleep: 11, 12, 13,14

Social: 15, 16, 17

Emotional: 18, 20

On first presentation to clinic patients had a full clinical assessment, completed the MSNOT-20 questionnaire and, if relevant, had skin prick test and nasal inspiratory peak flow. The management plan including pharmaceutical option was discussed; if eligible and clinically appropriate (using treatment guidelines and clinical experience) treatment was advised with the aforementioned combination nasal spray and, following informed consent, initiated as per manufacturers guidelines; 1 spray in each nostril twice a day in those over 12 years. Where needed patient information leaflet (Appendix 2) and clinical demonstration of the correct technique when using a nasal spray was discussed.

As this particular brand combination was initially not available at the index hospital a GP prescription was provided. After four weeks, patients were asked to repeat section two of the MSNOT-20 questionnaire again, results were sent back to the researchers.

Data was collated, statistical analysis was carried out and the results were represented through bar charts, graphs and tables.

Results

There were 53 eligible subjects in this study, 30 women 3 of whom had been pregnant within the last 12 months. The age range was 18-78 years with 83% of patients between 18-65 years of age; just under thirty percent of these were between the ages of 18-30, breakdown in Graph 1.

The majority of subjects described themselves as Caucasian/white, the ethnicity was distributed as shown in Graph 2.

Forty-nine percent of subjects were employed with occupations including office workers, banking staff, media industry and more. Thirteen percent were retired, eight percent were students, nine were housewives whilst the remaining were either unemployed or did not disclose their occupation.

Only 44 of the 53 had analysable responses to the question on accommodation. The majority lived in a house or bungalow, 33 of the 44, whilst the remaining 11 lived in a flat or maisonette.

Of the cohort eleven percent were current smokers, ranging from 1 to 20 cigarettes per day. The remaining had no smoking history and only one person did not answer the question.

Subjects were asked about family history of potentially atopic disease, as shown in Graphs 3a-3d. Statistical analysis showed that, in this sample, there was no significant correlation between symptom severity and family history of asthma/eczema/food allergy/hay fever, $p>0.1$.

The total MSNOT-20 score is the sum of the symptom severity rating from each of the 20 disease specific questions in section 2 of the questionnaire. There was a statistically significant ($p<0.05$) decrease in the total MSNOT-20 score following treatment, Graph 4 shows the improvement in total MSNOT-20 score after treatment for each subject whilst Graph 5 represents the overall mean and standard deviations for before and after treatment groups.

There was a statistically significant improvement following treatment in all subgroups except emotional, shown in Graph 6 and Table 1. Histograms 1a-1e show the proportion of the difference within the subgroup following treatment.

Subgroup	Before treatment Mean (Standard deviation)	After treatment Mean (Standard deviation)	P value
Nasal	17.49 (2.02)	6.72 (1.99)	P<0.05
Paranasal	7.91 (3.61)		2.62 (1.66)
Sleep	2.81 (3.80)	0.40 (1.23)	P<0.05
Social	1.04 (2.50)	0.11 (0.61)	P<0.05
Emotional	0.55 (1.35)	0.19 (0.56)	P=0.08

Table 1: Mean and standard deviation for each subgroup before and after treatment, with statistical significance. Each subgroup was composed of the following questions from section 2 of the MSNOT-20 questionnaire: Nasal: 1, 2, 3, 19; Paranasal: 5, 6, 7, 8, 9, 10; Sleep: 11, 12, 13,14; Social: 15, 16, 17; Emotional: 18, 20.

Correlation of the different subgroups using Spearman rank showed that the total MSNOT-20 score correlated most strongly with the nasal subgroup (R=0.5117, n=53, p<0.05). Subsequently the nasal group had strong correlation with paranasal (R=0.3868, p<0.05), sleep (R=0.3126, p<0.05) and social scores (R=0.3247, p<0.05). Emotional subgroup was seen to correlate strongest with the paranasal subgroup (R=0.4702, p<0.05).

Subjects were asked to highlight the most important symptoms for them, they were allowed to choose a maximum of 5 and their responses have been shown in Graph 7. The top 3 symptoms which patients ranked the highest were; need to blow the nose, ear pain and blocked nose.

When asked about duration of symptoms, everyone had had symptoms for more than 6 weeks, further breakdown shown in Graph 8. All patients had received treatment by the GP, just under half (24/53) had to consultant their GP 3 or more times (maximum number of consultation were 6). Thirty of the fifty-three patients enrolled also sought help from their Chemist whilst 4/53 had also tried alternative therapies. Forty percent had seen an Ear, Nose and Throat specialist in the past.

The types of treatment that patients had received have been outlined in Graph 9, however one third of patients (18/53) said that the treatment did not "work in any way" for their symptomatology.

Fifty-one percent of people used their treatment on most days. Twenty-six percent used their treatment once or twice a day whilst 17% used it once or twice a week. The remaining 6% only used their treatment once or twice a year. The financial burden on patients was significant. Sixty percent of patients spent between £5-£20 every month on treatment with 9% saying they had to spend more than £20 in a month, the highest monthly cost of treatment quoted by this cohort was £50.

Of all those enrolled onto the study, 17% had previously had an operation on their nose. Though their total MSNOT-20 score was, on average, higher than their counterparts who had not previously had a nose operation, this was not statistically significant (p=0.2).

Their symptoms meant that 90% of subjects (46 of the 51 analysable responses) had to take time off work or education because of their nose/sinus symptoms, with the numbers of days taken off ranging from between 2-15, breakdown shown in Graph 10.

Fifty-nine percent of subjects (31/53) had a positive skin prick test (SPT), 9 were negative on SPT and the remaining 15 subjects were not eligible for testing according to their initial referral, as per Trust protocol. The allergens patients were sensitive to are shown in Graph 11.

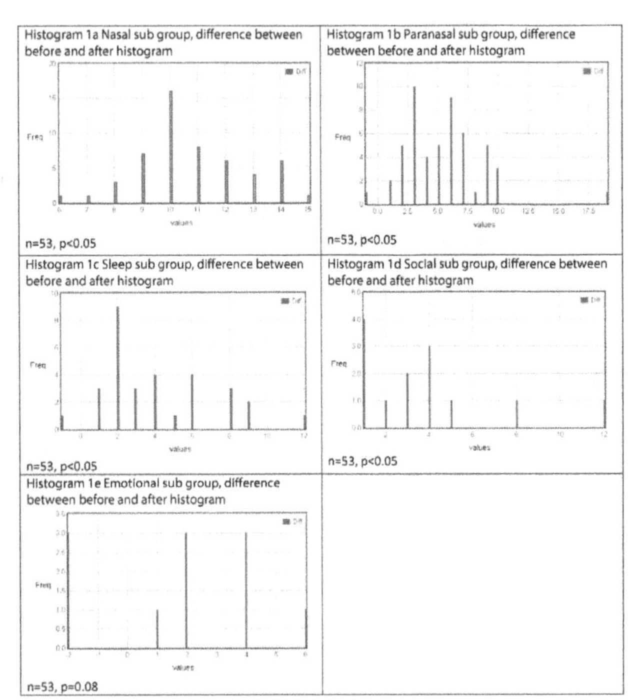

Histogram 1a-1e: Difference in before and after treatment values for each subgroup.

Treatment has been shown to be effective at improving symptomatology in each subgroup and the total MSNOT-20 score of all patients who had allergic rhinitis, as shown in Graphs 12a-12f, all of which were statistically significant except emotional subgroup.

A comparison of scores between skin prick test positive and negative, i.e., allergic and non-allergic patients, shown in Graph 13, showed that allergic patients had worse total MSNOT-20 score and also more severe symptomatology in all domains, however this was not deemed statistically significant, p>0.2.

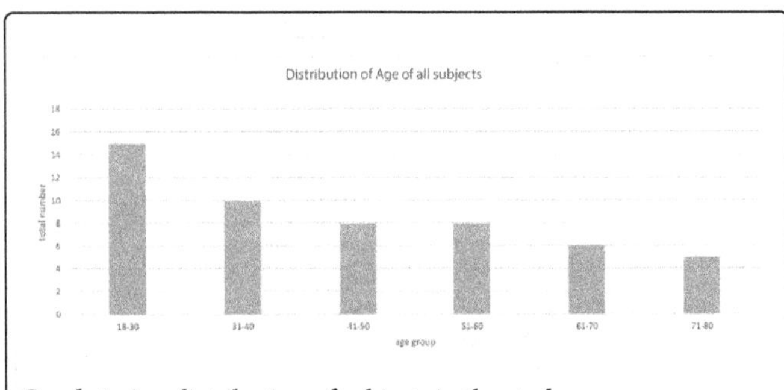

Graph 1: Age distribution of subjects in the study.

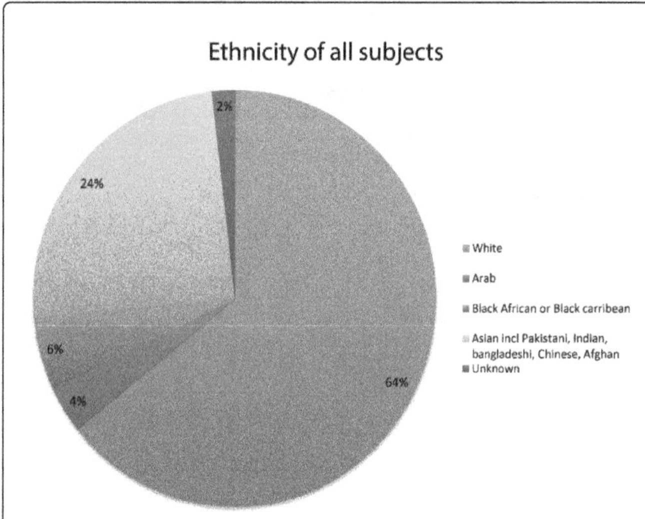

Graph 2: Ethnic distribution of subjects in the study.

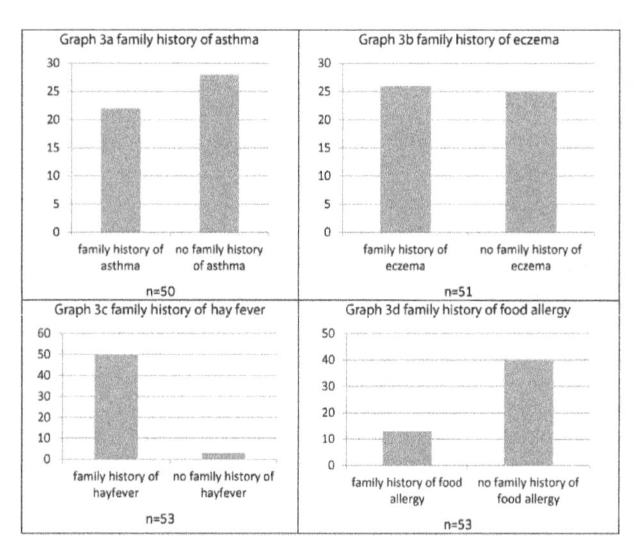

Graph 3a-3d: Family history of asthma, eczema, hay fever and food allergy respectively.

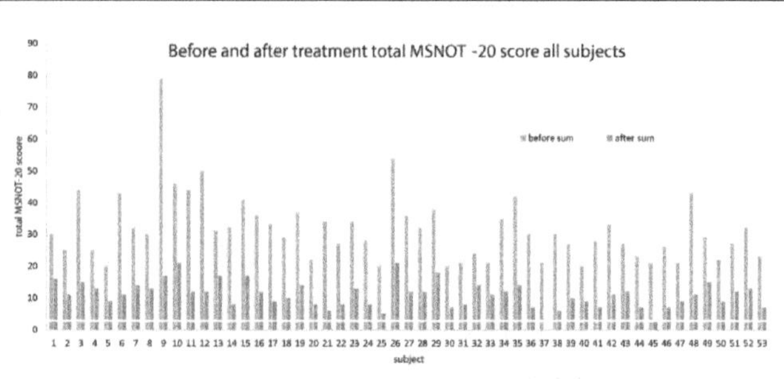

Graph 4: Total msnot-20 score before and after treatment for each individual.

The nasal inspiratory peak flow was analysable in 28 people, of which 61% had an abnormal reading. Unfortunately, there were not enough valid samples to analyse the peak flow values of patients.

Patients were asked to comment, should they wish, following one-month use of the spray. The following excerpts are quoted here, with consent:

One patient describing his condition in his own words prior to treatment: "very debilitating and persistent problem"

The following are the positive comments of using the therapy:

"very beneficial", the patient subsequently wrote how he has stopped using other non-steroidal symptomatic treatments

"having a positive effect on my allergy symptoms. It feels noticeably clear when (I) breath and the swelling seems to have subsided"

"quite effective and helped me a lot going through the spring hay fever season…it has also helped (in) improving my breathing condition… I would like to keep on taking 'Dymista' "

"was far more effective than [market competitor trade names quoted]"

"my nasal passages felt clearer and unblocked and the post nasal drip seems diminished"

A couple of patients mentioned the side effect they noted:

"the taste it leaves in my mouth…perhaps a more natural taste would give more confidence to me and others taking your medicine"

"the worst part was the taste"

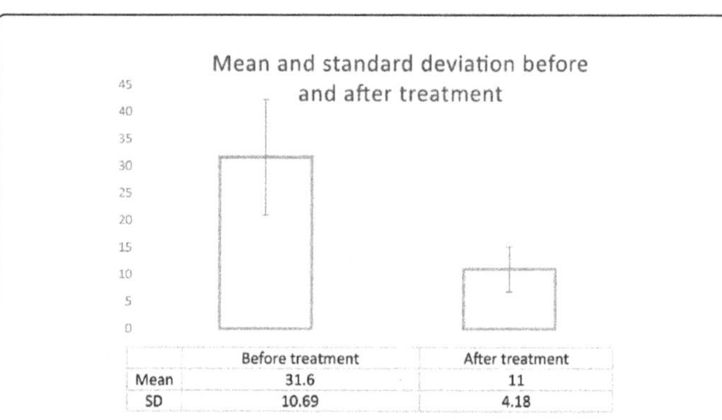

	Before treatment	After treatment
Mean	31.6	11
SD	10.69	4.18

Graph 5: Mean and standard deviation (SD) before and after treatment.

Discussion

This treatment can significantly improve symptomatology in those suffering with allergic rhinitis, improving both the total MSNOT-20 score and that of each of the five subgroups, however this is not statistically significant in the emotional subgroup, which maybe as a consequence of the reduced prevalence of these symptoms before treatment in our cohort.

The correlations between the total disease severity score and different subgroups were analysed, please note that the closer the correlation score is to 1, the stronger relationship [21]. Our study showed that the total MSNOT-20 score correlates strongest with the nasal subgroup implying how effective and targeted treatment at the nose can have a huge influence on the disease severity as a whole. In itself the nasal subgroup correlates with the paranasal (its strongest relationship) followed by sleep then social. This proves that vast impact that nasal symptoms have on different domains of a person's health. We found that emotional score was strongest associated with the paranasal subgroup highlighting this lesser recognised impact of dysfunction of the air sinus's and ear symptoms.

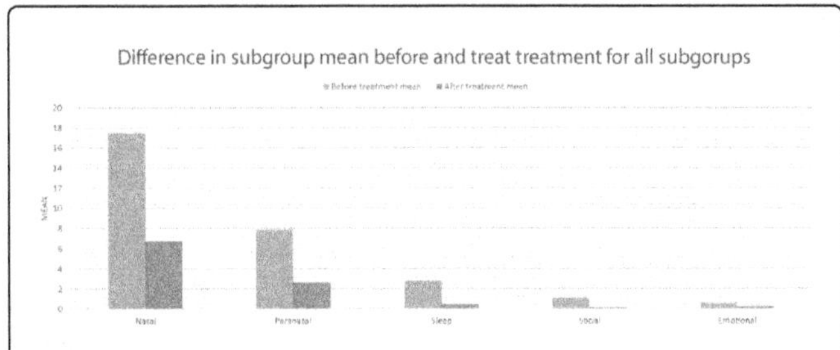

Graph 6: Comparison of improvement in all subgroups before and after treatment.

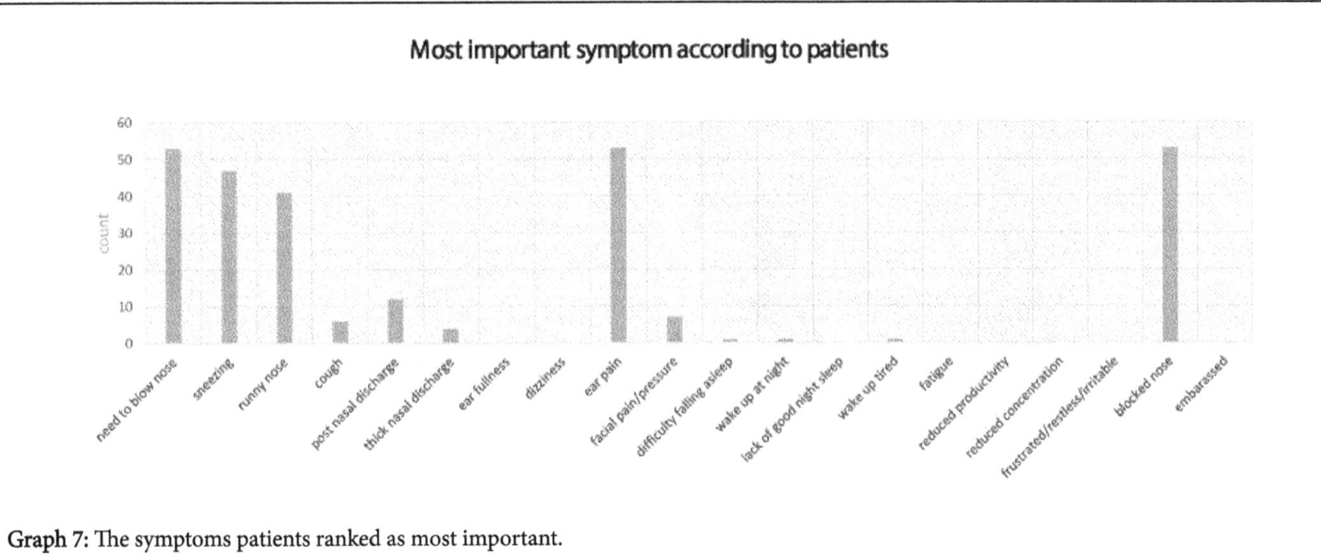

Graph 7: The symptoms patients ranked as most important.

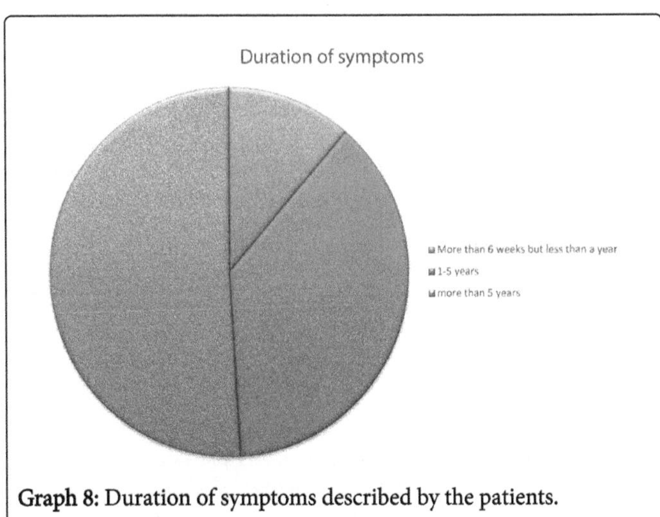

Graph 8: Duration of symptoms described by the patients.

We identified the top three allergens as grass, house dust mite and tree pollen which is similar to those found in a large international meta-analysis whose top three were house dust mite, grass and cat [11]. This shows that a significant number of our patients, hence indicative of the referrals to hospital received, suffer from allergic rhinitis and the need for effective treatment in our patients. In fact, we saw how allergic rhinitis patients had a worse severity score in each domain and in their total score also though this wasn't deemed statistically significant.

Our study supported the evidence that allergic rhinitis is a significant cause of presentation to the GP [8]. In our cohort all patients had consulted their GP about their condition with some having up to 6 consultations about their nasal and sinus symptoms. This condition is also a burden on specialist care services with 40% of our cohort having previously seen an Ear, Nose and Throat specialist prior to enrolment in this study.

It is interesting to note that 1 in 10 of our patients were current smokers. Smoking has been shown to be associated with high prevalence of chronic rhinitis at a dose dependant effect [22]. Even though we were not able to identify its correlation with symptom severity presently, this highlights the need to promote greater patient education and support in smoking cessation initiatives.

This study shows how sufferers are reduced to having to take time off work due to the nasal and/or sinus symptoms and as the majority of our cohort is within the working age bracket, this has significant consequences for both the individual and economy as a whole. This is not the only financial consequence, indeed 60% of patients had to spend £5-£20 a month on treatment with almost one in ten paying £20 or more per month, combine this with the fact that all the patients had had their symptoms for more than 6 weeks, hence unlikely acute infection, with the maximum duration of time quoted as >5 years, this proves the huge burden rhinitis has on its sufferers. It is also important to note that a third of patients said that the treatment they took did not work for them. Subsequent treatment with combination nasal spray was then proven to improve their symptoms and has been found in previous studies to be more convenient and effective when used by patients [18-20].

The top three symptoms that patients rated as the most troublesome were need to blow the nose, ear pain and blocked nose which shows the significance nasal symptoms have in the subjective disease experience, previous studies [15] have also proven how nasal disease impacts on quality of life including social limitation, time off school and reduced work productivity.

This study once again proved the useful tool of the MSNOT-20 in research into Rhinitis in identifying disease, quantifying its impact in different domains of health and health related quality of life and measuring response to treatment in all these domains.

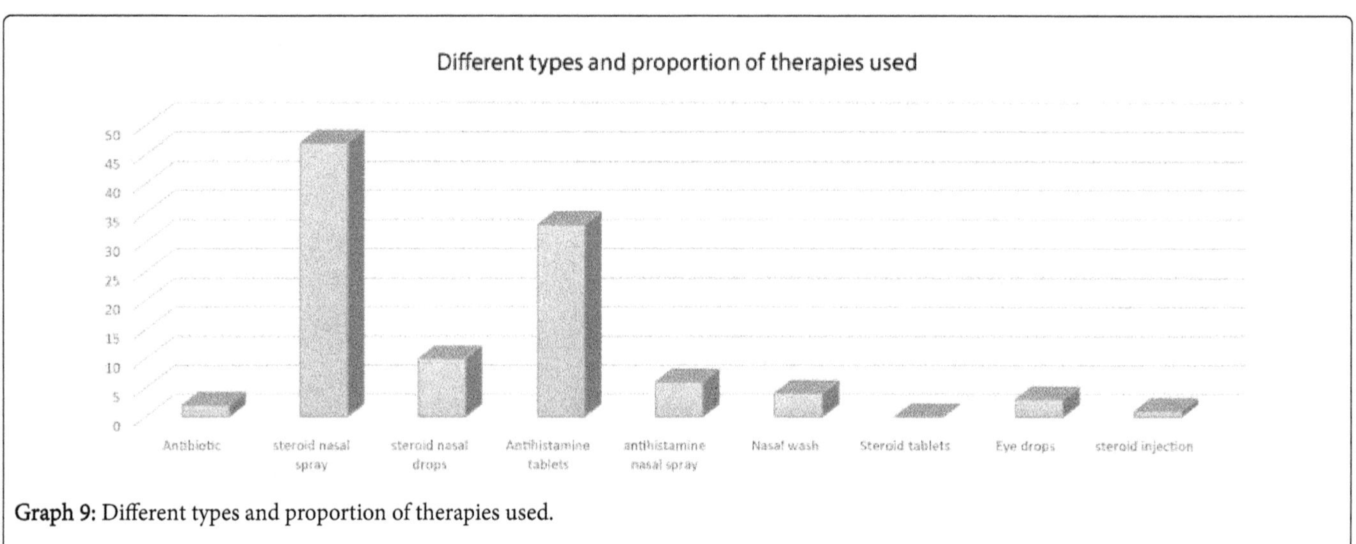

Graph 9: Different types and proportion of therapies used.

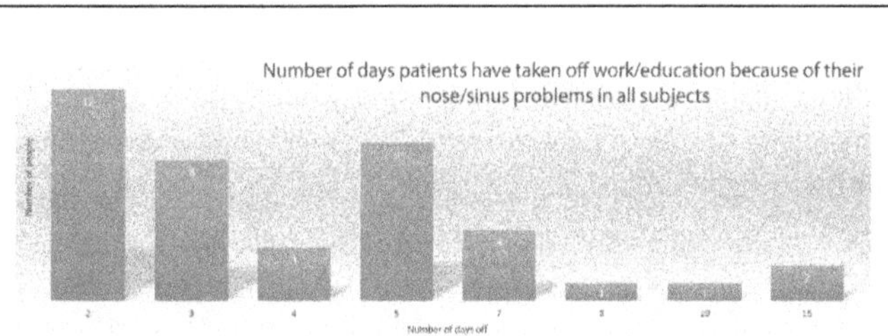

Graph 10: Number of days patients have had to take off work/ college/university because of your nose/sinus symptoms.

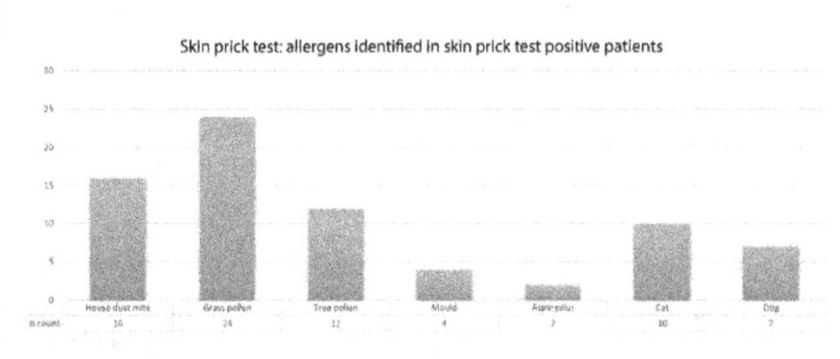

Graph 11: Allergens patients were positive to on skin prick testing.

Conclusion

This study has shown that combination of intranasal steroid with intranasal antihistamine in one novel spray improves symptoms of those suffering from allergic rhinitis in patients who have failed conventional primary care therapy. Patients felt this improvement and commented positively to this effect.

This study has also shown that rhinitis impairs quality of life, negatively impacting on education and/or work leading to patients taking up to 15 sick days as well as incurring significant financial cost.

The MSNOT-20 has been proven to be a quick, effective and reliable tool for exploring rhinitis, its effect on quality of life and having a multi-domain assessment of response to treatment.

Conflict of Interest

A.S.S received a financial grant from Meda Pharmaceuticals. Meda Pharmaceuticals had no role in study design, collection, analysis, interpretation of data, writing the report or decision to submit for publication.

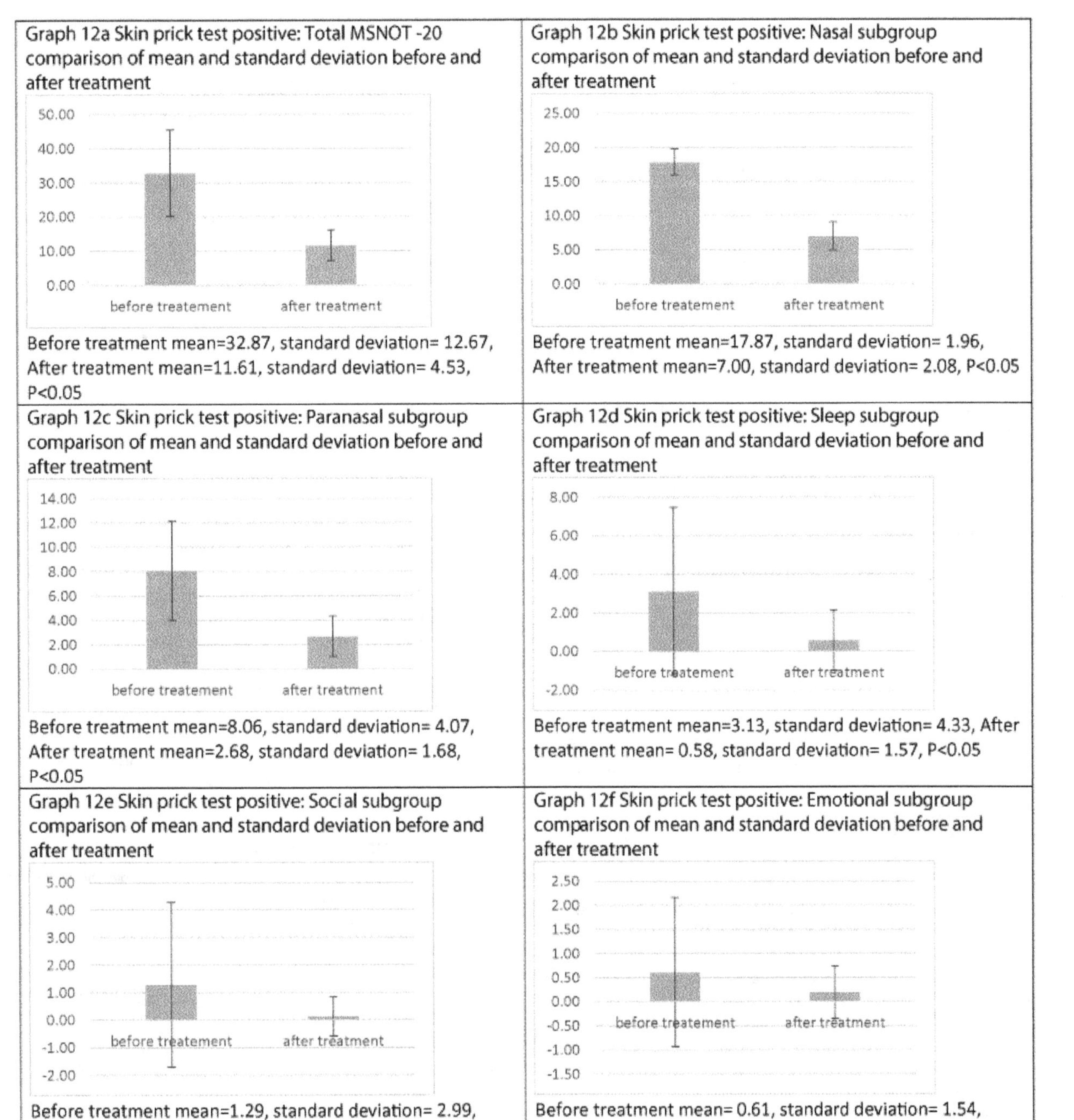

Graph 12: Skin prick test positive.

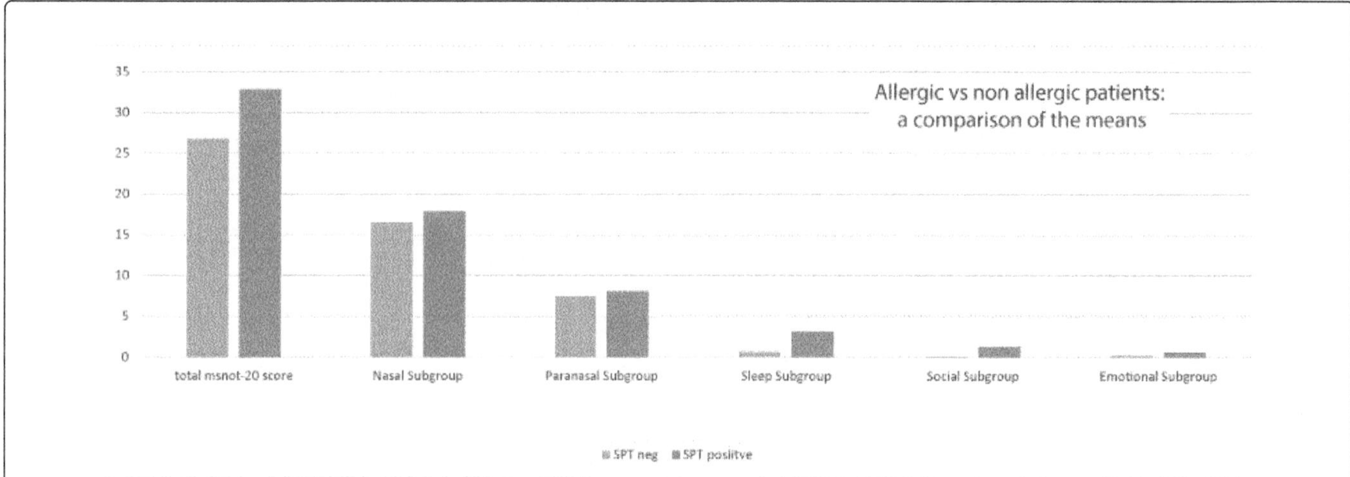

Graph 13: A comparison of the means of each subgroup and total msnot-20 score of skin prick test (SPT) positive and negative patients, allergic and non-allergic, respectively.

Acknowledgement

We would like to thank Dr Peter Nightingale, Statistician, University of Birmingham, for his help in the statistical analysis.

References

1. Sami A (2010) Epidemiology of rhinitis in secondary school children using MSYPQ and comparison with modified SNOT-20 used in adult community based survey. European Academy of Allergy and Clinical Immunology 25.
2. Kariyawasam HH, Scadding GK (2010) Seasonal allergic rhinitis: Fluticasone propionate and fluticasone furoate therapy evaluated. J Asthma Allergy 3: 19-28.
3. Emanuel M (1995) Hay fever, a post industrial revolution epidemic: A history of its growth during the 19th century. Clinical & Experimental Allergy 18: 295-304.
4. Strachan D (1995) Epidemiology of hay fever: Towards a community diagnosis. Clinical & Experimental Allergy 25: 296-303.
5. von Mutius E, Weiland SK, Fritzsch C, Duhme H, Keil U (1998) Increasing prevalence of hay fever and atopy among children in Leipzig, East Germany. Lancet 351: 862-866.
6. Fokkens W, Lund V, Mullol J (2007) European position paper on rhinosinusitis and nasal polyps group (2007) European position paper on rhinosinusitis and nasal polyps. Rhinol Suppl 1-136.
7. Lanza DC, Kennedy DW (1997) Adult rhinosinusitis defined. Otolaryngol Head Neck Surg 117: S1-7.
8. Bousquet J, Khaltaev N, Cruz AA, Denburg J, Fokkens WJ, et al. (2008) Allergic rhinitis and its impact on asthma (ARIA) 2008 update (in collaboration with the World Health Organization, GA(2)LEN and AllerGen). Allergy 63 Suppl 86: 8-160.
9. Canonica G, Bousquet J, Mullol J, Scadding G, Virchow J (2007) A survey of the burden of allergic rhinitis in Europe. Allergy 62: 17-25.
10. Smith HE, Hogger C, Lallemant C, Crook D, Frew AJ (2009) Is structured allergy history sufficient when assessing patients with asthma and rhinitis in general practice? J Allergy Clin Immunol 123: 646-650.
11. Bousquet P, Chinn S, Janson C, Kogevinas M, Burney P, et al. (2007) Geographical variation in the prevalence of positive skin tests to environmental aeroallergens in the European community respiratory health survey I. Allergy 62: 301-309.
12. Ryan D, van Weel C, Bousquet J, Toskala E, Ahlstedt S, et al. (2008) Primary care: The cornerstone of diagnosis of allergic rhinitis. Allergy 63: 981-989.
13. Greiner AN1, Hellings PW, Rotiroti G, Scadding GK (2011) Allergic rhinitis. Lancet 378: 2112-2122.
14. Brozek JL, Bousquet J, Baena-Cagnani CE, Bonini S, Canonica GW, et al. (2010) Allergic rhinitis and its impact on asthma (ARIA) guidelines: 2010 revision. J Allergy Clin Immunol 126: 466-476.
15. Sami AS, Scadding GK (2014) Rhinosinusitis in secondary school children-part 2: Main project analysis of MSNOT-20 Young Persons Questionnaire (MSYPQ). Rhinology 52: 225-230.
16. Sami AS, Scadding G (2013) Management of allergic rhinitis in schools. British Journal of School Nursing 8: 119-123.
17. Nathan RA (2008) The pathophysiology, clinical impact and management of nasal congestion in allergic rhinitis. Clin Ther 30: 573-586.
18. Carr W, Bernstein J, Lieberman P, Meltzer E, Bachert C, et al. (2012) A novel intranasal therapy of azelastine with fluticasone for the treatment of allergic rhinitis. J Allergy Clin Immunol 129: 1282-1289.
19. Sami AS, Ahmed N (2014) Dymista (c) nasal spray with multifocal analysis of its impact on the rhinitis disease experience. Otolaryngology: Open Access 4: 1-5.
20. Meltzer EO, LaForce C, Ratner P, Price D, Ginsberg D, et al. (2012) MP29-02 (a novel intranasal formulation of azelastine hydrochloride and fluticasone propionate) in the treatment of seasonal allergic rhinitis: A randomized, double-blind, placebo-controlled trial of efficacy and safety 33: 324-332.
21. Altman DG. Practical statistics for medical research (1990) CRC press.
22. Eriksson J, Ekerljung L, Sundblad BM, Lötvall J, Torén K, et al. (2013) Cigarette smoking is associated with high prevalence of chronic rhinitis and low prevalence of allergic rhinitis in men. Allergy 68: 347-354.

The Effects of N-Acetyl Cysteine on Nasal Mucociliary Clearance in Healthy Volunteers

Morvarid Elahi[1]* and Homayoun Elahi[2]

[1]General Practitioner, Firoozgar General Hospital, Iran University of Medical Sciences, Tehran, Iran
[2]Assistant Professor of Otolaryngology, Firoozgar General Hospital, Iran University of Medical Sciences, Tehran, Iran

Abstract

Background: Mucociliary clearance is an important host defense function of the upper respiratory tract that requires the coordinated beating of cilia and results in the transport of mucus to the oropharynx. N-Acetyl Cysteine is a mucolytic drug currently used in pulmonary diseases. In the present study we sought to assess the effects of N-Acetyl Cysteine nasal mucociliary clearance in healthy volunteers.

Methods: A total of 100 healthy individuals (55 male) with the mean age of 34.21 (± 12.63) years were included in the present randomized, double-blind and placebo-controlled study. Participants were assigned into two groups of case and control. The Mucociliary Clearance Time (MCT) was measured by saccharine test; measuring the time in minutes required for the subject to taste a saccharin particle placed on the inferior turbinate of the nasal. The variables studied were nasal MCT before and after taking the placebo or NAC, age, and sex. Data were analyzed using SPSS V.16.

Results: Wilcoxon signed ranks test demonstrated considerable different of Saccharine Test Time (STT) between before and after taking the NAC (p=0.021), and no significant different of STT between before and after taking the placebo (p=0.723).

Conclusion: N-Acetyl Cysteine exerts measurable effect on nasal mucociliary clearance in healthy volunteers; therefore may be beneficial in conditions associated with disruption of mucociliary clearance such as rhinitis and sinusitis. However, further studies are suggested to achieve more conclusive results.

Keywords: Mucociliary clearance; N-Acetyl cysteine; Saccharin test

Introduction

The respiratory system is constantly exposed to environmental pathogens and toxins, spread as aerosol in the environment. The mucociliary system is the first defense of airways against harmful particles and disruptive environmental triggers. Ingredients, bacteria and respiratory viruses are trapped by airways' mucosa and driven to the larynx by respiratory beats, ultimately egress due to swallowing or coughing [1]. Airways' clearance by the mucocilary system is the main host defense mechanism of upper or lower respiratory tracks. Defects in this process, either genetically or acquired, make an individual susceptible to contracting chronicnasal, paranasal sinuses' and airways' tracks chronic infections [2]. Nose is the major part of the respiratory system that transfers air into and out of the system, playing an important role in providing necessary humidity (100%) and temperature (37 degrees), local defense and filtration of ingredients and gases [3]. A variety of factors affect mucociliary clearance such as increasing age, smoking, chronic nasal and pulmonary diseases (rhinitis, asthma, bronchiectasis, and chronic bstructive pulmonary disease), and anatomical defects of the upper respiratory track (septal deviation, hypertrophy of the concha, etc.) and a history of nasal surgery or trauma. The role of defects in mucociliary function due to either genetic diseases (cystic fibrosis) or acquired (secondary to infection of erosive mucociliary system diseases) has been recognized in many chronic airways tracks' diseases [4]. For example, defects in one or more parts of mucociliary clearance (epithelium, mucosa and cilia) cause chronic rhinosinusitis and stasis rinosinusial discharges lead to chronic inflammations [5]. Today, respiratory inflammation diseases are at the top of primary referral reasons to clinics. Airways' discharges are treated using mucoactive drugs which accommodate airways' clearance. Mucoactive drugs are classified based on their mechanisms; one group directly affects the production and chemical composition of airways' discharges, resulting in high efficacy on mucociliary clearance. Another group, having no certain impact on mucosa, helps in treatment of unusual discharges by affecting airways' structures and functions and modifying pathopysiologic mechanisms [6]. The saccharin test is a valid and reliable technique to evaluate the amount of mucociliary clearance times [7]. The saccharin test and similar tests, such as Aspartame are very useful to evaluate the mucociliary system's function. These tests are simple without the need for complex equipments and do not cause any discomfort for the patient. Results of these tests are dependent on individual factors which are directly related to mucociliary clearance. Verifying the consistency between nasal mucociliary clearance and tracheobronchial tracks suggests qualification of mucociliary clearance by less invasive methods like the saccharin test.

Methods

This study was reviewed and approved by the Institutional Review Board at the Iran University of Medical Sciences, and written informed consent was obtained from all participants. Volunteers enrolled in this clinical trial were scheduled to receive the NAC or the placebo and do STT before and after it in Firoozrar general hospital, Tehran, Iran, from January 2012 to March 2012. All individuals were divided into case and control groups by double-blind method.

***Corresponding author:** Morvarid Elahi, Firoozgar General Hospital, Valiasr Square, Tehran, Iran; E-mail: morvarid.elahi@gmail.com

A total of 100 healthy volunteers (55 males and 45 females) with a mean age of 34.21 ± 12.63 y/o (ranging from 19 to 86) were included. Range of age for 71% of volunteers was 21-40 y/o, along with 3% under 20 and 3% above 60. The control group consisted of 24 men (48%) and 26 women (52%) with a mean age of 33.72 ± 14.40 y/o (ranging from 18 to 86), resulting in a normal distribution. The case group consisted of 31 men (62%) and 19 women (38%) with a mean age of 34.58 ± 10.75 y/o (ranging from 27 to 58). Although the median was 28.5 and had long distance to end of range (86 y/o), distribution of age data was not normal. Despite the mean age, the mean gender of the control group has a normal distribution, but the case group does not (Figure 1).

136 volunteers (double the required individuals) were selected to participate in the study, where 36 volunteers were excluded. The exclusion criteria consisted of any anatomical defects of the upper respiratory system (septal deviation, hypertrophy concha, etc), history of nasal surgery or trauma, history of chronic nasal and respiratory diseases (asthma, rhinitis, chronic obstructive pulmonary disease, nasal polyps), acute infection of respiratory diseases during the recent six weeks, gustatory defects, history of smoking or use of drug ("nonsmoker" was defined as a person who has never smoked or has given up smoking for five years), pregnancy and history of taking drugs that influence mucociliary clearance, such as antihistamines, adrenergic drugs, anticholinergic drugs, local and systemic anticongestants, mucolytics, corticosteroids and theophyllin.

The saccharin test was based on Anderson et al. method in 1974 [8]. Saccharin test was done for every individual before taking medication of the NAC or the placebo. Individuals did not need any preparation for STT. For each test, 50 mg of saccharin powder, made by Merk Company, was placed on inferior turbinate, 1 cm away from the tip. Since maximum dose of saccharin is 2.5 mg per kg per day, the amount used in this study was safe for the subjects. The researcher made sure saccharin was precisely located on mucosa, avoiding squamous cell epithelium. All the individuals were in sitting position, bending their heads slightly backwards and breathed normally. All individuals were asked to inform the researcher of sensing any new taste in their pharynx, where they were not aware of the sweet taste of saccharin to prevent false positives. Time measurements were done before and after taking NAC or the placebo. The highest NAC concentration in the mucosa is detected within 2-4 hours. The taste of saccharin powder requires 12-15 hours to be eliminated from the nasopharynx cavity, and doing the second saccharin test sooner than 15 hours could have interfered with the first one. As a result, the test was repeated after 18 hours to avoid overlaps and time measurements were done before and after taking NAC or the placebo.

Data analysis was completed using Statistical Package for Social Sciences version 16 software. For each measured variable, descriptive values are expressed as the mean-standard deviation. Analysis of quantitative variables was done using Wilcoxon signed ranked test. Categorical variables were compared using the Chi square test and relationships were assessed by Pearson. Reported p values are 2-tailed and p<0.05 is considered statistically significant.

Results

The mean Saccharin Test Time (STT) before taking the placebo or NAC in all 100 volunteers was 9':59" ± 6':06" (ranging from 2':00" to 14':00"). The mean time of sensing sweetness of saccharin in the control group before taking the placebo was 10':45" ± 7':13" (ranging from 2':00" to 14':00"), where the mean time of distinguishing saccharin taste in the control group after taking the placebo was 11':05" ± 7':46" (ranging from 1':30" to 17':00"). So, the mean time of the control group before and after showed only a 00:20" difference. In Wilcoxon Signed Ranks test of the control group, there were 3 individuals (6%) among 50 with no fluxion, 23 (46%) with negative fluxion and 24 (48%) with positive fluxion.

The mean time of sensing sweetness of saccharin in the case group before taking the NAC was 9':13" (rangeing from 3':00 "to 14':00"), where the mean time of distinguishing saccharin taste in the case group after taking the NAC was 8':07" (ranging from 1':00" to 15':00"). Therefore, the mean time of case group before and after taking NAC demonstrated a 00:54" difference. Wilcoxon Signed Ranks in case group showed 1 individual (2%) among 50 with no fluxion, 14 (28%) with negative fluxion and 35 (70%) with positive fluxion. There was no relationship between the age and the difference STT before and after taking the placebo and NAC in all 100 volunteers, where related analysis indicated 0.95% assurance (p=0.503) (Figure 2). There was no relationship between the age and the difference of STT before and after taking the placebo in control group (0.95% assurance (p=0.463)), as well as NAC in the case group (0.95% assurance (p=0.309)). There was no relationship between the genders and the difference of STT before and after taking the placebo or NAC in the 100 volunteers, where related analysis showed 0.95% assurance (p=0.153). There was no relationship between the genders and the difference of STT before and after taking the placebo in the control group, as well as NAC in case group with 0.95% assurance (p=0.271 and p=0.672, respectively).

Discussion

Respiratory system is tremendously resistant to environmental triggers in spite of being exposed to many types of pathogens and toxic chemical substances. Respiratory mucosa provides this highly effective defense by traping inspiratory and removing toxic ingredients from lungs using cilia movements, cilia beats and coughing [9]. Mucous is produced and excreted constantly where mucosa cilia frequency of 12-15 beats per minute rate is ensures clearance of mucosa layers at rate of one millimeter per minute [10]. The rate of clearance is increased by hydration, as well as higher rate of cilia beats due to adrenergic, cholinergic and adenosine agonist drugs [10,11]. Examination of

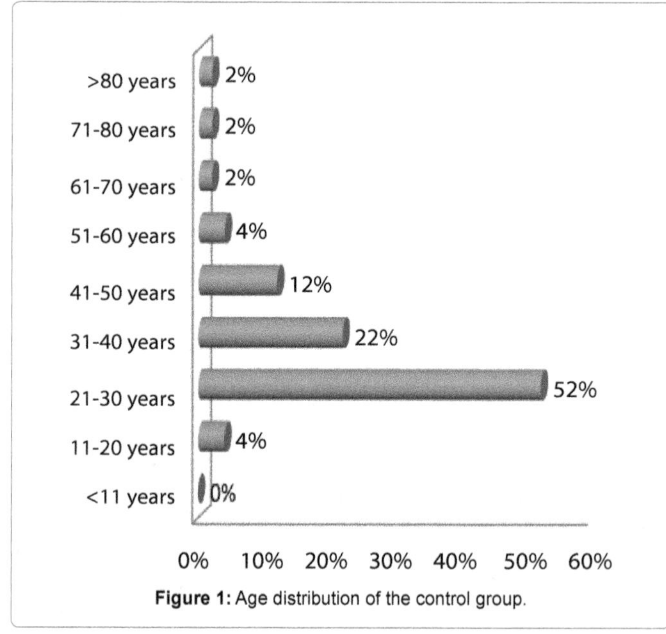

Figure 1: Age distribution of the control group.

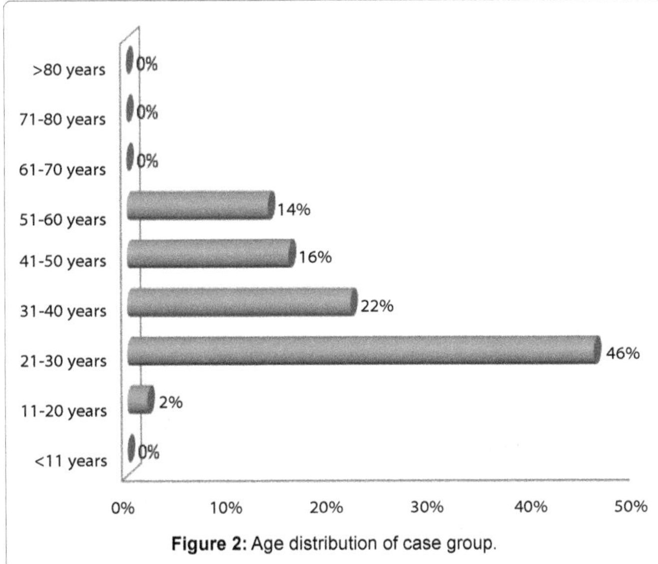

Figure 2: Age distribution of case group.

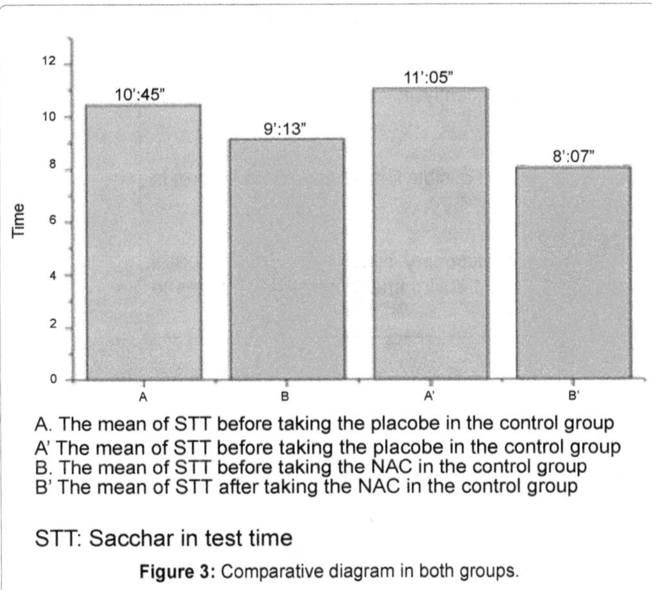

Figure 3: Comparative diagram in both groups.

mucociliary clearance can aid in screening respiratory diseases, where early diagnosis of low mucociliary function can result in faster and more effective treatments [12]. Studies have shown that using substances such as saccharin and aspartame for testing is easy to implement and analyze, without requiring complex equipments or causing discomfort for patients [13-15]. In current study saccharine test was used to evaluate the effect of NAC on mucociliary system. Maximum time of sensing sweet taste (14':00") was shorter than that reported by Rev med study (36':00") [16] which is explained by race and genetic differences as well as volunteers' younger age of the current study. Previous studies reported a meaningful relationship between demographic variants (age and gender) and saccharin test time [15,16]. In the current study, there was no relationship between age and the mean STT because there was no normal age distribution by chance. We can improve this error by bigger sample size (Figure 3).

Difference of 00:20" between the mean times of the control group before and after application of placebo indicates lack of distinction between them which was confirmed by Wilcoxon Signed Ranks. 48% of individuals who took the placebo sensed the saccharin taste sooner than the first time due to individuals' autosuggestion. There is no statistical relationship between these variants with 95% assurance (p=0.723). The mean times of case group before and after taking NAC showed a 00:54" difference, with a positive fluxion nearly three-fold compared to the control group. There was also a significant difference between STT before and after taking the NAC with 95% assurance (p=0.021), confirming the positive impact of NAC on nasal mucociliary clearance.

Conclusion

We conclude that N-acetyl Cysteine exerts measurable effect on nasal mucociliary clearance in healthy volunteers and therefore is beneficial in conditions associated with disruption of mucociliary clearance such as rhinitis and sinusitis diseases as much as pulmonary diseases as an adjuvant.

References

1. Reynolds HY (1994) Respiratory Host Defenses - Surface Immunity Original Research Article. Immunobiology 191: 402-412.
2. Sato S, Kiyono H (2012) The mucosal immune system of the respiratory tract. Current Opinion in Virology 2: 225-232.
3. Suarez CS, Dintzis SM, Frevert CW (2012) Respiratory Comparative Anatomy and Histology 54: 121-134.
4. Johnson-Delaney CA, Orosz SE (2011) Ferret Respiratory System: Clinical Anatomy, Physiology, and Disease. Veterinary Clinics of North America: Exotic Animal Practice 14: 357-367.
5. Kyd JM, RuthFoxwell A, Cripps AW (2001) Mucosal immunity in the lung and upper airway. Vaccine 19: 2527-2533.
6. Miyata T, Kai H, Isohama Y, Takahama K (1998) Current opinion of muco-active drug research: strategies and problems. Eur Respir J 11: 480-491.
7. Marttin E, Schipper NGM, Verhoef JC (1998) Nasal mucociliaryclearanceas a factor in nasal drug delivery. Adv Drug Deliv Rev 29: 13-38.
8. Andersen IB, Camner P, Jensen PI (1974) Acomparison of nasal and tracheobronchial clearance. Arch Environ Health 19: 290-293.
9. JanHolmgren (1991) Mucosal immunity and vaccination. FEMS Microbiology Letters 89: 1-9.
10. Salathe M (2007) Regulation of mammalianciliary beating. Annu Rev Physiol 69: 401-422
11. Thornton DJ, Sheehan JK (2004) From mucins to mucous: toward a more coherent understanding of this essential barrier. Proc Am Thorac Soc 32: 54-61.
12. Ellerman A, Bisgaard H (1997) Longitudinal study of lung function in acohort of primary ciliary dyskinesia. Eur Respir J 10: 2376-2379.
13. Canciani M, Barlocco EG, Mastella G (2005) The saccharin method for testing mucociliary function in patients suspected of having primary ciliarydyskinesia. Pediatric Pulmonology 5: 210-214.
14. Plaza Valia P, Carrion Valero F, MarinPardo J (2013) Saccharin test for the study of mucociliary clearance: reference values for a Spanish population. US National Library of Medicine. Archivos de Bronconeumologia 49: 131-175.
15. Rev med Brux (2011) Airway clearance techniques in chronic obstructive pulmonary syndrome 32: 381-387
16. Kenneth Yu, John R. Stram (1995) Nasal mucociliary clearance and the saccharin tablet test: What does it measure? Otolaryngology - Head and Neck Surgery 113: 170-171.

Tinnitus: An Evolutionary Symptom?

Sylvester Fernandes*

Department of Health Sciences, Newcastle University, Newcastle, Australia

***Corresponding author:** Sylvester Fernandes FRCSEd, FRACS, FACS, LLB, 46 Fairfax Road, Warners Bay, NSW 2282, Australia; E-mail: mdsfe@yahoo.com.au

Abstract

Introduction: The mechanism contributing to the causation of tinnitus continues to evade us. It is unlikely that our current thinking is progressing in the right direction. The literature on the subject is mounting but with no real insights into causation.

Objectives: To introduce, if possible, a paradigm shift that may produce a different trend in thinking and hopefully change our direction and lines of research.

Materials and methods: Herein is presented a hypothesis employing logical inductive reasoning aided by modern computer logic and also incorporating neuroscience, artificial intelligence, evolution and philosophy. This hypothesis attempts to employ a forensic methodology ("crime scene analysis" technique) and utilising the available evidence to build an aetiology, as other methods have not contributed significantly in deciphering causation. A pragmatic model incorporating the known features of tinnitus is thus available.

Results: A plausible explanation for the causation of tinnitus is offered with a possible link to its evasive nature, in our search for a cause.

Conclusion: The functional value of tinnitus may be provided by our evolutionary history. It is possible that tinnitus was a protective adaptive phenomenon in earlier forms but in our current environment merely contributes to nuisance value.

Keywords: Subjective tinnitus; Tinnitus mechanisms; Evolutionary symptoms

Introduction

Tinnitus is the perception of sound in the absence of an external source. It is described as 'subjective' when perceived by the patient and 'objective' when perceived in addition, by others. The vast majority of tinnitus is subjective. While the majority perceive tinnitus only as a mild symptom, many struggle with severe tinnitus that significantly impairs their quality of life. In such cases tinnitus can be a debilitating condition, that negatively impacts a patient's overall health and social well-being. Sometimes even moderate cases can interfere with the ability to work and socialize.

The U.S. Centers for Disease Control estimates that nearly 15% of the general public (over 45 million Americans) experience some form of tinnitus. Roughly 20 million people struggle with burdensome chronic tinnitus, while 2 million have extreme and debilitating problems [1]. Tinnitus is the leading service-related disability among U.S. veterans, with 9.7% of all veterans receiving service-related disability compensation [2]. An estimated one in five high schoolers suffer from tinnitus [3].

Thus tinnitus has huge negative costs, both in terms of human and economic impact. Apart from the suffering at the individual and his/her relationship level, these costs are also felt by the population at-large by way of compensation damages in associated industrial noise induced hearing loss and in war veterans. Sums are also invested in research to find a proximate cause and thus a cure.

The mechanism contributing to the causation of tinnitus continues to evade us to date and perhaps this may be related to the insistence of neuroscience on the search for proximate explanations based on mechanisms, but a full biological explanation may require an evolutionary explanation for the origin and function of tinnitus.

There is no known effective treatment for tinnitus. Relief most often comes through various methods of "managing" the condition [4].

This hypothesis proposes:

a. Tinnitus may have an evolutionary basis.

b. and instantiates at a "nagging center" with a "halting problem" possibly in the thalamic regions.

c. Tinnitus and hearing have separate paths. Hearing initiates peripherally and tinnitus initiates centrally.

d. that compete for attention at the consciousness level.

Materials and Methods

In the best quest of testing this hypothesis, and as tinnitus is presumed to be a "vigilance" signal for danger (see below), it was felt that it might be more plausible if we could find a subset of the human population who lacked tinnitus and were at greater risk, say, of injuring in bicycle accidents when hit from behind or the side by cars that they could not detect, as well as another with tinnitus, who were less at risk due to the persistent "cautionary signal" from tinnitus. There is no shortage of the former [5] and although the absolute absence of tinnitus was not confirmed, it is more likely than not, that they did not suffer from tinnitus, This may tentatively serve as the first arm of the quest. As expected, attempts to document the latter arm in the literature or on social media were futile.

However cycling accidents do increase as individuals grow older, with 10 to 15 year old riders being more at risk than other age groups up to about the age of 60 years, when the incidence falls [5]. This is more likely to indicate riskier behaviour by younger groups and a switch to motorised transport in the later years rather than an absolute relation to tinnitus, although such cannot be ruled out with certainty.

Faced with such circumstances, we undertook an open, self report study on 37 patients aged between 11 and 73 years and a significantly male predominance (29 males and 8 females) who were referred for the management of bothersome bilateral tinnitus, who were questioned directly about what effect tinnitus itself has on them when crossing a busy road. All of them said, that the presence of tinnitus causes them to be more "cautious/wary/tense/apprehensive/alert" and they have a tendency to check and recheck visually before crossing. Even after closer questioning, none of them admitted that it does not cause any concern on a busy road. They explained that the distraction caused by the tinnitus increases their wariness as they are aware of this distraction tendency and the disability it provokes in these and similar circumstances. When specifically propositioned that it may be their hearing loss rather than tinnitus that may be causing them concern, 34 insisted that they had considered hearing loss but felt that it was the tinnitus that caused the anxiety and the added vigilance under the circumstances. In other words, an undeniable "anxious vigilance" is maintained.

Results

None of them had an accident or any near misses supposedly due to the innate caution. Available statistics show that there were 174 pedestrian fatalities on Australian roads in 2012 [6]. The casualties were possibly much more.

Discussion

This study demonstrates:

1. A high level of alertness/vigilance in tinnitus. Such has also been reported by other authors [7]. No case of "untroubled by tinnitus" was noted.
2. The absences of any casualties. This denotes effective vigilance. (evolutionary type 1 error response. See below)

These findings lend significant weight to the validity of an evolutionary basis for tinnitus as explained above in Materials and Methods.

Nevertheless, it is accepted that one cannot convincingly test an ultimate adaptationist hypothesis only with proximate, mechanistic data. And it is also not convincing to imagine a past environment and endow it with features that support the hypothesis but that cannot be observed or measured. However it is not at all unreasonable to accept a predator/prey environment with evolutionary pressure for survival.

That tinnitus does occur in the absence of disease clearly implies that pathological causes are not absolutely necessary for its occurrence and when such do occur, they may only really be correlations and may imply that a proximate pathological cause may not be necessary and an adaptive or evolutionary mismatch hypotheses as indicated below, is probable.

Mechanics

In attempting the mechanics, it may benefit to visualize a three stage model:

1. Input
2. Mechanism
3. Output

Knowledge of any two of the above allows a pre/retro-diction or an explanation of the remnant component. However, when only one is known we need a hypothesis, which when confirmed by experimentation leads to a theory.

Thus, in the elucidation of tinnitus, it may benefit to visualize a three stage model thus:

1. Input (cause or stimulus) - a "halting problem" in the brain's connectome parallel processor (possibly the medial and dorsal parts of the thalamus).

2. Mechanism - separate paths for hearing and tinnitus conveying perception to conscious attention.

3. Output (effect) - tinnitus percept in consciousness.

Sensation along the hearing path is initiated by sound at the ear and finally perceived consciously by the brain. Tinnitus may initiate at a "iterative (nagging) center" (the site with the "halting problem", see below) and finally be perceived consciously, attention allowing, by the brain.

The facts [8,9] about tinnitus are:

- Tinnitus is a conscious central percept [10-13] and is not perceived during sleep or anesthesia.
- Tinnitus has several similarities with pain and the neuroses and possibly addiction [14-19].
- The qualia (subjective qualitative experience) of the tinnitus are private and privileged only to the sufferer. The point is made at this stage that tinnitus, like thoughts, feelings etc occupies the *phenomenal* consciousness domain, being private and individual.
- Functional MRIs tend to localize areas of activation in tinnitus [20-23].
- Tinnitus is best masked by incorporating the "dead" frequencies [24,25].

The following serve to elucidate the proposed hypothesis further:

Evolution

In the Heller and Bergman study [26], 94% of 80 normal individuals experienced tinnitus in quiet surroundings. Considering such a high proportion which is also available in other similar studies [27,28] including one with a placebo suggestion [28], the possibility that tinnitus may lie in our evolved cognitive architecture cannot be ruled out. Tinnitus possibly initiated as "siren" hearing, to warn the organism to be on guard constantly for predators. The "siren" sound creates an atmosphere of present-centeredness which may have adaptive value for the organism by forcing the recruitment of a broad network of task-related neural resources. The triggered limbic and autonomic events may be such ("fight or flight") responses. The oft-noted association of tinnitus with the limbic/autonomic response is thus easily explained.

Such a natural "siren" may be comparable in computer terms to the "halting problem" of the Turing machine (see below). As evolution proceeded, and possibly to reduce energy consumption, a higher expenditure of cognitive resources and related energetics, 'normal hearing' evolved with cortical representation. With the evolution of 'normal hearing' the evolutionary alertness advantage of tinnitus was not required and was hence subjugated to the subcortex, with access to conscious attention. This inference also helps to support the concept of separate paths for hearing and tinnitus, having evolved at different times for different needs.

As per our hypothesis, tinnitus initiated at the time when 'normal hearing' was not available. It is quite possible that this situation reverts back to that initial stage with the advance of a hearing loss causing a pre-normal hearing scenario again.

The experimental animal models support that tinnitus exists in our common ancestor species, at least as far back as rodents [29,30].

Another path that may point to the ancient and primal aspect of tinnitus and its evolution is its rhythmic quality. Rhythm is the systematic patterning of events in terms of timing accent and grouping. "Systematic patterning" distinguishes rhythmic patterns from random patterns of events in time. Rhythm can be periodic, like the beat of music or it may be non-periodic, like the sound of a morse code message (which manifests temporal structure without periodicity). In other words, all periodic patterns are rhythmic, but not all rhythmic patterns are periodic.

Rhythm is fundamental to the nervous system which abounds in rhythms, including the heartbeat and the rhythmic oscillations of electrical potentials in the brain (also found in numerous species of mammals including rodents, rabbits, dogs, cats, bats, and marsupials). These latter brain wave oscillations manifest different patterns.

Pulsatile tinnitus manifests a periodic rhythmic pattern and non-pulsatile tinnitus manifests a non-periodic rhythmic pattern which involves grouping or phrasing, which is the (perceptual) segmentation of events into chunks. Rhythm may thus suggest a link to the evolutionary status of tinnitus.

The acoustic element of tinnitus is tonally very basic, again suggesting an early appearance in evolution. Even birdsong is more complex suggesting a later evolution and the possibility that tinnitus emerged prior to the emergence of vocalisation is thus a distinct possibility.

Due to the eons of time involved, this a priori evolution cannot be subjected to falsifiability. Such may not matter in this case as this is a historical hypothesis about the causes of traits in current populations.

It thus appears that animals can experience tinnitus but the human characteristics of language and narrative; the tendency to attribute causes to events in the world; and perhaps the ability to experience emotions like awe make tinnitus a concern for some individuals.

Halting problem

As neurons have threshold firing only, tinnitus is most likely to be a "halting problem", where the input of the causative signal/code is subject to an infinite loop of causation and effect.

The senses employ a form of multi-layer nets subcortically in perception which are also good at pattern recognition. In tinnitus such a layer of neurons may be subject to the above "halting problem".

As the brain is a massively parallel processor, the term is used here in comparison to the "halting problem" of the Turing machine which in computer language is a program that will not halt on a particular contributing input. Computer scientists are able to build such machines that can mimic human abilities and still not understand the mechanism of those abilities.

As such, the exact mechanism of the "halting problem" of the Turing machine (a mathematical concept) still remains an enigma. Nevertheless it is useful to incorporate the concept into our argument as it allows us an explanation of the repetitive nature of the phenomenon of tinnitus at a computational level by the brain (thalamus).

Separate paths

At this stage of our knowledge, it is admitted that this is subject to confirmational empiricism. The following pointers however may suffice to suggest the plausibility that the hearing and tinnitus pathways may be separate:

1. Tinnitus can occur in the presence of normal hearing [26], indicating that separate pathways are highly probable.

2. Only some patients with hearing loss develop tinnitus.

3. Absence of both hearing as well as tinnitus is plausible with separate paths.

4. Somatosensory tinnitus occurs in the absence of a hearing loss.

5. If ototoxic drugs and excessive noise damage the hearing pathway then it is unlikely that tinnitus will travel the same functionally damaged path to produce a sensation of sound.

6. Cochlear implants (may) work in some cases [31] of tinnitus as they possibly repopulate the hearing pathway.

7. Support for such dual pathways is also provided by the existing concepts of a classical (lemniscal) and non-classical (extralemniscal) auditory pathway.

Consciousness

The absolute attention workspace may be occupied by one of several options to include sense data, thoughts, tinnitus etc. and the competition for this workspace is like radio channels competing for a narrow frequency band with a "winner take all" equilibrium [32].

Counselling aids the patient to take control of this space and oust the negative intruders by introducing positive thoughts ("voluntary" top-down attention) and as this space is limited, this can work. Sound therapy (masking) also works ("reflexive" bottom-up attention) by attempting to occupy this space.

The cognitive component of tinnitus is essentially the remnant of the type 1 error (false positive) response which was the more reliable interpretation necessary for the survival of our ancestors when a predator clue emerged. Imagine an ancestor interpreting an unfamiliar sound as nonthreatening (false negative or type 2 response). Not many such interpreters would survive and reproduce. The type 1 error (false positive) response is thus etched into our constitution.

Extinction of this basic response is the aim of Cognitive Behavioural Therapy (CBT).

Evolutionary (Ultimate) Substantiation

Tinnitus is a uniform trait in mammals and possibly pre-mammals, possibly emanating from the need for predator vigilance in the need for survival [33]. This concept may also bear an evolutionary similarity to saccadic vision (employed for tracking moving prey or predators by our ancestors). Prior to the long period of evolution of the basic tasks required of an auditory system, to include acoustic feature discrimination, sound source localization, frequency analysis, and auditory scene analysis, this "siren" sound may have had survival value. Subsequently, with the evolution of the ear and normal hearing, and possibly to conserve energy this trait is suppressed but re-accessible with the loss of serviceable hearing. Another way of looking at this would be that tinnitus is genetic and hearing loss provides an epigenetic footing.

Essentially heuristic behaviours, which were quite adaptive during the earlier parts of human evolutionary history are no longer adaptive, given the current environments in which we find ourselves (mismatch) and are hence now considered (medical) neuroses. Neuroses also occur over a continuum spectrum, and like emotions are not easily subject to voluntary cortical control and are therefore available only to therapy which lies in the domain of the psychiatrist/psychologist (e.g. cognitive behavioural therapy).

Proximate Substantiation

To date fMRI is the only non invasive investigation available for the investigation of tinnitus. These studies have provided inconsistent and contradictory results and "a vague picture of the neuronal correlates of tinnitus" [34].

What is the function of tinnitus?

Tinnitus is a repetitive sound. All physical and emotional signals like pain, hunger, anxiety, etc. have a repetitive nature, thus attempting to gain attention and keep it, and thus serving a survival need. Repetitive stimuli, like flickering lights, smoke alarms create an urgency of response but once the absence of danger is realised, only serve to create an annoyance. The fact that sufficient neural machinery has evolved to create this attention seeking and a response mechanism, may denote its importance as a "warning alarm" in survival.

Perception of tinnitus in a very quiet environment may be related to the fact that tinnitus acquires a non-competitive access to consciousness in this situation and also such an environment may promote anxiety which may facilitate access [35].

Why a "siren" sound?

Ultimately survival and reproduction is the objective of every organism. To this end every (evolutionary) adaptive mechanism is dedicated. In a predator coexisting environment, a method of surveillance is essential. These methods essentially only depend on the basic available perceptory armamentarium i.e. the senses, for an immediate response as opposed to the 'learned' response.

Some evolutionary pressure considerations may provide a clue:

1. The visual sensation is actually the most reliable for survival and only a 360 degree vision in all axes, at all times, would be helpful but this is a physical unreality under available anatomical constraints and any other misinterference with vision would itself threaten survival. Some organisms may have followed this path with extinction consequences.

2. The olfactory sensation is the most unreliable for survival and hence the most likely to be ignored by the organism. The smell sense is more primitive in evolution, with individual (not species) specific preferential links (and related only to specific odorants) to the limbic/autonomic systems [36]. Thus it is unlikely to create an atmosphere of urgency. Also, in the competition for attention, hearing trumps olfaction. In falling to sleep (losing consciousness) hearing is the last sensation to disappear. Also, because of the paucity of spatial localisation, olfaction cannot be concerned with precise environmental details. Chemical sensitivity is the oldest response of animals to the environment and with the development of the neopallium, it appears that auditory and visual sensations gained prominence [37]. It is a common experience of pet owners that unfamiliar smells provoke curiosity and unfamiliar sounds provoke caution. Nevertheless, in earlier times, some organisms may have followed this path to extinction.

3. The touch and taste sensations are "too close for comfort "under predator supervision. Again, this path may have been followed by some organisms with guaranteed extinction.

A further consideration

Working memory (and "attention") were initially explored by Alan Badderly with the concept of the "Central Executive (CE)" [38]. With the plethora of information available, entry into "attention" occurs after filtration by the CE conglomerate of the prefrontal cortex (PFC) and the basal ganglia (BG). Essentially PFC allows prioritisation of current task goals (maintaining focus) and BG provide the mental muscle to block out information that does not match these goals. Emotional stimuli dependent on Darwinian hierarchy for survival gain most priority. In other words, evolutionarily, the brain is always on high alert for perceived threats. The emotional salience of tinnitus is undoubted.

There is a time delay between conscious awareness and the emotion. Similar delays between spontaneous voluntary acts and "readiness potentials" are available elsewhere in cognitive neurophysiology [39].

It is plausible that there is a persistent pre-tinnitus activity (innate evolutionary) that is filtered into awareness as tinnitus when there is malfunction of the central executive blocking mechanism (BG). Such occurrences have been documented [40,41].

Predictions

1. Due to the proximity/commonality (cf. also quantum computation possibility) of the prefrontal – limbic path in these afflictions, it is likely that tinnitus may be co-morbid with anxiety, depression, chronic pain, sleep disorders and perhaps addiction including gambling [42]. A genetic linkage may also contribute.

2. Being an evolutionary phenomenon, it is more likely that tinnitus may only succumb to psychotherapy in some cases [4].

3. The most effective curative (as opposed to management) therapy is Cognitive Behavioural Therapy (CBT) [43-45].

Tinnitus is annoying and unmanageable only when the limbic and autonomic systems are recruited. The measured loudness of tinnitus is maximally within 30 to 40 dB of threshold, which by itself is not significantly loud but the associated limbic and autonomic system recruitment provoke anxiety and depression at a subcortical level. CBT is helpful as it attempts to alter the subcortical response but does not affect the acoustic component of tinnitus thereby rendering it impotent and nonreactive [46].

4. The probability of success of any CBT may be made available by prior assessment of prefrontal (control) testing by using the Stroop Color-Word Interference Task or similar tasks.

5. Drug therapy must aim at cognition-altering or attention- altering medication without affecting reason/consciousness. It may also be possible in future to provide BG neuroreceptor exo-agonists to mount an effective blockage to innate tinnitus/anxiety/depression/chronic pain/addiction and deny entry to limbic and consciousness paths. Such endo-neurotransmitters (cf. endomorphins provoked by belief) may possibly be contributing to the minor reported successes, and are essentially a "placebo effect".

Conclusion

A credible mechanism for tinnitus must conclusively explain how tinnitus occurs in the absence of a hearing loss. It must also explain why tinnitus only occurs in some but not all cases of hearing loss.

It is proposed here that tinnitus is a maladaptive evolutionary trait that in humans resulted from phylogenetic inertia [47], and in the modern human constitutes a mismatch between a slow-evolving organism and a changing environment [33].

It is also proposed that hearing and tinnitus occupy separate proximate paths competing for conscious 'attention'.

Further discussion including challenges to current concepts is available elsewhere [48]. Similar to the pragmatic solar model of the atom and the double helix structure of the DNA molecule, this hypothesis awaits empiric confirmation which in this case may be available with advances in technology, to detect the tiny sequential changes that occurred over millions of generations that have resulted in partially differentiated components, that may serve many functions in parallel [33,42].

References

1. National Health and Nutrition Examination Survey (2011-2012) U.S centers for disease control.
2. Annual Benefits Report (2012) US department of veterans affairs.
3. Gilles A, Van Hal G, De Ridder D, Wouters K, Van de Heyning P (2013) Epidemiology of noise-induced tinnitus and the attitudes and beliefs towards noise and hearing protection in adolescents. PLoS One 8: e70297.
4. Folmer RL, Theodoroff SM, Martin WH, Shi Y (2014) Experimental, controversial and futuristic treatments for chronic tinnitus. J Am Acad Audiol 25: 106-125.
5. Reported Road Casualties Great Britain, 2013: Main Results (2014) Department for transport. Collisions involving cyclists on britain's roads: Establishing the causes.
6. Australian road deaths database. Department of infrastructure and transport's online.
7. Andersson G, McKenna L (2006) The role of cognition in tinnitus. Acta Otolaryngol Suppl : 39-43.
8. Tyler RS (2006) Neurophysiological models, psychological models and treatments for tinnitus. In: Tyler RS (eds.) Tinnitus treatment: Clinical protocols (1-22). New York: Thieme
9. Møller AR, Langguth B, De Ridder D, Kleinjung T (2011) Textbook of tinnitus. Springer.
10. Eggermont JJ, Roberts LE (2004) The neuroscience of tinnitus. Trends in Neurosciences 27: 676-682.
11. Eggermont JJ (2003) Central tinnitus. Auris Nasus Larynx 30 Suppl: S7-12.
12. Langers DR, de Kleine E, van Dijk P (2012) Tinnitus does not require macroscopic tonotopic map reorganization. Front Syst Neurosci 6: 2.
13. Adjamian P, Hall DA, Palmer AR, Allan TW, Langers DR (2014) Neuroanatomical abnormalities in chronic tinnitus in the human brain. Neuroscience and Biobehavioral Reviews 45C: 119-133.
14. Møller AR (2007) Tinnitus and pain. Prog Brain Res 166: 47-53.
15. Flor H, Nikolajsen L, Staehelin Jensen T (2006) Phantom limb pain: A case of maladaptive CNS plasticity? Nat Rev Neurosci 7: 873-881.
16. King T, Vera-Portocarrero L, Gutierrez T, Vanderah TW, Dussor G, et al. (2009) Unmasking the tonic-aversive state in neuropathic pain. Nat Neurosci 12: 1364-1366.
17. Folmer RL, Griest SE, Martin WH (2001) Chronic tinnitus as phantom auditory pain. Otolaryngol Head Neck Surg 124: 394-400.
18. Koob GF (2000) Neurobiology of addiction. Toward the development of new therapies. Ann N Y Acad Sci 909: 170-185.
19. Simpson RB, Nedzelski JM, Barber HO, Thomas MR (1988) Psychiatric diagnoses in patients with psychogenic dizziness or severe tinnitus. J Otolaryngol 17: 325-330.
20. Melcher JR, Sigalovsky IS, Guinan JJ Jr, Levine RA (2000) Lateralized tinnitus studied with functional magnetic resonance imaging: Abnormal inferior colliculus activation. J Neurophysiol 83: 1058-1072.
21. Lanting CP, De Kleine E, Bartels H, Van Dijk P (2008) Functional imaging of unilateral tinnitus using fMRI. Acta Otolaryngol 128: 415-421.
22. Smits M, Kovacs S, de Ridder D, Peeters RR, van Hecke P, et al. (2007) Lateralization of functional magnetic resonance imaging (fMRI) activation in the auditory pathway of patients with lateralized tinnitus. Neuroradiology 49: 669-679.
23. Golm D, Schmidt-Samoa C, Dechent P, Kröner-Herwig B (2013) Neural correlates of tinnitus related distress: An fMRI-study. Hear Res 295: 87-99.
24. Meikle MB, Vernon J, Johnson RM (1984) The perceived severity of tinnitus: Some observations concerning a large population of tinnitus clinic patients. Otolaryngology Head Neck Surgery 92: 689-696
25. Norena A, Micheyl C, Chéry-Croze S, Collet L (2002) Psychoacoustic characterization of the tinnitus spectrum: Implications for the underlying mechanisms of tinnitus. Audiology Neurootology 7: 358–369.
26. Heller MF, Bergman M (1953) Tinnitus aurium in normally hearing persons. Ann Otol Rhinol Laryngol 62: 73-83.
27. Tucker DA, Phillips SL, Ruth RA, Clayton WA, Royster E, et al. (2005) The effect of silence on tinnitus perception. Otolaryngol Head Neck Surg 132: 20-24.
28. Del Bo L, Forti S, Ambrosetti U, Serena C, Mauro D, et al. (2008) Tinnitus aurium in persons with normal hearing: 55 years late. Otolaryngology-Head and Neck Surgery 139: 391-394.
29. Kaltenbach JA (2011) Tinnitus: Models and mechanisms. Hear Res 276: 52-60.
30. von der Behrens W (2014) Animal models of subjective tinnitus. Neural Plast 2014: 1-13.
31. van Zon A, Smulders YE, Ramakers GG, Stegeman I, Smit AL et al. (2015) Effect of unilateral and simultaneous bilateral cochlear implantation on tinnitus: A randomized controlled trial. Laryngoscope 126: 956-951.

32. Baars BJ, Franklin S, Ramsøy TZ (2013) Global workspace dynamics: Cortical "binding and propagation" enables conscious contents. Frontiers Psychology 4:200.

33. Nesse RM (2011) Ten questions for evolutionary studies of disease vulnerability. Evol Appl 4: 264-277.

34. Schecklmann S, Lehner A, Poeppl TB, Timm, Peter K, et al. (2013) Auditory cortex is implicated in tinnitus distress: A voxel-based morphometry study. Brain Structure and Function 218: 1061–1070.

35. Lang PJ, Davis M (2006) Emotion, motivation, and the brain: Reflex foundations in animal and human research. Prog Brain Res 156: 3-29.

36. Zald DH, Pardo J (1997) Emotion, olfaction and the human amygdala: Amygdala activation during aversive olfactory stimulation. Procedings of the Natural Academy of Science 94: 4119-4124.

37. Wenzel BM (1974) The olfactory system and behavior in Limbic and Autonomic Nervous Systems Research. Springer.

38. Badderly A (1996) Exploring the central executive. The Quarterly Journal of Experimental Psychology 49:5-28

39. Libet B (2004) Mind time. The temporal factor in consciousness, Harvard University Press.

40. Larson PS, Cheung SW (2012) Deep brain stimulation in area LC controllably triggers auditory phantom percepts. Neurosurgery 70: 398-405.

41. Larson PS, Cheung SW (2013) A stroke of silence: Tinnitus suppression following placement of a deep brain stimulation electrode with infarction in area LC. Journal of Neurosurgery 118: 192-194.

42. Satinover J (2001) The quantum brain. John Wiley, pp: 173-189

43. Canals P, Pérez Del Valle B, Lopez F, Marco A (2016) The efficacy of individual treatment of subjective tinnitus with cognitive behavioural therapy. Acta Otorrinolaringol Esp 67: 187-192.

44. Moschen R, Riedl D, Schmidt A, Kumnig M, Bliem HR, et al. (2015) The development of acceptance of chronic tinnitus in the course of a cognitive-behavioral group therapy. Psychosomatic Medicine and Psychotherapy 61: 238-246.

45. Malinvaud D, Londero A, Niarra R, Peignard P, Warusfel O, et al. Auditory and visual 3D virtual reality therapy as a new treatment for chronic subjective tinnitus: Results of a randomized controlled trial. Hearing Research 333: 127-135.

46. Fernández MM, Shin J, Scherer RW, Murdin L (2015) Interventions for tinnitus in adults: An overview of systematic reviews. Cochrane ENT Group.

47. Blomberg SP, Garland Jr T (2002) Tempo and mode in evolution: Phylogenetic inertia, adaptation and comparative methods. Journal of Evolutionary Biology 15: 899-910.

48. Fernandes S (2015) Deciphering tinnitus from the shoulders of giants: A Kuhnian shift may be required. Otolaryngol (Sunnyvale) 5: 205. Available at bit.ly/1OHNSKd Accessed on December 30, 2015.

Utilizing Dehydrated Human Amnion/Chorion Membrane Allograft in Transcanal Tympanoplasty

Griffith S Hsu*

DuPage Medical Group, Department of Otolaryngology-Head and Neck Surgery, Illinois, USA

Abstract

Objective: To evaluate the utility and effectiveness of dehydrated Human Amnion/Chorion Membrane (dHACM) in transcanal tympanoplasty.

Patients: A retrospective analysis of 14 patients (8 adults and 4 children) with stable tympanic membrane perforations for greater than 6 months.

Intervention: Transcanal tympanoplasty performed by a single surgeon utilizing a dHACM allograft.

Main outcome measures: Operative time, pain, graft success and audiologic improvement.

Results: At the 6 week post-operative visit a decrease in perforation size was noted in 8 patients (57.1%) and complete closure of the perforation occurred in 6 (42.9%). For patients without tympanosclerosis (n=10) complete closure was achieved in 5 patients (50%) and complete or partial success in 7 patients (70%). Mean air bone gap decreased from a pre-operative measurement of 23.0 ± 10.1 dB to 16.8 ± 7.4 dB at 6 weeks after tympanoplasty. The technique was well tolerated. Using the transcanal method and dehydrated amnion/chorion membrane allograft, the mean operative time was 13.3 ± 0.10 minutes.

Conclusions: Commercially available dHACM appears to be a safe, viable graft material for transcanal tympanoplasty.

Keywords: Allograft; Amniotic membrane; Tympanoplasty

Introduction

Tympanoplasty is a surgical procedure used in patients to repair defects in the tympanic membrane and restore or maintain hearing function [1]. A wide variety of autologous grafting materials have been used for tympanoplasty, including cartilage, perichondrium, and loose areolar tissue, fat and most commonly, temporalis fascia [2]. Recently, commercially available allograft materials such as Alloderm (LifeCell Corp., Branchburg, NJ) derived from donated skin from human cadavers has been used as an alternative to autologous tissue in efforts to reduce scarring, infection and pain, as well as operative time [2]. Although, this material may provide a suitable grafting option, it's acellular characteristic only serves as a scaffold or template for ingrowth, which may limit its long-term success.

Human amniotic membrane has been considered to be an ideal biological dressing in that it promotes epithelialization and reduces pain while having antibacterial properties [3]. Biochemical properties of amniotic membrane help to reduce inflammation and enhance soft tissue healing [3]. Growth factors including EGF, TGF-β, FGF and PDGF A and B are present in human amniotic tissue and not only self-signaling but also mediate the tissue repair process [4]. Basic scientific research has suggested growth factor involvement in accelerating or enhancing healing of tympanic membrane [5,6]. In addition to growth factors, human amniotic membrane contains extracellular architectural elements including collagens type IV, V and VII. These materials form an important substrate and scaffold within various tissues which is needed for advanced wound healing and ingrowth of cells. The extracellular matrix of amniotic membrane is also comprised of other structural materials including fibronectin, laminins, proteoglycans and glycosaminoglycans, all which may promote the wound healing process.

A commercially available dehydrated Amnion/Chorion Membrane (dHACM) allograft (EpiFix®, MiMedx Group, Inc., Marietta, GA) is created through a proprietary PURION® process which cleans, dehydrates and sterilizes human amniotic/chorionic membrane while preserving key attributes of natural amniotic membrane. Scientific studies have demonstrated that dHACM is composed of extracellular matrix materials, growth factors, and cytokines in essentially the same amount and in a preserved state when compared with natural amniotic membrane tissue [7]. The composition of the allograft has been demonstrated both qualitatively with specific immunohistochemical testing and quantitatively with ELISA testing to document this equivalence [7].

Use of natural human amniotic membrane for tympanoplasty has been reported in studies conducted outside the United States, with positive results [8-11]. The purpose of the present analysis was to evaluate the utility and effectiveness of dHACM in patients residing in the United States undergoing transcanal tympanoplasty.

Materials and Methods

A clinical evaluation of the dHACM allograft for tympanic membrane repair was conducted. All transcanal tympanoplasties were performed by a single surgeon in an outpatient surgical setting and

***Corresponding author:** Griffith S Hsu, DuPage Medical Group, 430 Pennsylvania Avenue, Suite 330, Glen Ellyn, IL 60137, USA, E-mail: griffith.hsu@dupagemd.com

utilized dHACM for the primary graft. Clinical records were reviewed from patients with stable tympanic membrane perforation of greater than 6 months in duration undergoing transcanal tympanoplasty between November 2009 and November 2010. An Investigational Review Board (Western IRB) reviewed the project summary and determined that the project met the conditions for exemption under 45 CFR 46.101(b) [4].

Surgical technique and procedure

The procedure was performed at one of two outpatient surgical centers. Subjects underwent general anesthesia and followed standard sterile prepping technique. An operative microscope was used to perform the operation. 1% lidocaine with 1:100,000 epinephrine was infiltrated in the external auditory canal. Sterile saline was used to irrigate the ear canal. After the size of the perforation was noted the timing of the procedure was then initiated. The edges of the perforation were freshened with a straight pick and cupped forceps. The middle ear was then packed with gel foam soaked with saline until the space immediately behind the perforation was obliterated.

An appropriate sized graft of dHACM was then fashioned to cover the perforation. The size of the graft was designed to slightly overlap the size of the perforation so that there would be no visible defect. The dHACM was then hydrated with sterile saline for 30 seconds, and then placed on the lateral surface of the tympanic membrane. The edges were smoothed, allowing continuity of the graft and the native tympanic membrane. Operative photography was taken of the initial perforation and then with the graft in position. Additional saline-soaked gel foam was then placed carefully over the graft, over the borders and the central portion of the graft until the graft was not visible and to secure its position. Once completed, timing was then halted.

Data collection and analysis

Medical record review was conducted to collect patient demographics, clinical presentation at time of surgery, duration of surgery, results of audiometric testing and results of surgery, including documented patient satisfaction. Post-operative office visits were conducted at 1, 3, and 6 weeks after surgery. Audiometric testing was conducted preoperatively and at the 6 week follow-up visit. Outcomes assessed included closure of perforation at 6 weeks, reduction in size of perforation, pain or swelling at the operative site, auditory response, length of operation, and patient and clinician satisfaction with the product.

Results

Over the one year period, dHACM was utilized in 14 patients undergoing transcanal tympanoplasty. Other than all patients presenting with tympanic rupture of at least 6 months duration, patients had different clinical presentations, which is tabulated in Table 1.

Post-operative observations at weeks 1, 3 and 6 are presented in Table 2. Drainage was reported by two patients at week one and three, though this is believed to be related to the gel foam that was used to secure the graft in position. No infections or other adverse events were identified. By post-op week 6, all 14 patients (100%) reported return of hearing. Audiometric testing was performed prior to surgery and at 6 weeks post-op. Overall, mean air bone gap decreased from a pre-op measurement of 23.0 ± 10.1dB to 16.8 ± 7.4dB at 6 weeks post-op (two-tailed p value of 0.058). The eight patients with improved audiometric scores had a mean difference of 13.6 ± 8.9dB between pre-op and 6 week post-op mean air bone gap measurements.

	N=14
Mean Age (years)	42.8 ± 22.5 (9,79)
>18 years	10 (71.4%)
≤ 18 years	4 (28.6%)
Male gender	7 (50%)
Cholesteatoma	1 (7.1%)
Tympanosclerosis	4 (28.6%)
Prior surgery on ear	2 (14.3%)
Size of perforation:	
<25%	9 (64.3%)
25-50%	3 (21.4%)
>50%	2 (14.3%)

Data presented as n (%) as indicated

Table 1: Clinical presentation.

	Week 1 (n=14)	Week 3 (n=14)	Week 6 (n=14)
Pain at surgical site	1 (7.1%)	1 (7.1%)	1 (7.1%)
Swelling	1 (7.1%)	0	0
Drainage	2 (14.3%)	2 (14.3%)	0
Infection	0	0	0
Auditory response	9 (75%)	13 (92.9%)	14 (100%)

Data presented as n (%) as indicated

Table 2: Post-operative observations.

Overall, complete closure of the tympanic membrane occurred in 6 of the 14 patients (42.9%), complete or partial closure occurred in 8 patients (57.1%). Of the 8 patients with continued perforation at 6 weeks post-op, 4 (50%) had tympanosclerosis, 2 were children, and 4 had >25% perforations at time of surgery. Of the 2 patients with prior surgery of the affected ear, one had successful healing and one did not. For those patients without tympanosclerosis (n=10) complete success was achieved in 5 patients (50%) and complete or partial success in 7 patients (70%).

Mean duration of surgery was 13.3 ± 0.10 minutes (range 9.1-23.7 minutes), median 12.2 minutes. Overall, 11 patients reported satisfaction with the procedure and 13 of 14 patients would opt to use the material and operative technique again if future surgery in either ear was required.

Discussion

Investigations conducted outside the United States have reported on the use of natural human amniotic membrane for tympanoplasty [8,9]. Harvinder et al. [9] compared human amniotic membrane and temporalis fascia graft for underlay myringoplasty, concluding that amniotic membrane was a suitable graft material for repairing perforated tympanic membranes. Permeatal, endaural or postauricular approach was used and final outcome was assessed after 6 months. Successful closure was achieved in 13 of 20 (65%) of patients in the amniotic membrane group and in 17 of the 30 (56.7%) of the temporal fascia group. Difficulty in obtaining human amniotic membrane and issues with cleaning and sterilizing the tissue were noted. An Egyptian study by Fouad et al. [8] included 64 patients age 18-50 without cholesteatoma, infection, or prior surgery, reported similar success rates in the temporal fascia group and amniotic membrane groups of 87.5% and 84.4% respectively, although mean operative time was significantly reduced with the use of amniotic membrane [10]. This is an important observation in that avoiding a separate incision to harvest graft material results in reduced operative time, patient discomfort and scarring, and eliminates risk for infection of the harvest site. In the

Fouad study a postauricular approach was used and final outcome was assessed after 3 months. In the present evaluation of dHACM applied via transcanal approach, and including patients with cholesteatoma, tympanosclerosis, and prior surgery, complete closure was observed in 42.9% of patients and partial or complete closure in 57.1%. As differences in surgical approach, patient history and timing of follow up exist between the current study and previous reports results are not comparable.

For over a century, human amniotic membrane has been used in the treatment of various types of wounds [12]. Historically, widespread use of human amniotic membrane has been limited due to issues related with tissue preparation, stabilization and storage. Derived from placentas, human amniotic membranes are often difficult to obtain, prepare and store. The PURION process allows for the creation of a dHACM allograft available in multiple sizes with a shelf life of 5 years at ambient temperature. This is the first evaluation on the use of dHACM to repair tympanic membrane perforations in the United States.

Weaknesses of the present study are those characteristic of retrospective studies and small study samples. The small numbers of patients preclude evaluation of factors that may impact treatment success such as presence of tympanosclerosis, size of perforation, medical history, age, and tobacco use. The lack of controls eliminates the ability to compare results to other treatment modalities. Variable surgical methods, and underlay vs. overlay technique may also contribute to successful closure, but this cannot be assessed with the current data. In addition, patients were only followed for 6 weeks after surgery, a longer follow-up period may allow for better assessment of graft effectiveness.

Although further studies are needed to determine efficacy of dHACM for tympanoplasty and which types of patients may most benefit from its use, the current evaluation provides useful preliminary information and suggests that dHACM may be an acceptable, safe and well tolerated graft material in patients requiring tympanoplasty, especially those where a shorter operative time and/or avoidance of additional graft-harvesting wound is desired.

Source of Study Funding: MiMedx Group, Inc.

References

1. Adams ME, El-Kashlan HK (2010) Tympanoplasty and ossiculoplasty. In: Otolaryngology: Head & Neck Surgery. Cummings CW, Flint PW, Haughey BH, et al. (Edr). (5th Edn), Mosby Elsevier, Philadelphia.
2. Haynes DS, Vos JD, Labadie RF (2005) Acellular allograft dermal matrix for tympanoplasty. Curr Opin Otolaryngol Head Neck Surg 13: 283-286.
3. Ravishanker R, Bath AS, Roy R (2003) "Amnion Bank"--the use of long term glycerol preserved amniotic membranes in the management of superficial and superficial partial thickness burns. Burns 29: 369-374.
4. Parolini O, Solomon A, Evangelista M, Soncini M (2010) Human term placenta as a therapeutic agent: from the first clinical applications to future perspectives. In: Berven E. editor. Human Placenta: Structure and Development. Nova Science Publishers: 1-48.
5. Kato M, Jackler RK (1996) Repair of chronic tympanic membrane perforations with fibroblast growth factor. Otolaryngol Head Neck Surg 115: 538-547.
6. Ma Y, Zhao H, Zhou X (2002) Topical treatment with growth factors for tympanic membrane perforations: progress towards clinical application. Acta Otolaryngol 122: 586-599.
7. Koob TJ, Rennert R, Zabek N, Massee M, Lim JJ, et al. (2013) Biological properties of dehydrated human amnion/chorion composite graft: implications for chronic wound healing. Int Wound J 10: 493-500.
8. Fouad T, Rifaat M, Buhaibeh Q (2010) Utilization of amniotic membrane graft for repair of the tympanic membrane perforation. EJENTAS 11:31-34.
9. Harvinder S, Hassan S, Sidek DS, Hamzah M, Samsudin AR, et al. (2005) Underlay myringoplasty: comparison of human amniotic membrane to temporalis fascia graft. Med J Malaysia 60: 585-589.
10. Shojaku H, Takakura H, Okabe M, Fujisaka M, Watanabe Y, et al. (2011) Effect of hyperdry amniotic membrane patches attached over the bony surface of mastoid cavities in canal wall down tympanoplasty. Laryngoscope 121:1953-1957.
11. Turan E, Onerci M, Hosal S, Akdas F (1990) Use of liyofilized human amniotic membrane as lining the tympanic cavities. J Islamic Academy Sciences 1:66-69.
12. John T (2003) Human amniotic membrane transplantation: past, present, and future. Ophthalmol Clin North Am 16: 43-65, vi. t

Variables that Effect Psychophysical Parameters and Duration to Stability in Cochlear Implant Mapping

Maria CS[1*] and Maria PLS[2]

[1]*Department of Ear Sciences, The University of Western Australia, Nedlands, Western Australia, Australia*

[2]*Ear Science Institute Australia, Subiaco, Western Australia, Australia*

[*]**Corresponding author:** Chloe Santa Maria, Department of Ear Sciences, The University of Western Australia, 4th Floor, Harry Perkins Medical Research Institute, QEII Medical Campus, Hospital Ave, Nedlands, WA, 6000, Australia, E-mail: chloesantamaria1@gmail.com

Abstract

The process of rehabilitation after cochlear implant surgery involves programming the psychophysical parameters of the implant in a process called mapping. The audiology appointments involved in the mapping process are large contributors to cost of implant rehabilitation. The map is defined as stable when there is little variation over time. Once an implant map is stable there is reduced need for intensive rehabilitation and an increase in implant patient satisfaction. A literature search was conducted using the terms "map cochlear implant", "mapping cochlear implant", "psychophysical cochlear implant" with a date range from August 1957 to February 2016. A total of 560 articles were identified and 29 articles were retrieved for detailed evaluation. The most important factor identified, that determines map stability, is the patient's subjective implant experience. Patient demographics and implant variables have not been identified as significant. The second side implant in bilateral implantation has been shown to have significantly less time to map stability. There is a need for further studies to examine relationships between preoperative variables and the mapping process, rather than applying a "one size fits all approach", which is the current standard of care. This is of particular need in the setting of the second side in bilateral implantation.

Introduction

Hearing and speech perception for sensorineural hearing loss sufferers have been improved significantly since the advent of cochlear implantation [1]. Patients are required to perform audiological rehabilitation post implantation in order to achieve the best hearing outcomes. The process of rehabilitation and cochlear implant programming involves a process called mapping.

Mapping involves the measurement of a patient' physical responses to audiological stimuli with the resultant psychophysical profile termed the map. This involves generating a noise and asking patients whether they can hear it and to what degree. The psychophysical parameters that are measured include Threshold (T) scores, Comfort (C) scores and the Dynamic Range (DR) [2].

The T score is the quietest sound detectable that always produces a response by a given patient, the C score is the loudest sound that they can tolerate without discomfort for a sustained period of time, and the DR is the difference between these two values [2]. Psychophysical parameters are measured for each portion of the cochlear implant electrode array (the basal, medial and apical regions). This mapping stage is known to be a period of high variability in audiological responses, and requires close follow up by an audiologist with an average of 6 visits in the first year, with some institutions advocating for up to ten [3-5].

Map stability occurs when there is little variation in these parameters over time, and is assessed through audiological graphing of the data. Once a cochlear implant map is stable there is reduced need for ongoing rehabilitation, reduced need for intensive monitoring and an increase in implant satisfaction. Typically this period of variability requires six weeks to six months to become stable [3,6-9].

Patient audiological benefits are often balanced with the costs associated with cochlear implantation to justify the health economics, many such analyses take into account the direct and indirect surgical and device costs but do not directly evaluate the costs associated with rehabilitation afterwards [10-13].

Literature examining the duration of audiological rehabilitation and efficiency in cochlear implants have found the average duration of audiological visit to be 93 minutes, and given the frequency of visits post implantation, these costs are significant [14]. The time to achieve map stability directly impacts the number of post implantation audiological reviews and so it is important to identify what variables influence this. An understanding of the factors that affect map stability helps to inform decision making during the perioperative period and may also provide some cost efficiency with regards to rehabilitation.

Methods

A pubmed search using terms "map cochlear implant", "mapping cochlear implant" and "psychophysical cochlear implant" was performed with a date range of August 1957 to February 2016. A total of 560 articles were identified. Articles were screened for title and abstract only with a total of 29 articles retrieved for a more detailed evaluation. Articles reviewed were limited to the English language.

Discussion

Most cochlear implant centers apply a "one size fits all approach" to the mapping process [5]. This leads to a failure to identify, and potentially address, outliers until they are failing to stabilize within the usual time. Very few studies report on medium to long term psychophysical characteristics of cochlear implant audiological rehabilitation which limits the ability to understand the true effect of variables on the mapping process. Factors that have been examined in the literature in relation to map stability include subjective patient feedback, age, gender, etiology of deafness, duration of deafness, array type, and sequence in bilateral sequential cochlear implantation.

Subjective patient feedback

Most centers rely mainly on the patient's subjective feedback as a basis for the mapping changes, which is interesting considering most clinicians do not believe the patient's subjective experience leads to optimal cochlear implant performance [5]. In a global survey of cochlear implant center mapping practices, it was found that the average center schedules three sessions in the first three months, three sessions in the following nine months, and another one annual session thereafter [5]. The majority of time, in these appointments, is spent with verification and adjustments to optimize loudness. Most centers rarely spend time adjusting map parameters other than minimum and maximum levels in follow up appointments. The most important factor that determines map stability is the patient's subjective implant experience. This of course is difficult to quantify but there are a number of potential factors discussed below that contribute to this.

Age

Age, as a predictor of cochlear implant audiological outcomes, is reported in the literature with different effect. Some of the published literature indicate that older age at implantation relates to poorer audiological outcomes [15,16]. Most studies examining the specific effect of age however have not shown any significant effect [4,17,18]. One study suggested a difference between adults and children in the first six months, with comfort levels showing significant change but beyond six months the levels were stable [19]. This did not change the overall time to map stability and was thought to be due to the fitting method used in children rather than actual psychophysical differences. It is possible that the effect of age at implantation on audiological outcomes in the studies mentioned above, may be in part reflecting a longer duration of deafness rather than a pure effect of age on outcome. From the information in the literature it seems that while age may contribute to the audiological outcome of the cochlear implant, it has little long term effect on the mapping process.

Gender

From examining the few studies that have examined the relationship between gender and audiological outcomes, psychophysical parameters and stability duration, there is no significant effect of gender [4,17].

Etiology of deafness

Establishing an effect of etiology of deafness and psychophysical parameters and stability is often challenging, given that frequently the cause of deafness is unknown. Because of the lack of most studies to differentiate etiology, there is yet to be any identified conditions that definitively have a significant effect [3,4,20]. A few specific conditions have been identified as likely having particular effects on elements of the psychophysical parameters. The T score has been associated with the presence and type of tissue present within the cochlear, with pathological tissue growth within the cochlear being associated with increased T scores and a reduced DR score [21,22]. Conditions associated with ganglion cell survival may show a relationship between number of surviving neurons and improved C scores [20]. The degree to which pathological tissue or nerve cell survival impacts on duration to stability however has not been assessed.

Duration of deafness

It is well established that the longer the duration of deafness the poorer the audiological outcomes with cochlear implantation [16,17,23-25]. Prolonged auditory deprivation has been considered to be a significant factor in reducing the benefit potentially received by cochlear implantation, and is the foundation for the recommendation of preoperative hearing aids [26]. Dynamic ranges have been found to be reduced with deafness greater than 10 years, which may influence satisfaction with the implant [20]. Duration of deafness has not been shown as a significant variable for time to map stability [4].

Array type

One small study compared perimodiolar arrays to straight electrode arrays in the same individuals who had bilateral implantation first with one and then another electrode array type. As might be expected, compound action potential thresholds, T levels and C levels were lower in perimodiolar arrays but there was not any significant difference in dynamic range [27]. This study did not follow patients for long enough to comment on timing for stability, but given the lack of difference in dynamic range between array types, it would be unlikely to be an important variable for map stability.

The second side in bilateral cochlear implantation

In the current health economic climate of first world countries, many researchers are investigating to justify the cost effectiveness of bilateral cochlear implantation. Bilateral implantation have added benefits (over unilateral) to recipients with bilateral profound hearing loss including improved sound localization and speech perception in noise [28,29]. This follows on to provide improved quality of life in a way that can be measured as a positive over the economic cost [10-13]. A randomized control trial on cost utility of bilateral implants concluded that bilateral implants is cost effective if the patient has a life expectancy of five to ten years or longer [30]. Interestingly, the majority of cost analyses of bilateral implantation are yet to incorporate the costs associated with implant rehabilitation and mapping. When examined as a primary outcome, the time for map stability has been defined as significantly shorter on the second side [4]. There was a reduced time to achieve stability on average by 36 days in the second implant (87 days for first implant and 51 days for the second implant) [4]. Potential explanations for faster duration to achieve stability include faster neural pathways and neuroplasticity resulting from prior experience and practice relating to the first implant mapping process. Prior learning has been shown to be fundamental in the development of new neural pathways [31]. Other proposed mechanisms include patients being more familiar with the process and what auditory stimuli sound like. It is recognized that initial auditory stimuli is often labelled as uncomfortable or not tolerable relating to inexperience and unfamiliarity with tones, and that with experience these tones become recognized as acceptable [32]. All these potential explanations tie back to the patient's subjective experience being the most likely factor affecting time of map stability. Despite this significantly reduced duration and the costs associated with audiology follow up, many institutions do not alter the mapping process for the second side in bilateral implantation.

With consideration to mapping, a unique issue to the second implanted side is that of the user needing to fuse the information of both implants into a single sound stimuli. Failure to do this by the patient leads to sounds seeming unbalanced with a single sound source being perceived as separate [33]. Balancing not only involves loudness but also localization of the sound source. Fusion of the sound information can take time, although how long is needed is undefined. There has been a suggestion that new mapping procedures and signal processing strategies are needed, for the second implant in bilateral implantation, to allow for better fusion between them [33-35]. Another potential for delay in the second side is that electrodes mapped to the same frequency range in each ear may stimulate different locations in each cochlea due to an insertion depth difference of each electrode array. This also can account for poor sound image fusion [36]. It is recognized that the timing of the second implant, particularly in pre lingual children, is important for outcomes including central processing and language development [37]. It has not been reported whether this translates into comparably longer mapping times for the second implant. If these factors where adapted into a mapping process designed for the second side in bilateral implantation, the time for map stability could even be potentially shorter.

As described above, since the patient's subjective feedback is the major tool in an audiology mapping session, it seems plausible why only limited variables have been directly linked to timing for map stability and that in the case of the second implant a patient benefits from having already experienced a first implant [4].

Other potential variables

A number of other factors have been identified as effecting the audiological outcomes of cochlear implantation including pre-lingual compared to post-lingual deafness, the presence of residual hearing, the coding strategy used and the implant manufacturer [38-39]. These have yet to be examined with regards to mapping and would benefit from being investigated in future research.

Conclusion

The time it takes to map stability contributes greatly to the cost of post-operative rehabilitation in cochlear implantation. The greatest factor in determining map stability is the patient's subjective experience. Because this is difficult to quantify, there is a need for further studies to examine relationships between preoperative variables and the mapping process so that these can be factored into the mapping planning, rather than applying a "one size fits all approach", which is the current standard of care. This is of particular need in the setting of the second side in bilateral implantation.

References

1. Russell JL, Pine HS, Young DL (2013) Pediatric cochlear implantation: expanding applications and outcomes. Pediatr Clin North Am 60: 841-863.
2. Shapiro WH, Bradham TS (2012) Cochlear implant programming. Otolaryngol Clin North Am 45: 111-127.
3. Walravens E, Mawman D, O'Driscoll M (2006) Changes in psychophysical parameters during the first month of programming the nucleus contour and contour advance cochlear implants. Cochlear Implants Int 7: 15-32.
4. Domville-Lewis C, Santa Maria PL, Upson G, Chester-Browne R, Atlas MD (2015) Psychophysical Map Stability in Bilateral Sequential Cochlear Implantation: Comparing Current Audiology Methods to a New Statistical Definition. Ear Hear 36: 497-504.
5. Vaerenberg B, Smits C, De Ceulaer G, Zir E, Harman S, et al. (2014) Cochlear implant programming: a global survey on the state of the art. ScientificWorldJournal 2014: 501738.
6. Schmidt M, Griesser A (1997) Long-term stability of fitting parameters with the COMBI 40. Am J Otol 18: S109-110.
7. Brown CJ, Hughes ML, Luk B, Abbas PJ, Wolaver A, et al. (2000) The relationship between EAP and EABR thresholds and levels used to program the nucleus 24 speech processor: data from adults. Ear Hear 21: 151-163.
8. Franck KH, Norton SJ (2001) Estimation of psychophysical levels using the electrically evoked compound action potential measured with the neural response telemetry capabilities of Cochlear Corporation's CI24M device. Ear Hear 22: 289-299.
9. Vargas JL, Sainz M, Roldan C, Alvarez I, de la Torre A (2012) Long-term evolution of the electrical stimulation levels for cochlear implant patients. Clin Exp Otorhinolaryngol 5: 194-200.
10. Summerfield AQ, Lovett RE, Bellenger H, Batten G (2010) Estimates of the cost-effectiveness of pediatric bilateral cochlear implantation. Ear Hear 31: 611-624.
11. Kuthubutheen J, Mittmann N, Amoodi H, Qian W, Chen JM (2015) The effect of different utility measures on the cost-effectiveness of bilateral cochlear implantation. Laryngoscope 125: 442-447.
12. Chen JM, Amoodi H, Mittmann N (2014) Cost-utility analysis of bilateral cochlear implantation in adults: a health economic assessment from the perspective of a publicly funded program. Laryngoscope 124: 1452-1458.
13. Crathorne L, Bond M, Cooper C, Elston J, Weiner G, et al. (2012) A systematic review of the effectiveness and cost-effectiveness of bilateral multichannel cochlear implants in adults with severe-to-profound hearing loss. Clin Otolaryngol 37: 342-354.
14. Shapiro WH, Huang T, Shaw T, Roland JT Jr, Lalwani AK (2008) Remote intraoperative monitoring during cochlear implant surgery is feasible and efficient. Otol Neurotol 29: 495-498.
15. Gantz BJ, Tyler RS, Knutson JF, Woodworth G, Abbas P, et al. (1988) Evaluation of five different cochlear implant designs: audiologic assessment and predictors of performance. Laryngoscope 98: 1100-1106.
16. Blamey PJ, Pyman BC, Gordon M, Clark GM, Brown AM, et al. (1992) Factors predicting postoperative sentence scores in postlinguistically deaf adult cochlear implant patients. Ann Otol Rhinol Laryngol 101: 342-348.
17. Green KM, Bhatt Y, Mawman DJ, O'Driscoll MP, Saeed SR, et al. (2007) Predictors of audiological outcome following cochlear implantation in adults. Cochlear Implants Int 8: 1-11.
18. Shea JJ, Domico EH, Orchik DJ (1990) Speech recognition ability as a function of duration of deafness in multichannel cochlear implant patients. Laryngoscope 100: 223-226.
19. Molisz A, Zarowski A, Vermeiren A, Theunen T, De Coninck L, et al. (2015) Postimplantation changes of electrophysiological parameters in patients with cochlear implants. Audiol Neurootol 20: 222-228.
20. Shim Y, Kim H, Chang M, Kim C (1995) Map dynamic ranges versus duration of hearing loss in cochlear implantees. Ann Otol Rhinol Laryngol Suppl 166: 178-180.
21. Busby PA, Plant KL, Whitford LA (2002) Electrode impedance in adults and children using the Nucleus 24 cochlear implant system. Cochlear Implants Int 3: 87-103.
22. Kawano A, Seldon HL, Clark GM, Ramsden RT, Raine CH (1998) Intracochlear factors contributing to psychophysical percepts following cochlear implantation. Acta Otolaryngol 118: 313-326.
23. Gantz BJ, Woodworth GG, Knutson JF, Abbas PJ, Tyler RS (1993) Multivariate predictors of audiological success with multichannel cochlear implants. Ann Otol Rhinol Laryngol 102: 909-916.
24. Kileny PR, Zimmerman-Phillips S, Kemink JL, Schmaltz SP (1991) Effects of preoperative electrical stimulability and historical factors on performance with multichannel cochlear implant. Ann Otol Rhinol Laryngol 100: 563-568.

25. Waltzman SB, Fisher SG, Niparko JK, Cohen NL (1995) Predictors of postoperative performance with cochlear implants. Ann Otol Rhinol Laryngol Suppl 165: 15-18.

26. Mosnier I, Bebear JP, Marx M, Fraysse B, Truy E, et al. (2014) Predictive factors of cochlear implant outcomes in the elderly. Audiol Neurootol 19: 15-20.

27. Jeong J, Kim M, Heo JH, Bang MY, Bae MR, et al. (2015) Intraindividual comparison of psychophysical parameters between perimodiolar and lateral-type electrode arrays in patients with bilateral cochlear implants. Otol Neurotol 36: 228-234.

28. Tyler RS, Dunn CC, Witt SA, Noble WG (2007) Speech perception and localization with adults with bilateral sequential cochlear implants. Ear Hear 28: 86S-90S.

29. Basura GJ, Eapen R, Buchman CA (2009) Bilateral cochlear implantation: current concepts, indications, and results. Laryngoscope 119: 2395-2401.

30. Smulders YE, van Zon A, Stegeman I, van Zanten GA, Rinia AB, et al. (2016) Cost-Utility of Bilateral Versus Unilateral Cochlear Implantation in Adults: A Randomized Controlled Trial. Otol Neurotol 37: 38-45.

31. Eggermont JJ (2008) The role of sound in adult and developmental auditory cortical plasticity. Ear Hear 29: 819-829.

32. Sun JC, Skinner MW, Liu SY, Huang TS (1999) Effect of speech processor program modifications on cochlear implant recipients' threshold and maximum acceptable loudness levels. Am J Audiol 8: 128-136.

33. Fitzgerald MB, Kan A, Goupell MJ (2015) Bilateral Loudness Balancing and Distorted Spatial Perception in Recipients of Bilateral Cochlear Implants. Ear Hear 36: e225-236.

34. Fitzgerald MB, Sagi E, Morbiwala TA, Tan CT, Svirsky MA (2013) Feasibility of real-time selection of frequency tables in an acoustic simulation of a cochlear implant. Ear Hear 34: 763-772.

35. Goupell MJ, Kan A, Litovsky RY (2013) Mapping procedures can produce non-centered auditory images in bilateral cochlear implantees. J Acoust Soc Am 133: EL101-107.

36. Kan A, Litovsky RY, Goupell MJ (2015) Effects of interaural pitch matching and auditory image centering on binaural sensitivity in cochlear implant users. Ear Hear 36: e62-68.

37. Santa Maria PL, Oghalai JS (2014) When is the best timing for the second implant in pediatric bilateral cochlear implantation? Laryngoscope 124: 1511-1512.

38. van Schoonhoven J, Sparreboom M, van Zanten BG, Scholten RJ, Mylanus EA, et al. (2013) The effectiveness of bilateral cochlear implants for severe-to-profound deafness in adults: a systematic review. Otol Neurotol 34: 190-198.

39. Gaylor JM, Raman G, Chung M, Lee J, Rao M, et al. (2013) Cochlear implantation in adults: a systematic review and meta-analysis. JAMA Otolaryngol Head Neck Surg 139: 265-272.

Approach to the Patient with External Laryngeal Trauma: The Schaefer Classification

Omakobia E* and Micallef A

Department of ENT and Head & Neck Surgery, University College Hospital, London

Corresponding author: Omakobia E, Senior House Officer in ENT and Head & Neck Surgery, University College Hospital, 235 Euston Road, London, NW1 2BU, E-mail: eugeneomakobia@doctors.org.uk

Abstract

Although not a common presentation, laryngeal trauma can be a potentially life-threatening injury and therefore warrants close attention by relevant clinicians including general practitioners, emergency department practitioners and otolaryngologists. In our experience, since such cases are not frequently encountered, knowledge of optimal assessment and management is highly variable. In this article, we present a further case of laryngeal trauma, emphasizing the importance of a clear and structured management approach including the use of a classification system for injury severity. We hope that this will serve as a useful aide-mémoire to clinicians thus improving patient survival and long-term functional outcomes, specifically relating to breathing, speech and swallowing.

Introduction

Laryngeal trauma is an uncommon presentation to the otolaryngologist usually via the emergency department and rarely via a general practitioner. However, due to the potentially life-threatening nature of such injuries, it is crucial that relevant clinicians are aware of key principles surrounding initial assessment and management. Since such cases are infrequently encountered, confidence in managing these cases is variable. There is a wide range of presenting signs and symptoms, which may not correlate with severity of injury; hence severe injuries may be missed. Here we present a further case of laryngeal trauma which was successfully managed conservatively. We emphasise the importance of a structured management plan for the various types of laryngeal trauma, and the use of a classification system for severity of injury. Such measures have been shown to increase patient survival and improve long-term functional outcomes, pertaining to breathing, speech and swallowing.

Case Report

A 46 year old female presents to the emergency department having been held in a strangle hold by a prisoner for approximately ten minutes during her work as a prison nurse. On arrival, she complains of difficulty breathing, a hoarse voice and anterior neck discomfort. She is promptly assessed by emergency department clinicians who deem her airway to be stable as she has no stridor and is maintaining oxygen saturations of 96-98% on room air. She is then referred to the otolaryngology (ENT) team for further assessment. On examination by the ENT team, mild bruising is noted overlying the left side of the thyroid cartilage but the normal anatomical landmarks of the neck are preserved. Flexible endoscopic examination of the larynx revealed mild oedema and bruising of the vocal cords which were otherwise mobile; consistent with a Schaefer type 1 laryngeal injury. A Computerised Tomography (CT) scan was organised which ruled out laryngeal fracture and showed no mucosal disruption. The patient was then treated with intravenous dexamethasone (with proton pump inhibitor cover to prevent further laryngeal irritation), nebulised adrenaline and humidified oxygen as required, antibiotics and voice rest. She was observed on the ward for 48 hours and clinically improved. She was then safely discharged and at 2 week follow up in the laryngology outpatient clinic, her voice and airway were found to be markedly improved with no swallowing difficulties.

Discussion

What are the broad types of external laryngeal trauma?

Two broad categories of external laryngeal trauma are recognised, namely penetrating or blunt injuries [1]. Common mechanisms resulting in blunt laryngeal trauma include motor vehicle accidents, physical assault (as in the reported case) or sports injuries. Penetrating laryngeal trauma may arise following knife, gunshot and blast injuries [2]. Laryngeal trauma is thought to account for less than 1% of all cases seen at major trauma centres and constitutes approximately 1 in 30'000 emergency department visits [3]. Schaefer SD reviewed cases of laryngeal trauma over a 27 year period and noted increasing rates of penetrating neck injuries, whilst blunt laryngeal injuries appear to be declining. This appeared to be a consistent finding throughout the literature [3,4].

Whilst this report primarily focuses on external laryngeal trauma, it is important to note that iatrogenic internal injury, in particular intubation trauma, is a significant aetiological factor not to be overlooked. Notably, the most common cause of arytenoid cartilage dislocation cited in the literature is intubation trauma, accounting for 80% of cases, followed by external trauma, implicated in 15% of cases [5].

How do patients present?

A key factor to note from the outset when assessing patients who have suffered laryngeal trauma is that no single symptom correlates well with injury severity. Indeed, laryngeal trauma may initially go unnoticed as patients may appear deceptively asymptomatic in the early hours after injury [6]. Common presenting symptoms include dysphonia, neck pain and/or bruising, dyspnoea, aphonia, haemoptysis and odynophagia. Common signs of laryngeal injury include stridor, subcutaneous emphysema, loss of normal anatomical landmarks of the neck, neck tenderness or bruising, loss of laryngeal crepitus, vocal cord paralysis and airway obstruction [7-9].

It is worth noting that whilst laryngeal trauma is an uncommon presentation in adult patients, the incidence of paediatric laryngotracheal injuries is even lower. This is thought to be attributable to several factors. Firstly, children are less likely to be involved in violent altercations and road traffic accidents. Secondly, the paediatric larynx is more pliable and anatomically located higher in the neck, allowing more protection from the mandible in comparison to adults; thereby decreasing the likelihood of fracture. However, by virtue of its narrower lumen and looser mucosal attachments to underlying cartilage, the paediatric larynx is more predisposed to soft tissue injury, including oedema and haematoma formation, resulting in life-threatening airway obstruction [10]. This is an important concept to be aware of at initial presentation as it can be seen that the age of the patient can affect the likelihood of specific types of laryngeal injury. A high index of clinical suspicion is required for early diagnosis.

What are the priorities in initial assessment?

The Advanced Trauma Life Support (ATLS) protocol is indicated for any individual who is severely injured. In keeping with this protocol, the initial priority is to assess and secure the airway in any patient who has suffered laryngeal trauma [11]. Once deemed stable, the airway should be further evaluated using flexible fibreoptic laryngoscopy to assess the extent of laryngeal injury. This is a critical step in the initial assessment of patients who have experienced laryngeal trauma.

Additionally, cervical spine injuries must be excluded in all cases of laryngeal trauma [12]. Due to the likelihood of concurrent injuries, a complete trauma assessment must be performed in keeping with ATLS principles. In a large case series of 392 patients over a 5 year period, associated injuries included skull base or intracranial injury (13%), open neck injury (9%), cervical spine injury (8%) and oesophageal or pharyngeal injury (3%) [12].

When should patients be referred to ENT?

Emergency department clinicians and rarely general practitioners are usually the first to assess patients who have experienced laryngeal trauma. Such patients should be referred to an ENT specialist for airway assessment and flexible fibreoptic laryngoscopic examination. In our experience, some clinicians felt that very minor cases of laryngeal trauma e.g., sports injuries could be discharged home without ENT input.

However, it is widely reported in the literature that although patients may sometimes appear asymptomatic, there may be a severe underlying laryngeal injury [6]. Atkins et al. suggest that up to a third of cases may initially present without symptoms in the first 24-48 hours post injury [13]. Hence, we would argue that some form of early ENT input would be prudent for all cases of laryngeal trauma.

What investigations are required?

If the airway stable, it is widely accepted that Computerised Tomography (CT) remains the gold standard for assessing the extent of laryngeal injury. CT imaging also helps to rule out cervical spine injuries. Most studies report high sensitivity and specificity, although stated absolute values were not found in the literature [14]. Hence, most patients with laryngeal injury undergo CT imaging as a first line imaging investigation.

However, in paediatric patients, where laryngeal cartilages are not ossified and consequently not well visualised on CT, MRI (Magnetic Resonance Imaging) is advisable as a suitable second line imaging investigation [15]. Indeed, Duda Jr et al. report that by virtue of its superior contrast resolution, MR imaging may be preferable in detecting epiglottic injuries, including avulsion in the subacute or chronic setting [16]. Furthermore, CT imaging may miss laryngeal fractures and cartilage avulsions. In cases, where there is clinical suspicion of laryngeal fracture but no definitive CT findings, MRI should be considered to aid in diagnosis.

Obviously, if the airway is not stable and cannot be managed safely, CT scanning is inadvisable. In these cases, it may be necessary to proceed directly to neck exploration as the risks to the patient outweigh the benefits of imaging [11].

Is there a classification system for severity of injury?

The Schaefer Classification System for categorising the severity of laryngeal injury is the most widely used [3]. Through this system, laryngeal injuries are divided into five categories of increasing severity, outlined in Table 1 below.

Groups	Severity of injury in ascending order
Group 1	Minor endolaryngeal hematomas or lacerations without detectable fractures
Group 2	More severe edema, hematoma, minor mucosal disruption without exposed cartilage, or nondisplaced fractures
Group 3	Massive edema, large mucosal lacerations, exposed cartilage, displaced fractures, or vocal cord immobility.
Group 4	Same as group 3, but more severe, with disruption of anterior larynx, unstable fractures, two or more fractures lines, or severe mucosa! Injuries.
Group 5	Complete laryngotracheal separation.

Table 1: Schaefer classification system [3].

Schaefer SD looked at a large case series of 139 consecutive patients with laryngeal trauma over a 27 year period. A particular emphasis was placed on patient management and the findings were used to devise a classification system for injury severity. Whilst each laryngeal injury is unique and must be managed on its own merit, categorisation of injuries into an organised system assists clinicians in determining a structured management plan.

How are patients managed?

Patients are managed according to the severity of injury; hence the Schaefer classification system serves as a useful guide. Management ranges from adjunctive medical treatment for mild injuries e.g., humidification, steroids, antibiotics and anti-reflux agents to surgical treatments including direct laryngoscopy, pharyngo-oesophagoscopy, tracheotomy and open repair with or without stenting for progressively more severe injuries. Suggested management for each type of injury is best summarised in Table 2 below.

Type	Management
1	Observation, humidification, antibiotics, steroids, anti-reflux medications, voice rest
2	Tracheotomy/intubation, panendoscopy, antibiotics, steroids
3	Panendoscopy, open surgical repair with or without stenting and with or without tracheotomy
4	Panendoscopy, open surgical repair with stenting, with tracheotomy
5	Tracheotomy/intubation, panendoscopy, reconstruction, restoration, or resection with end-to-end anastomosis with or without stenting

Table 2: Suggested management for each type of laryngeal injury [17].

It is important to note that laryngeal trauma infrequently occurs as an isolated injury and there may be concomitant injuries. If there is associated facial trauma, this poses additional difficulties in securing the airway as there may be oedema, bleeding, secretions or loss of bony support, complicating face mask ventilation [18]. Once intubation is considered, the aim is to pass the endotracheal tube across the injured area without precipitating more injury.

Alternatively, tracheostomy aims to gain airway access distal to the site of injury. As in the reported case, Schaefer type 1 minor endolaryngeal injuries can be managed conservatively with antibiotics, steroids, voice rest and anti-reflux medications. However, for more severe Schaefer type 3-5 injuries, open surgical repair will be required to secure a definitive airway. Thus, a systematic classification and management approach is crucial in guiding early decision-making and improving patient outcomes.

Are there any long-term complications?

In studies involving both penetrating and blunt laryngeal trauma, complication rates with regard to chronic airway obstruction have been estimated to be as high as 15-17%, whilst voice compromise occurs in up to 21-25% of cases [12]. There is evidence to suggest that early treatment within 48 hours improves patient outcomes in terms of voice and airway function when compared to delayed treatment. In a reasonable size case series of 112 patients with laryngeal trauma, Butler et al. reported that 28% had good voice outcome with 73% having good airway function in the delayed treatment group. In comparison, significantly better outcomes were noted in the early treatment group, with 78% having good voice outcome and 93% having good airway function [14] and 99% of all patients reported normal swallowing after laryngeal injury.

Key Points

Very mild initial signs and symptoms may occasionally mask a very severe laryngeal injury, ultimately leading to airway compromise or obstruction.

The immediate priority in the treatment of laryngeal injuries is to establish and maintain a stable airway.

Airway evaluation should include flexible fibreoptic laryngoscopy and imaging to allow classification of injury severity; thus guiding treatment planning to improve patient outcomes.

References

1. Ballenger JJ (1985) Diseases of the Nose, Throat and Ear, Head and Neck (13th ed.) Philadelphia, Pa: Lea and Febiger pp: 432-453.
2. Sniezek JC, Thomas RW (2012) Resident Manual of Trauma to the Face, Head, and Neck, American Academy of Otolaryngology-Head and Neck Surgery pp: 177.
3. Schaefer SD (1992) The acute management of external laryngeal trauma. A 27-year experience. Arch Otolaryngol Head Neck Surg 118: 598-604.
4. Gussack GS, Jurkovich GJ, Luterman A (1986) Laryngotracheal trauma: a protocol approach to a rare injury. Laryngoscope 96: 660-665.
5. Teng Y, Wang H, Lin Z (2014) Arytenoid Cartilage Dislocation from External Blunt Laryngeal Trauma: Evaluation and Therapy without Laryngeal Electromyography. Med Sci Monit 20: 1496-1502.
6. Myers EM, Iko BO (1987) The management of acute laryngeal trauma. J Trauma 27: 448-452.
7. Levine RJ, Sanders AB, La Mear WR (1995) Bilateral vocal cord paralysis following blunt trauma to the neck. Ann Emerg Med 25: 253-255.
8. Goldenberg D, Golz A, Flax-Goldenberg R, Joachims HZ (1997) Severe laryngeal injury caused by blunt trauma to the neck: a case report. J Laryngol Otol 111: 1174-1176.
9. Oh JH, Min HS, Park TU, Lee SJ, Kim SE (2007) Isolated cricoid fracture associated with blunt neck trauma. Emerg Med J 24: 505-506.
10. Chatterjee D, Agarwal R, Bajaj L, Teng SN, Prager JD (2016) Airway management in laryngotracheal injuries from blunt neck trauma in children. Paediatr Anaesth 26: 132-138.
11. Schaefer SD (2014) Management of acute blunt and penetrating external laryngeal trauma. Laryngoscope 124: 233-244.
12. Jewett BS, Shockley WW, Rutledge R (1999) External laryngeal trauma analysis of 392 patients. Arch Otolaryngol Head Neck Surg 125: 877-880.
13. Atkins BZ, Abbate S, Fisher SR, Vaslef SN (2004) Current management of laryngotracheal trauma: case report and literature review. J Trauma 56: 185-190.
14. Butler AP, Wood BP, O'Rourke AK, Porubsky ES (2005) Acute external laryngeal trauma: experience with 112 patients. Ann Otol Rhinol Laryngol 114: 361-368.
15. Becker M, Burkhardt K, Dulguerov P, Allal A (2008) Imaging of the larynx and hypopharynx. Eur J Radiol 66: 460-479.
16. Duda JJ, Lewin JS, Eliachar I (1996) MR evaluation of epiglottic disruption. AJNR Am J Neuroradiol 17: 563-566.
17. Lee WT, Eliashar R, Eliachar I (2006) Acute external laryngotracheal trauma: diagnosis and management. Ear Nose Throat J 85: 179-184.
18. Jain U, McCunn M, Smith CE, Pittet JF (2016) Management of the Traumatized Airway. Anesthesiology 124: 199-206.

Advanced Bionics® Cochlear Implants in Patients with Prelingual Hearing Loss

Henrique Furlan Pauna[1]*, Guilherme Machado de Carvalho[2], Alexandre Caixeta Guimarães[3], Luiz Henrique Schuch[3], Eder Barbosa Muranaka[2], Walter Adriano Bianchini[4], Agrício Nubiato Crespo[5], Edi Lucia Sartorato[6] and Arthur Menino Castilho[4]

[1]*Resident at Otolaryngology, Head and Neck Department, UNICAMP, Brazil*
[2]*MD, ENT Doctor at Otolaryngology, Head and Neck Department, UNNICAMP, Brazil*
[3]*ENT Doctor at Otolaryngology, Head and Neck Department, UNICAMP, Brazil*
[4]*ENT Doctor, Otologist, MD, PhD, Head Otology, Audiology and Implantable Ear Prostheses, UNICAMP, Brazil*
[5]*ENT Doctor, MD, PhD, Head of Otolaryngology, Head and Neck Department, UNICAMP, Brazil*
[6]*PhD, Head of CBMEG, UNICAMP, Brazil*

Abstract

Introduction: Cochlear Implants (CI) have become standard in the treatment of prelingual, postlingual and perilingual deafness in children. Bilateral implants are considered standard for bilaterally affected children. Studies also find that the CI provides better access to speech for most children, and this access results in improved speech perception. In earlier times children who did not react to acoustic stimuli and were neither able to understand speech nor to acquire it spontaneously encountered severe discrimination, being dismissed as simple-minded or worse. Different studies broadly agree that one or two of every 1000 newborns have a hearing impairment that on current evidence warrants treatment or observation, i.e., permanent hearing loss with a lowering of the absolute threshold of hearing for speech perception by at least 35 dB. Approximately 50% of severe hearing impairments arising in the inner ear are thought to be hereditary in origin. When new Cochlear Implant (CI) sound processors are being introduced by the manufacturers, usually the newest generation implants benefit first from the new technology in order to release the full potential of the new hardware.

Objective: Evaluate the improvement of speech language and sound perception in patients with prelingual deafness that underwent cochlear implant using Advanced Bionics® device.

Method: Retrospective study of the medical records of the patients fitted with Advanced Bionics® cochlear implant in our institution between 2011 and 2012.

Results: Sixteen patients underwent to cochlear implantation using Advanced Bionics® devices. There were 43,75% prelingual and 43,75% postlingual patients with bilateral hearing loss. Mean age at implantation in the prelingual group was 3.6 years (ranged from 2 to 6 years). There was one case with medical history of deafness in family. All prelingual patients used hearing devices before the cochlear implant. The hearing levels improved after CI in all patients.

Conclusion: This study evaluated patients with pre-lingual deafness using the Advanced Bionics® cochlear implants demonstrated significant gains in neural stimulation and language development in children.

Introduction

Cochlear Implants (CI) have become the standard treatment of prelingual, postlingual and perilingual deafness and hearing loss in children and it is a revolutionary yet time-sensitive treatment for deaf children that must be performed within a critical window time for maximum benefit. Sensorineural hearing impairment alters speech perception in a complex nonlinear manner [1,2].

Reports on the speech of deaf children examined differences in the speech of deaf children as a function of hearing loss and/ or perceptual abilities; differences in the speech of deaf children as a function of hearing device via hearing aid or cochlear implants; longitudinal changes in the speech of deaf children; or deviation of speech acoustics of deaf children comparing to those of normal hearing children [1].

Cochlear implants have enabled a number of severely hearing impaired individuals to access auditory information and improve speech perception as well as speech production skills. Several studies demonstrate that multi-channel cochlear implants also promote the development of speech perception and speech production in prelingually deafened children.

Many factors such as sociocultural characteristics, teaching methodology, language skill, and phonological awareness contribute to the development of the ability to read in children with normal hearing [3]. Children with prelingual, profound hearing loss who use CIs tend to perform better on closed and open set word-identification tasks than their peers with profound hearing loss who use hearing aids [3]. It is vital that all newborn children undergo hearing screening to identify deaf children at birth [2]. Children with both postlingual and prelingual deafness and cochlear implants can acquire auditory–visual and visual–visual conditional discriminations using discrimination training regimens that were similar in character to those used with hearing populations, and subsequently exhibit both cross-modal (i.e. auditory-visual) and intramodal equivalence relations [4].

***Corresponding author:** Henrique Furlan Pauna, Otology, Audiology and Implantable Ear Prostheses, Ear, Nose, Throat and Head & Neck Surgery Department, PO BOX 6111, Postal Code: 13081-970, São Paulo, Brazil; E-mail: h_pauna@hotmail.com

The skills involved in functional reading literacy include the following: a) reading lengthy, complex, abstract prose texts as well as synthesizing information and making complex inferences; b) integrating, synthesizing, and analyzing multiple pieces of information located in complex documents; and c) locating more abstract quantitative information and using it to solve multistep problems when the arithmetic operations are not easily inferred and the problems are more complex [5].

This manuscript aims to evaluate the improvement of sound perception in patients with prelingual deafness that underwent cochlear implant using Advanced Bionics® device.

Methods

Retrospective study of the medical records of the patients implanted with Advanced Bionics® cochlear implant in our institution between November, 2011 and November, 2012.

Device

For this study, we used the Advanced Bionics® devices (the HiFocus®1j electrode and the HiRes 90K® implant).

The HiFocus® 1j electrode consists of a fantail, electrode lead, and HiFocus 1j electrode array. The electrodes, composed of platinum-iridium alloy, are housed in a silicone carrier and extend from the titanium case. The HiFocus® 1j intra cochlear electrode array is designed to be inserted approximately 25 mm into a normally patent cochlea. It consists of 16 planer contacts arranged along the medial (or inside) surface of the electrode array for stimulation of discrete segments of the cochlea. The electrode contacts are numbered 1 through 16 from apex to base. The neck refers to the jog at the proximal end of the array that transitions the array to the lead. The fantail is directly connected to the electronic implant. The lead, which extends from the fantail, refers to the silicone carrier in which the electrode wires are enclosed [6].

The HiRes 90K® implant has 16 independent output circuits with bi-directional communication link of telemetry, the information update rate is 90kHz, a stimulation rate up to 83,000 pulses per second, weights 12 grams and has an impact resistance value of 6 joules [6].

Subjects

There were 16 patients that underwent to a cochlear implant using the Advanced Bionics® devices. The selected patients were informed about the surgery risks and benefits and postoperative expectations and signed an informed consent form. All ethical guidelines established by the institution were respected. The study was approved by the institution's Medical Ethics Committee (004/2013).

Inclusion criteria

The following criteria are based on the guidelines of the Brazilian Otolaryngology Association (ABORL-CCF) aiming to guide medical professionals and standardize criteria for cochlear implantation:

- Severe or deep sensorineural bilateral hearing loss;
- Patient without benefit after experience with the use of Hearing Aids (HA) for a minimum period of 3 months in severe hearing loss;
- Proper motivation of the family to use the cochlear implant and to develop intervention; and
- Presence of linguistic code established and properly rehabilitated by the oral method.

Exclusion criteria

- Appropriate gain after fitting a hearing aid;
- Improperly rehabilitation by the oral method;
- Absence of cochlea and cochlear nerve; and
- Unfavorable psychological assessment.

Audiological tests

Included subjects were tested before implantation with and without their HAs and four months after CI activation.

PTAs

Preoperative PTAs were performed in free field conditions, with and without HAs, as well as postoperative using CI. Measures were performed for 250, 500, 1000, 2000, 3000, 4000, 6000 and 8000 Hz using the AC30-SD25 audiometer calibrated according to ISO 389/64.

Data analysis and statistic

The limited number of patients required the use of non-parametric statistics for all variables. Wilcoxon tests for paired samples were used to compare the SP results obtained pre and post CI surgery. The cut-off level for statistical significance was set at 0.05.

Results

Sixteen patients underwent to cochlear implantation using Advanced Bionics® devices (Table 1). There were seven (43.75%) prelingual, two (12.5%) perilingual and seven (43.75%) postlingual patients with bilateral hearing loss. Mean age at implantaion was 3.6 years (range 2 to 6 years) in the prelingual group. There was one case with medical history of deafness in family. All prelingual patients used hearing device before the cochlear implant. We compared the hearing levels before and after the cochlear implantation and observed the improvement of hearing levels after the procedure in all patients (Chart 1 and 2). In this study, 43.75% of the patients were diagnosed with hearing loss since birth (after Universal Newborn Hearing Screening was performed).

There were no technical difficulties during the cochlear implantation and only one patient referred local pain after the procedure. In this study, ten (62.5%) of the cases had an unknown etiology for the hearing loss after the investigation.

Only one male patient underwent to a surgical procedure.

Discussion

Cochlear implants have been approved for use in profoundly deaf children as young as 1 year of age. Longitudinal studies of outcomes in deaf children have established that a Cochlear Implant (CI) leads to gains in spoken language [7]. Since the approval by the Food and Drug Administration in 1984, the communicative benefits provided by Cochlear Implants (CIs) to postlingually deafened adults have been well documented [8].

Profound hearing loss affects people of all ages. For children, hearing is central to neurocognitive development, since sound deprivation early in life degrades the multiplicity of neural circuits that are responsible for information processing, especially those involved in the acquisition of speech and language [9]. Despite objections from the deaf community, thousands of prelingually deaf children have also received CIs, and many have shown excellent outcome on a wide range

Subject	Gender	Age	Lingual	OFL	Cause	PST pre-CI	Side of CI
1	F	11	Pre	Y	Rubeola	0%	Left
2	F	66	Post	Y	-	0%	Right
3	F	31	Peri	Y	Meningitis	0%	Right
4	F	22	Post	Y	-	0%	Right
5	F	18	Post	Y	-	0%	Right
6	F	57	Peri	Y	-	26%	Left
7	F	50	Post	Y	Trauma	0%	Left
8	F	60	Post	Y	-	14%	Right
9	F	17	-	Y	-	0%	Right
10	F	24	Post	Y	Mondini dysplasia	26%	Left
11	F	21	Post	Y	-	0%	Right
12	F	2	Pre	N	-	Child	Right
13	F	2	Pre	N	-	Child	Left
14	F	5	Pre	Y	Congenital rubeola	Child	Right
15	M	2	Pre	N	-	Child	Right
16	F	4	Pre	Y	Premature	Child	Right

Table 1*:* Subjects by gender, age, type of hearing loss (pre, peri or postlingual), orofacial language, cause of hearing loss, PST before CI and side of CI.

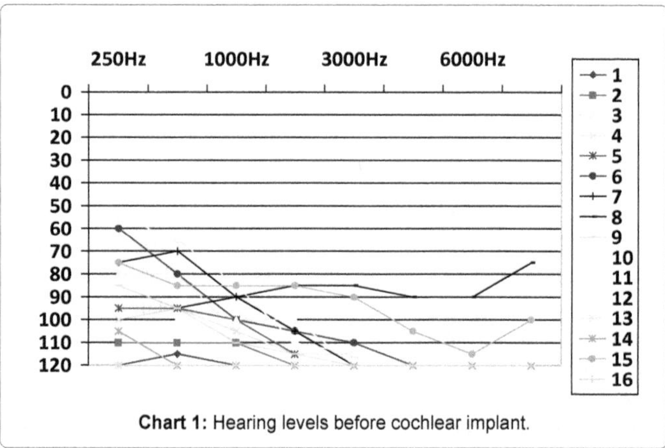

Chart 1: Hearing levels before cochlear implant.

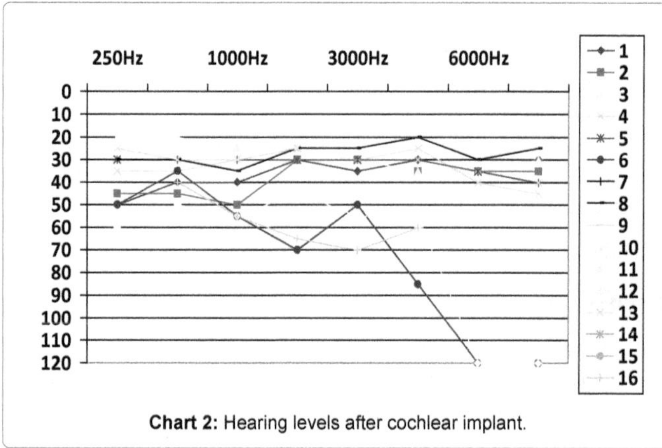

Chart 2: Hearing levels after cochlear implant.

of measures of hearing, speech, and language. Using auditory inputs from their CIs, some prelingually deafened pediatric CI users have been able to acquire spoken language at a pace that is similar to normal-hearing children [8].

The 1990s heralded major advances in speech-encoding strategies for cochlear implants, offering speech recognition without lip reading to the majority of recipients [9]. Several recent studies have suggested that the latest implant technology could indeed provide some open-set speech perceptual abilities to these patients. These conclusions, however, are based on analyses of results obtained with only a very small number of patients, and the data often showed enormous variability among individuals, making the true assessment of their effectiveness an exceedingly difficult task [8].

It appears that the deafness-induced changes along the entire auditory pathway, including the degeneration of the auditory nerve, the alteration of synaptic structures in the midbrain, and the failure to establish appropriate intracortical projections in the auditory cortex, all contribute to the gradual deterioration of auditory performance with increasing duration of auditory deprivation [10]. Different studies broadly agree that one or two of every 1000 newborns have a hearing impairment that on current evidence warrants treatment or observation, i.e., permanent hearing loss with a lowering of the absolute threshold of hearing for speech perception by at least 35 dB [11].

As with other sensory impairments, there is hereditary and non-hereditary or congenital and pre-, peri-, or postnatal causes of hearing disorders. While the cause of conductive hearing loss can usually be identified relatively simply (e.g., by means of otoscopy in the case of tympanic effusion or accumulation of earwax), even thorough diagnostic investigation fails to uncover the reason for around half of the cases of inner ear hearing impairment in childhood. Approximately 50% of severe hearing impairments arising in the inner ear are thought to be hereditary in origin (Table 2).

The realization that children who had been born deaf could also derive substantial benefit, with some developing speech and language trajectories similar to those of their hearing peers, was transformational for childhood deafness, making mainstream schooling a viable option for many deaf children [9]. The benefits for speech and language development, as well as speech intelligibility brought by CI-enabled hearing are greatest if these are received as soon after diagnosis as possible. Continued improvements in preoperative diagnostics, electrode design, speech coding strategies and surgical techniques, have broadened the CI applications spectrum. Nowadays-with the exception of cochlear- and cochlear nerve aplasia-almost all malformations are manageable with CIs [12].

Conclusion

For this study we evaluated patients with prelingual, perilingual and postlingual deafness using the Advanced Bionics® cochlear implants and have demonstrated significant gains in hearing levels in both children and adults.

Hearing impairment in early childhood: signs and risk factors – Ptok, 2011.
• Concern on the part of parents/guardians regarding the hearing, speech development, or general development of their child
• Family history of permanent hearing impairment in childhood
• Stay of more than 5 days in the neonatal intensive care unit, possibly including the need for ventilation, extracorporeal membrane oxygenation, assisted breathing, administration of ototoxic drugs or loop diuretics, and hyperbilirubinemia requiring transfusion
• Intrauterine infections such as cytomegalovirus, herpes, rubella, syphilis, and toxoplasmosis
• Craniofacial anomalies, including malformation of the earlobe, auditory canal, or auricular appendages and anomalies of the auditory pit and petrosa
• External signs that may indicate a syndrome involving sensorineural hearing loss or permanent conductive hearing loss, e.g., a white forelock
• Syndromes involving immediate, progressive, or late-onset hearing loss, such as neurofibromatosis, osteopetrosis, and Usher syndrome; other complexes associated with hearing disorders are Waardenburg, Alport, Pendred, and Jervell-Lange-Nielsen syndromes
• Neurodegenerative diseases such as Hunter syndrome or sensorimotor neuro - pathies such as Friedreich ataxia and Charcot-Marie-Tooth syndrome
• Demonstration in culture of infections associated with sensory hearing loss, including bacterial or viral (especially herpes or varicella) meningitis
• Head injury, particularly fractures of the skull base or petrosa requiring inpatient treatment
• Chemotherapy
• Otitis media recurring frequently or persisting for more than 3 months

Table 2: Hearing impairment in early childhood: signs and risk factors – Ptok, 2011.

References

1. Kant AR, Patadia R, Govale P, Rangasayee R, Kirtane M (2012) Acoustic analysis of speech of cochlear implantees and its implications. Clin Exp Otorhinolaryngol 5 Suppl 1: S14-18.
2. Russell JL, Pine HS, Young DL (2013) Pediatric cochlear implantation: expanding applications and outcomes. Pediatr Clin North Am 60: 841-863.
3. Spencer LJ, Oleson JJ (2008) Early listening and speaking skills predict later reading proficiency in pediatric cochlear implant users. Ear Hear 29: 270-280.
4. Almeida-Verdu AC, Huziwara EM, de Souza DG, De Rose JC, Bevilacqua MC, et al. (2008) Relational learning in children with deafness and cochlear implants. J Exp Anal Behav 89: 407-424.
5. Spencer LJ, Tomblin JB (2009) Evaluating phonological processing skills in children with prelingual deafness who use cochlear implants. J Deaf Stud Deaf Educ 14: 1-21.
6. Technical Specifications HiRes 90K® Implant, HiResolution® Bionic Ear System, Advanced Bionics, 2011.
7. Horn DL, Pisoni DB, Sanders M, Miyamoto RT (2005) Behavioral assessment of prelingually deaf children before cochlear implantation. Laryngoscope 115: 1603-1611.
8. Teoh SW, Pisoni DB, Miyamoto RT (2004) Cochlear implantation in adults with prelingual deafness. Part I. Clinical results. Laryngoscope 114: 1536-1540.
9. O'Donoghue G (2013) Cochlear implants--science, serendipity, and success. N Engl J Med 369: 1190-1193.
10. Teoh SW, Pisoni DB, Miyamoto RT (2004) Cochlear implantation in adults with prelingual deafness. Part II. Underlying constraints that affect audiological outcomes. Laryngoscope 114: 1714-1719.
11. Ptok M (2011) Early detection of hearing impairment in newborns and infants. Dtsch Arztebl Int 108: 426-431.
12. Mlynski R, Plontke S (2013) [Cochlear implants in children and adolescents]. HNO 61: 388-398.

Auditory Brainstem Response Characteristics of Children with Cerebral Palsy: Clinical Utility and Prognostic Significance

Mohammad Shamim Ansari[1*], Rangasayee Raghunathrao[2], Mohammad A Hafiz Ansari[3]

[1]*Department of Speech and Hearing, Ali Yavar Jung National Institute for the Hearing Handicapped, K.C. Marg, Bandra (W), Mumbai-40050.Maharashtra, India*

[2]*Technical Department, Dr. S.R. Chandrasekhar Institute of Speech and Hearing, Hennur Main Road, Lingarajapuram, Bnagalore-560084. Karnataka, India*

[3]*Department of Physiology, Grant Medical College and Sir J. J. Groups of Hospital, Mumbai-400008, India*

[*]**Corresponding author:** Mohammad Shamim Ansari, Lecturer, Department of Speech and Hearing, Ali Yavar Jung National Institute for the Hearing Handicapped, K.C. Marg, Bandra (W), Mumbai-40050.Maharashtra, India; E-mail: msansari5000@yahoo.com

Abstract

Background: Cerebral palsy affects body muscle and movement coordination due to organic complications in the peripheral and central nervous systems and therefore often accompanied by other disorders of cerebral function. CP with additional impairment of hearing results in severe developmental deficits in communication, speech and language and cognitive skills. Thus it is important to examine the auditory nervous system to identify the complications caused by the hidden hearing loss. Auditory Brainstem Responses (ABR) provides objective measure of auditory system function and can be an important adjunct to the clinical neurophysiologic examinations. However, there is scanty information about the neurophysiologic investigations in children with spastic cerebral palsy.

Aim: To investigate whether the children affected with spastic CP exhibit distinct neural responses than the age matched normal hearing children.

Methodology: ABR measures were obtained for 50 children with spastic CP in the age range 3 to 12 years. The results were subsequently correlated with birth weight, gestational age, etiology and type of CP, neuroradiological findings, additional impairments and disabilities (including the ability to walk independently). 50 typically normal hearing children served as reference group for comparisons of neurophysiologic measures of auditory brainstem responses.

Results: A significant difference was found in the ABR latencies between the children with cerebral palsy and atypical children. Abnormal ABR measures in children with spastic CP demonstrated a correlation with the presence of moderate to severe developmental delay.

Conclusion: It can be concluded that ABR measures of CP group revealed a statistical difference with that of the typically developing children and it has demonstrated a statistically significant correlation with the presence of neurological deficits. Therefore, Auditory Brainstem Response measurement being a non-invasive neurophysiologic investigation can serve as important tool in the diagnostic work up of spastic CP.

Keywords: Spastic cerebral palsy; Additional impairment; Hearing loss; Peripheral auditory system; Click evoked auditory brainstem response

Abbreviations:

ABR: Auditory Brainstem Response; CP: Cerebral Palsy

Introduction

Cerebral palsy (CP) is a group of non-progressive neurological disorders [1,2] which affects body muscle tone and movements coordination [3]. CP occurs due to abnormal development of the cerebral motor cortex during fetal growth (embryonic period) or due to injury to the motor control centers of the developing brain during birth or after birth up to age about 2-3 years [4,5].

The four major subtypes of Cerebral palsy are spastic, athetoid, ataxic and mixed cerebral palsy. The spastic form of CP is the most commonly occurring in 65% of cerebral palsied population [5]. Prevalence of Cerebral palsy is increasingly encountered in neonatal clinics since more number of premature infants survives because of advance neonatal care and better medical facilities for treatment of perinatal infections.

Cerebral palsy is often accompanied by other disorders and problems of cerebral function, in particular intellectual impairment, speech and language deficits, epilepsy, vision and hearing disorders [6,7]. Recent studies have shown that hearing impairment occurs in 4 to 25% of children with CP [6]. These children with additional impairment of hearing presents ranges of special educational and psychological needs, to an even greater degree than for children with single disability [7].

Presence of reduced hearing acuity during infancy and early childhood in children with CP may have more deleterious effect on communication abilities, speech and language and cognitive development that can severely interfere with their psycho-, difficulties in parent-child and peer-child interactions, low self-esteem, linguistic and educational development [8]. However, a child's overall future and success can be improved greatly through the early identification of hearing loss, establishment of its site of lesion, and subsequent institution of intervention strategies may improve learning and language development [6,9].

Children with cerebral palsy have an organic complication in the peripheral and central nervous systems [7-9]. Thus it is important to examine the auditory nervous system to identify and reduce complications of hidden hearing loss. Although clinical evaluation may suggest hearing loss, a definitive diagnosis requires an audiological assessment [9].

Auditory Brainstem Response (ABR) measurements is an non invasive and objective method [8-10], can be used to assess hearing capabilities in infants younger than 6 months of age and in older children who are unable to perform conventional or conditioned play audiometry due to motor or intellectual problems [7-9].

ABRs are electrical potentials that are produced in response to a brief stimulus like click and are recorded from disk electrodes attached to the scalp. The early potentials reflect electrical activity at the cochlea, 8th cranial nerve, and brain stem levels and may be analyzed to estimate the magnitude of hearing loss and to differentiate among cochlea, 8th nerve, and brainstem lesions [7-9]. Therefore, ABR can be an important adjunctive diagnostic tool for the clinical neurophysiologic examinations of hearing loss in children with cerebral palsy.

In recent years, the neurophysiologic examination of children with Cerebral palsy has been of increasing interest to audiologists, otologists, pediatricians and other researchers to evaluate normal physiological maturation and integrity of the auditory system, in the screening of hearing impairments of infants, to diagnose and demonstrate brainstem damage and to provide prognosis for the patients with various neurological disorders [8,9].

In a retrospective study of 75 children with spastic cerebral palsy (CP), 17 (22.7%) had abnormal ABR waveform [10-12]. Another study concluded that one of the specific feature i.e., sensorineural hearing loss in athetoid CP caused by kernicterus can be identified by the ABR [13]. These authors concluded that ABR can provide new insights into mechanisms of brain damage and neural plasticity in children with cerebral palsy. In spite ABR being very promising diagnostic tool in assessment of hearing in difficult to test populations including the children with cerebral palsy, very fewer studies on auditory brainstem responses are available Indian literature.

Hence the present study was undertaken to characterize the electrophysiological findings in children with spastic cerebral palsy and correlate with their clinical features.

Materials and Methods

Research design

This prospective survey was done at our institute's electrophysiological laboratory in accordance with Institutional ethical norms. The necessary informed consent by the parents of the children was obtained.

Participants

Total 100 participants of both the sexes in the age range 3–10 years (mean=6.6 years, SD=2.12 years) were recruited for the study. The subjects were divided into two groups. The Group A consisted of 50 subjects with spastic cerebral palsy (37 male and 23 females with mean age of 6.8 years, SD=1.92 years) diagnosed by pediatrician and Group B included 50 normal hearing children (33 male and 27 female with mean age of 5.9 years, SD=2.32 years) with no known history of neurological, psychiatric and otological disease or trauma.

Demographic data of confirmed spastic CP and typically developing children were collected through medical reports, parental interview, case histories about age, prenatal, perinatal and postnatal events, and history of epilepsy. Group B subjects evidenced normal peripheral hearing sensitivity, defined as pure-tone thresholds (≤ 25 dB HL, re: ANSI, 1996) for each ear at octave frequencies between 250 and 8000 Hz. Normal middle-ear admittance and presence of acoustic reflexes at 500 and 1000 Hz for all subjects were confirmed by means of immittance measures.

Stimuli and recording parameters

ABRs were elicited by an acoustic 100 μs click stimulus. Responses were recorded via four Ag-AgCl surface electrodes having absolute contact impedance of <5 kΩ with no more than 3 kΩ difference between each of the two electrodes. Before connecting the electrodes, the skin was cleaned thoroughly to ensure good contact between the skin and the electrode surfaces. Non inverting electrode was positioned centrally on the scalp at Cz, two inverting electrodes were placed behind the mastoid (A1 and A2) and ground electrode was attached at forehead (FPz).

Monaural auditory stimulus consisting of alternating polarity clicks were delivered into the ear at a rate of 11.1/s at intensity level of 80 dBnHL through electrically shielded insert earphones (ER-3). The sampling rate was 20000 Hz and responses were online band passed filtered from 100 to 3000 Hz. Artifacts greater than ± 35 μV were rejected online. Two traces of 2000 sweeps were collected at alternating polarity. Responses of alternating polarities were added together to minimize contributions from the cochlear micro phonic responses [12]. Responses to 2000 click presentations were averaged for 12 ms. During testing, the children were in the supine position with eyes closed.

Result analysis

In 50 children with spastic cerebral palsy (CP), Auditory Brainstem Responses (ABRs) were recorded and subsequently correlated with birth weight, gestational age, etiological factors and additional impairments and disabilities (including the ability to walk independently).

Identification of brainstem recorded wave by the click stimulus was done based on the conventional clinical analysis. The peaks were marked by the two independent observers. The identities and the diagnostic categorizations of the children were blinded to the observers. The observers were also requested to rate the individual wave morphology as poor, fair and good.

ABR measures like absolute peak latencies of I, III, V waves, inter-peak latencies of I-III, III-V, and I-V were considered for comparison between the two groups. The mean, median, standard deviation, minimum, and maximum values for normal distribution of responses were calculated for the sample. An independent t-test was used to compare the mean value of the results. One way ANOVA was studied at significance levels of 5% (P<0.05) to find the association between ABR abnormalities and clinical features, additional impairment and risk factors. For statistical analysis, SPSS.16 software was used.

Results

The current study was designed to assess and compare the brainstem responses to click stimuli in children with spastic cerebral palsy and typically normal hearing and healthy developing children. The Group A included 50 children suffering from spastic CP consisted of 14 spastic tetraplegic, 17 spastic diplegic, 11 left side hemiplegic and 8 right side hemiplegic (Figure 1).

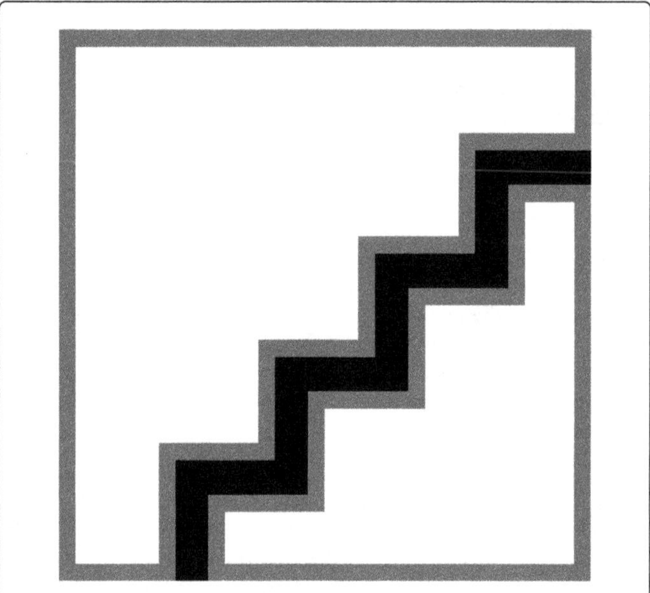

Figure 1: Showing sub-types of spasticity and severity of Group A.

	Absolute Latencies mean (SD) in ms			Inter-peak Latencies mean (SD) in ms		
	I	III	V	I-III	III-V	I-V
Group A	1.6	3.83	5.77	2.23	1.94	4.17
	± 0.09	± 0.14	± 0.10	± 0.13	± 0.11	± 0.10
Group B	1.5	3.61	5.54	2.11	1.91	4.04
	± 0.06	± 0.13	± 0.20	± .15	±.20	± 0.18
p-value at <0.05	0.01*	0.01*	0.02*	0.43*	0.7	0.02*

Table 1: Showing means and SD (in parenthesis) of absolute latency (ms) of wave peaks I, III, V and Inter-peaks latency (ms) I-III, III-V and I-V of click evoked ABR measures of Group A and Group B.

The ABR wave morphology in clinical population was rated as 67% poor, 31% fair and 2% good whereas normal hearing children were rated as having 3% poor 19% fair and 78% good wave morphology by the peak observers. The neurophysiologic responses to click generated waves I, III and V were analyzed based on the conventional clinical analysis of the absolute latencies and inter-peak latencies for both groups. Table 1 indicating mean and standard deviation of absolute and inter peak latencies and p-values between the groups.

The notable ABR abnormalities in CP children were prolongation of absolute latency of peak, III & V, inter-peak latencies of I-III and III–V. Figure 2 showing the absolute peak latency and inter-peak latency in both the groups. The means of Group A for ABR parameters were statistically significant from the Group B at significance level of p<0.05.

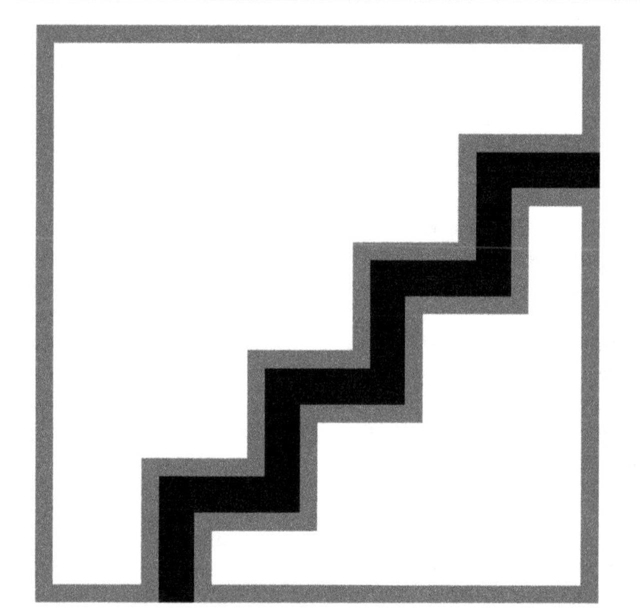

Figure 2: Showing click evoked mean absolute peak latencies and inter-peak latencies for Group A and B.

Out of the total 50 subjects, 31 children with spastic CP presented with associated clinical features and abnormalities such as microcephaly, mental retardation, delayed development and other risk factors. The percentage of abnormal auditory brainstem responses along with clinical feature of ABR findings are elucidated in Table 2.

Clinical Features/Risk Factors	N	Abnormal ABR %
Normal Developmental Milestone	7	2 (28%)*
Communication and Speech delay	31	31 (100%)**
Mental retardation/ Microcephaly	11	4 (36%)*
Global delay	12	10 (75%) **
Developmental Delay	7	4 (46%)*
Low birth weight	9	2 (40%)*
Prematurity+LBW	9	3 (50%)*
Bilateral Sensorineural hg loss	4	4 (100%)**
Birth asphyxia , Seizures/Epilepsy	8	4 (50%)*

Neonatal Jaundice/ Encephalitis	16	8 (50%)*

Table 2: Depicting clinical features, associated abnormalities and risk factors in children with spastic cerebral palsy, ** Statistically significant correlation at p value 0.01, * Statistically significant correlation at p value 0.05.

Abnormal ABR in children with spastic cerebral palsy demonstrated a statistically significant correlation at p value 0.001 with the presence of global developmental delay and additional disability of hearing loss, whereas prematurity, neonatal jaundice and encephalitis etc have statistically significant correlation at p value 0.05.

Discussion

The ABR results were primarily analyzed for the presence of the waves I, III and V. Wave I, or latency I is based on the transformation of tone-specific responses in the hair cells into impulses travelling along the auditory nerve, and after passing the cochlear nucleus of the brainstem, the impulse reaches the superior olivary complex, forming wave III or latency III [14,15]. Wave V is then produced in the inferior colliculus, and finally the temporal auditory cortex is reached [15-21].

The study faithfully characterizes the electrophysiological responses to click stimuli in children with spasticity and typically developing. It can be observed from Tables 1 and 2 that the children with CP who had other associated neurological symptoms showed statistically significant deviation from the regular pattern of ABR waveforms for absolute peak latencies I, III and V and inter-peak latency between I-III and III-V.

Most of the children with neurosensory disability, except one spastic CP with microcephaly, had bilaterally absent or delayed responses in ABR components. 31 of 50 CP children with clinical features, additional impairment and risk factors (Table 2), 17 had abnormality in wave I, 14 in wave III, 29 in wave V, 23 in IPL between wave I–V, 19 in IPL III–V (Table 1).

This is in consonance with the reports of previous works which reports that children with CP have abnormalities of the auditory sensory pathways at greater rates than found in the neurologically normal children [16,17]. These researches concluded that an abnormal ABR, manifested as an absence or prolongation of latencies have positive association with adverse neurological development in children [16,17].

The prolongation of the IPL I–V and IPL III–V conduction times has been found in high-risk preterm infants with a transient neurological abnormality [17,20,22]. A bilateral abnormality in a pre-discharge ABR examination of a VLBW infant has been shown to correlate with an adverse outcome in intelligent quotient, language and academic achievements [15,22].

Further, increased IPL III–V and IPL I–V conduction times have also been shown to be significant prognostic indicator for delayed motor development and abnormal neurological findings [15]. Abnormal or repeatedly absent ABR during the neonatal period have been correlated closely with the hearing impairment and psychomotor development deficits [15,22]. The studies also reported that abnormal ABRs in prematurely born children with spastic CP are indicative of poor prognosis and positive associated with a "multihandicap state" of the children [12,18,19].

The findings of the current study as elucidated in Table 2. Wherein 31 (62%) subjects had communication and speech problems, 12 (24%) had mental retardation, 19 (38%) had Global developmental delay, 13 (26%) were unable to walk independently and 4 (8%) had hearing loss. There was a statistically significant association between abnormal ABR recordings and preterm delivery, perinatal etiology of CP, hearing, speech and myoskeletal impairments, epilepsy and mental retardation ($p<0.001$). These findings are in concurrence with previous reports. Though, the exact etiology of abnormal ABR remains to be unleashed through this study. Hence, further research in this area is recommended.

However, it can be concluded that abnormal ABR recordings in children with spastic CP probably can be linked to the neurological deficits in the light of earlier reports. Thus, it is suggested that ABR testing should be incorporated in the diagnostic assessment of all children with spastic CP referred to Neurodevelopment Centers to plan holistic intervention strategies including amplification devices.

Conclusion

The study concludes that ABR measurement in spastic CP revealed marked differences with that of the typical children, delay in the absolute latency as well as inter-peak latency differences are indicative of neurological deficits. The clinical features, additional disabilities and risk factors have demonstrated a statistically significant correlation with the presence of abnormal ABR and thus neurological deficits.

ABR examinations can detect lesions that may be asymptomatic and subtle to preclude the optimal development of the child. The hearing impairment is frequent in children with cerebral palsy and causes severe deficits in communication, development of speech & language and cognitive skills. Thus it is important to examine the auditory nervous system to identify and reduce the complications caused by the hidden hearing loss.

Despite limitations of ABRs as time consuming tool, ABR is important tool to determinate the functional integrity of the auditory tract and evaluation of hearing thresholds in patients with cerebral palsy. Further, to conclude, since ABR measurement is non-invasive and objective neurophysiologic investigations, it can serve as important adjunct to the clinical examinations and diagnostic work up of spastic cerebral palsy.

References

1. Morris C (2007) Definition and classification of cerebral palsy: A historical perspective. Dev Med Child Neurol Suppl 109: 3-7.
2. Surveillance of Cerebral Palsy in Europe (2000) Surveillance of cerebral palsy in Europe: a collaboration of cerebral palsy surveys and registers. Surveillance of Cerebral Palsy in Europe (SCPE). Dev Med Child Neurol 42: 816-824.
3. Ghai OP (2004) Central nervous system. In: Ghai OP (eds.) Essentials paediatrics. New Delhi pp: 540-549.
4. Odding E, Roebroeck ME, Stam HJ (2006) The epidemiology of cerebral palsy: Incidence, impairments and risk factors. Disabil Rehabil 28: 183-191.
5. Rosenbaum P, Paneth N, Leviton A, Goldstein M, Bax M, et al. (2007) A report: The definition and classification of cerebral palsy April 2006. Dev Med Child Neurol Suppl 109: 8-14.
6. Kolker IA (2004) Hearing function and auditory evoked potentials in children with spastic forms of cerebral palsy. Neurophysiology 36: 270-275.

7. Sano M, Kaga K, Kitazumi E, Kodama K (2005) Sensorineural hearing loss in patients with cerebral palsy after asphyxia and hyperbilirubinemia. Int J Pediatr Otorhinolaryngol 69: 1211-1217.

8. Joint Committee on Infant Hearing (2007) Year 2007 position statement: Principles and guidelines for early hearing detection and intervention programs. Suppl Audiology Today 120: 1-29

9. Fowler KB, Boppana SB (2006) Congenital cytomegalovirus (CMV) infection and hearing deficit. J Clin Virol 35: 226-231.

10. Kaplan M, Hammerman C (2005) American Academy of Pediatrics guidelines for detecting neonatal hyperbilirubinaemia and preventing kernicterus. Arch Dis Child Fetal Neonatal Ed 90: 448-449.

11. Kohelet D, Arbel E, Goldberg M, Arlazoroff A (2000) Brainstem auditory evoked response in newborns and infants. J Child Neurol 15: 33-35.

12. Zafeiriou DI, Andreou A, Karasavidou K (2000) Utility of brainstem auditory evoked potentials in children with spastic cerebral palsy. Acta Paediatr 89: 194-197.

13. Morales Angulo C, Azuara Blanco N, Gallo Terán J, González Aledo A, Rama Quintela J (2006) [Sensorineural hearing loss in cerebral palsy patients]. Acta Otorrinolaringol Esp 57: 300-302.

14. Raj H (2004) Evoked potentials in preterm and term neonates with their relevance in hypoxic-ischemic insult. Journal of Neonatology 18: 34-39.

15. Markand ON (1994) Brainstem auditory evoked potentials. J Clin Neurophysiol 11: 319-342.

16. Majnemer A, Rosenblatt B, Riley PS (1990) Prognostic significance of multimodality evoked response testing in high-risk newborns. Pediatr Neurol 6: 367-374.

17. Kitamoto I, Kukita J, Kurokawa T, Chen YJ, Minami T, et al. (1990) Transient neurologic abnormalities and BAEPs in high-risk infants. Pediatr Neurol 6: 319-325.

18. Cox C, Hack M, Aram D, Borawski E (1992) Neonatal auditory brainstem response failure of very low birth weight infants: 8-year outcome. Pediatr Res 31: 68-72.

19. O'Shea TM (2008) Diagnosis, treatment and prevention of cerebral palsy. Clin Obstet Gynecol 51: 816-828.

20. Pike AA, Marlow N (2000) The role of cortical evoked responses in predicting neuromotor outcome in very preterm infants. Early Hum Dev 57: 123-135.

21. KuÅ‚ak W, Sobaniec W, Kuzia JS, BoÄ‡kowski L (2006) Neurophysiologic and neuroimaging studies of brain plasticity in children with spastic cerebral palsy. Exp Neurol 198: 4-11.

22. Venkateswaran S, Shevell MI (2008) Comorbidities and clinical determinants of outcome in children with spastic quadriplegic cerebral palsy. Dev Med Child Neurol 50: 216-222.

Permissions

All chapters in this book were first published in OTOLARYNGOLOGY, by OMICS International; hereby published with permission under the Creative Commons Attribution License or equivalent. Every chapter published in this book has been scrutinized by our experts. Their significance has been extensively debated. The topics covered herein carry significant findings which will fuel the growth of the discipline. They may even be implemented as practical applications or may be referred to as a beginning point for another development.

The contributors of this book come from diverse backgrounds, making this book a truly international effort. This book will bring forth new frontiers with its revolutionizing research information and detailed analysis of the nascent developments around the world.

We would like to thank all the contributing authors for lending their expertise to make the book truly unique. They have played a crucial role in the development of this book. Without their invaluable contributions this book wouldn't have been possible. They have made vital efforts to compile up to date information on the varied aspects of this subject to make this book a valuable addition to the collection of many professionals and students.

This book was conceptualized with the vision of imparting up-to-date information and advanced data in this field. To ensure the same, a matchless editorial board was set up. Every individual on the board went through rigorous rounds of assessment to prove their worth. After which they invested a large part of their time researching and compiling the most relevant data for our readers.

The editorial board has been involved in producing this book since its inception. They have spent rigorous hours researching and exploring the diverse topics which have resulted in the successful publishing of this book. They have passed on their knowledge of decades through this book. To expedite this challenging task, the publisher supported the team at every step. A small team of assistant editors was also appointed to further simplify the editing procedure and attain best results for the readers.

Apart from the editorial board, the designing team has also invested a significant amount of their time in understanding the subject and creating the most relevant covers. They scrutinized every image to scout for the most suitable representation of the subject and create an appropriate cover for the book.

The publishing team has been an ardent support to the editorial, designing and production team. Their endless efforts to recruit the best for this project, has resulted in the accomplishment of this book. They are a veteran in the field of academics and their pool of knowledge is as vast as their experience in printing. Their expertise and guidance has proved useful at every step. Their uncompromising quality standards have made this book an exceptional effort. Their encouragement from time to time has been an inspiration for everyone.

The publisher and the editorial board hope that this book will prove to be a valuable piece of knowledge for researchers, students, practitioners and scholars across the globe.

List of Contributors

Zahra Sarafraz, Mohammad Hossein Azaraein, Mansour Moghimi and Seyyed Ali Musavi
Faculty of Medicine and Health Sciences, Unit of Otolaryngology Medicine, Department of Otolaryngology, Yazd University of Medical Sciences, Yazd, Iran

Boutemeur S, Ramoul S, Azouani Y, Kabir A and Ferdjaoui A
Department of Oral and Maxillo-facial Surgery, Mustapha Pacha Hospital, Algiers, Algeria

Mouhannad Abdulber Fakoury
Department of ENT, Dubai Hospital, Dubai, UAE

Jyotiranjan Das and Ajay Manickam
Department of ENT, RG Kar Medical College, Kolkata, India

Jayant Saha and Shantanu Dutta
ILS Hospitals, Dumdum, West Bengal, India

Richard A Marshall, Peter M Som, Livnat Uliel, Neetha Gandikota, Idoia Corcuera-Solano and Lale Kostakoglu
Department of Radiology, The Mount Sinai Medical Center, One Gustave L. Levy Place, New York, USA

Eric Genden and Brett Miles
Department of Otolaryngology, The Mount Sinai Medical Center, One Gustave L. Levy Place, New York, USA

Andrew G. Sikora
Department of Otolaryngology, The Mount Sinai Medical Center, One Gustave L. Levy Place, New York, USA
The Tisch Cancer Institute, One Gustave L. Levy Place, Icahn Building, New York, USA
Department of Otolaryngology - Head and Neck Surgery, Baylor College of Medicine, Houston, TX, USA

Michael Buckstein and Vishal Gupta
Department of Radiation Oncology, The Mount Sinai Medical Center, One Gustave L. Levy Place, New York, USA

Krzysztof Misiukiewicz
Department of Hematology and Medical Oncology, The Mount Sinai Medical Center, One Gustave L. Levy Place, New York, USA

Sethu T Subha
Department of Surgery/ENT, Faculty of Medicine & Health Sciences, University Putra Malaysia, Malaysia

Loy Heng She
Canberra Hospital, Yamba drive, Garran, Australia

Wong Shew Fung
Department of Pathology, International Medical University, Malaysia

Davendralingam Sinniah
Department of Paediatrics, International Medical University, Clinical School Seremban, Malaysia

Valuyeetham Kamaru Ambu
Department of ENT, Hospital Tuanku Jaafar Seremban, Ministry of Health Malaysia, Seremban, Malaysia

Sylvester Fernandes
Department of Health Sciences, Newcastle University, Australia

Hermann Simo
The University of Toledo College of Medicine & Life Sciences, The University of Toledo Medical Center, Toledo, OH 43614, USA

Louis De Las Casas and Vasuki Anandan
Department of Pathology, The University of Toledo Medical Center, The University of Toledo Medical Center, Toledo, OH 43614, USA

Michal Preis
Department of Otolaryngology, Maimonides Medical Center, The University of Toledo Medical Center, Toledo, OH 43614, USA

Reginald Baugh
Department of Surgery, Division of Otolaryngology, Head & Neck Surgery, University of Toledo Medical Center, The University of Toledo Medical Center Toledo, OH 43614, USA

Jorge Paredes Vieyra, Ricardo Machado, Francisco Javier Jiménez Enriquez and Fabian Ocampo Acosta
Universidad Autónoma de Baja California, campus Tijuana, USA

Elliot Regenbogen
Division of Otolaryngology Head and Neck Surgery, Stony Brook University Medical Center, HSC T19-065, Stony Brook, NY 11794-8191, USA

Slawomir P. Oleszak
Division of Cardiothoracic Anesthesiology, Stony Brook University Medical Center, Stony Brook, NY 11794-8191, USA

Thomas Corrado
Division of Neuroanesthesia/ENT Anesthesia, Stony Brook University Medical Center, Stony Brook, NY 11794-8191, USA

A. Laurie W. Shroyer
Department of Surgery, Stony Brook University, School of Medicine, Stony Brook, NY 11794-8191, USA

Elizabeth Vanner
Departments of Pathology and Bioinformatics, Stony Brook University School of Medicine, Stony Brook, NY 11794-8691, USA

Jordan Goldstein
Stony Brook University School of Medicine, Stony Brook, NY 11794-8191

Michael L. Pearl
Division of Gynecologic Oncology, Stony Brook University Medical Center, Stony Brook, NY 11794-8191, USA

Yu Yoshizumi, Ayako Nakane, Haruka Tohara and Shunsuke Minakuchi
Gerodontology and Oral Rehabilitation, Department of Gerontology and Gerodontology, Graduate School of Medical and Dental Sciences, Tokyo Medical and Dental University, Japan

Shinya Mikushi
Department of Special Care Dentistry, Clinic for Oral Health Care and Dysphagia Rehabilitation, Nagasaki University Hospital, Japan

Irit Duek, Moran Amit and Ziv Gil
Department of Otolaryngology Head and Neck Surgery, Rambam Health Care Campus, Haifa, Israel
The Laboratory for Applied Cancer Research, the Clinical Research Institute, Rambam Health Care Campus, The Technion, Haifa, Israel

Gill E Sviri
Department of Neurosurgery, Rambam Health Care Campus, Haifa, Israel

Tomonori Terada, Nobuo Saeki, Nobuhiro Uwa, Kousuke Sagawa and Masafumi Sakagami
The Department of Otolaryngology, Hyogo Medical University, Japan

Takeshi Mohri
The Department of Otolaryngology, Hyogo Medical University, Japan
The Departments of Otolaryngology, Osaka Medical Center for Cancer and Cardiovascular Diseases, Japan

Takashi Fujii
The Departments of Otolaryngology, Osaka Medical Center for Cancer and Cardiovascular Diseases, Japan

Yasuhiko Tomita, Miki Tomoeda and Shota Kotani
The Departments of Pathology, Osaka Medical Center for Cancer and Cardiovascular Diseases, Japan

Rosa Carrieri Rossi
Division of Paediatric Otolaryngology, Federal University of Sao Paulo- UNIFESP SP, Brazil

Nelson Jose Rossi and Nelson Carrieri Rossi
Professor of Postgraduate of Orthodontics, North of Minas Foundation- FUNORTE, Brazil

Reginaldo Raimundo Fujiya and Shirley Nagata Pignatari
Associate Professor, Division of Paediatric Otolaryngology, Department of Otolaryngology and Head and Neck Surgery, Federal University of Sao Paulo- UNIFESP, Brazil

Diom ES
Otolaryngologist, Dakar, Senegal

Fagan JJ
Professor and Chairman, Division of Otolaryngology, University of Cape Town, Cape Town, South Africa

Dhirendra Govender
Professor and Chairman, Division of Anatomical Pathology University of Cape Town, Cape Town, South Africa

Sara Safar AlShehri and Kamal-Eldin Ahmed Abou-Elhamd
Department of ENT Surgery, College of Medicine, King Faisal University, Al-Ahsa, Saudi Arabia

Lawson Afouda Sonia, Avakoudjo François and Adjibabi Wassi
Ear Nose Throat Department at Hubert Koutoukou Maga National Teaching Hospital of Cotonou, Benin

Hounkpatin Spéro
Ear Nose Throat Department at Borgou Regional Teaching Hospital, Benin

Brun Luc
Pathology Department at Borgou Regional Teaching Hospital, Benin

Shingo Umemoto, Satoru Kodama, Takashi Hirano, Kenji Noda and Masashi Suzuki
Department of Otolaryngology, Oita University Faculty of Medicine 1-1 Idaigaoka, Hazama-cho, Yufu, Oita 879-5593, Japan

Bibek Gyanwali, Hongquan Wu, Meichan Zhu and Anzhou Tang
Department of Otolaryngology-Head and Neck Surgery, The First Affiliated Hospital of Guangxi Medical University, Nanning Guangxi, People's Republic of China

Bunu Karmacharya
Department of Radiology, The First Affiliated Hospital of Guangxi Medical University, Nanning Guangxi, People's Republic of China

Marianna Trignani, Angelo Di Pilla, Albina Allajbej and Domenico Genovesi
Department of Radiation Oncology, G. DAnnunzio University of Chieti, SS. Annunziata Hospital, Chieti, Italy

Melissa Laus, Valentina Mastronardi, Olga Leone, Marilina De Rosa, Giulio Campitelli and Adelchi Croce
Department of Otorhinolaryngology, G. DAnnunzio University of Chieti, SS. Annunziata Hospital, Chieti, Italy

Giuseppe Santarelli
Department of Nutrition, SS. Annunziata Hospital, Chieti, Italy

Ambra Pamio
Department of Hygiene and Public Health, G. DAnnunzio University, Chieti, Italy

Suat Bilici, Gulben Erdem Huq, Ahmet Volkan Sunter, Ozgur Yigit and Muhammmet Yıldız
Istanbul Education and Research Hospital, Istanbul, Turkey

Myriam Jrad, Asma Ben Mabrouk, Aymen Ben Othmen, Anis Zaidi and Habiba Mizouni
Department of Radiology, La Rabta Hospital, Jabberi 1017, Tunis, Tunisia

Jihene Marrakchi, Rym Zainine and Ghazi Besbes
Department of ENT, La Rabta Hospital, Tunis, Tunisia

Virangna Taneja
University Hospital Coventry and Warwickshire NHS Trust, Masonway, Birmingham B152EE, United Kingdom
Department of Otolaryngology and Head, Neck Surgery MAM College and association LN Hospital, Delhi, India

Shelly Khanna Chadha, Achal Gulati and Ankush Sayal
Department of Otolaryngology and Head, Neck Surgery MAM College and Association LN Hospital, Delhi, India

Motoharu Uehara
Uehara Otolaryngology Clinic, showaminami-3-10-12, kushiro city, Hokkaido 0840909, Japan

Hiroyuki Hirai
Advanced Medical Technology and Development Division, BML, Japan

ABI AAD Lamia and Dany Joseph Daou
Dental Public Health Department, Lebanese University, Hadath, Hadath Lebanon

Pauline Castelnau-Marchand, Eleonor Rivin del Campo and Yungan Tao
Department of Radiation Oncology, Gustave-Roussy, Paris Sud University, Villejuif, France

Guzide Ayse Ocak, Irem Hicran Ozbudak and Havva Serap Toru
Akdeniz University School of Medicine, Department of Pathology, Antalya/Turkey

Alper Tunga Derin
Akdeniz University School of Medicine, Department of Ear Nose Throat Head and Neck Surgery, Antalya/Turkey

Max Stanley Chartrand
DigiCare Behavioral Research, 820 West Cottonwood Lane, Suite #6, Casa Grande, Arizona, USA

Robert Mlynski
Department of Otorhinolaryngology, Head and Neck Surgery, Otto Körner, Rostock University Medical Center, Germany

Michael Ziese
University Clinic Magdeburg A.ö.R., University Clinic for Otolaryngology, Germany

Thorsten Rahne
Universitätsklinik und Poliklinik für Hals-Nasen-Ohrenheilkunde, Kopf- und Hals-Chirurgie, Hallesches Hör- und ImplantCentrum (HIC), Deutschland, Germany

Joachim Müller-Deile
Universitätsklinikum Schleswig-Holstein, Campus Kiel, Klinik für Hals-, Nasen-, Ohrenheilkunde, Kopf- und Halschirurgie, Deutschland, Germany

Gray MR
Progressive Healthcare Group, Benson, Arizona, USA

Thrasher JD
Retired, Consultant to Progressive Healthcare Group, Benson Arizona, USA

Dennis Hooper
Laboratories, Carrollton, Texas, USA

Dumanov MJ
Mycological Institute Subclinical Research Group, USA

Cravens R
Tucson Ear, Nose and Throat, Tucson, USA

Mitat Arıcıgil, Mehmet Akif Alan, Fuat Aydemir and Suayp Kuria Aziz
Department of Otorhinolaryngology, Meram Faculty of Medicine, Necmettin Erbakan University, Turkey

Abitter Yucel
Department of Otorhinolaryngology, Horasan State Hospital, Erzurum, Turkey

Amy L Rutt, James P Dworkin and Noah Stern
Department of Otolaryngology Head and Neck Surgery, Detroit Medical Center/Michigan State University, USA

Kiyoaki Tsukahara, Kazuhiro Nakamura, Ray Motohashi and Hiroki Sato
Department of Head and Neck Surgery, Tokyo Medical University Hachioji Medical Center, Tokyo 193-0998, Japan

Mamoru Suzuki
Department of Otolaryngology, Tokyo Medical University, sinjyukuku Tokyo, 160-0023, Japan

Arıcıgil M
Department of Otorhinolaryngology, Necmettin Erbakan University, Turkey

Yaser Najaf
Zain & Al-Sabah Hospital, Al-Jabriyah, Kuwait

Abdulmohsen AlTerki
Chairman of ENT College, Postgraduate Training, Kuwait Institute of Medical Specialization, Head of Unit & Consultant, ENT Department, Zain & Al-Sabah Hospitals, Kuwait

Adel Al-Buluoshi
Consultant Ophthalmologist and Oculoplastic and Reconstructive Surgery, Al Bahar Eye Center, Kuwait

Yusuf Muhammed Durna, Ozgur Yigit and Engin Acioglu
Department of Otorhinolaryngology, Istanbul Research and Training Hospital, Istanbul, Turkey

Feray Gunver
Department of Pathology, Istanbul Research and Training Hospital, Istanbul, Turkey

Ismail Önder Uysal and Kerem Polat
Cumhuriyet University Medical School, Department of Otolaryngology, Sivas, Turkey
Department of Microbiology, Cumhuriyet University, Sivas, Turkey

Elif Bilge Uysal
Department of Microbiology, Cumhuriyet University, Sivas, Turkey

Sema Koç
Department of Otorhinolaryngology, Gaziosmanpasa, University School of Medicine, Tokat, Turkey

Amtul Salam Sami
ENT and Allergy department, Royal National Throat, Nose and Ear Hospital, UK

Nida Ahmed
Acute Medicine, Ealing Hospital, UK

Sabahat Ahmed
Guys, Kings College and St Thomas's School of Medical Education, King's College, UK

Morvarid Elahi
General Practitioner, Firoozgar General Hospital, Iran University of Medical Sciences, Tehran, Iran

Homayoun Elahi
Assistant Professor of Otolaryngology, Firoozgar General Hospital, Iran University of Medical Sciences, Tehran, Iran

Sylvester Fernandes
Department of Health Sciences, Newcastle University, Newcastle, Australia

Griffith S Hsu
Du Page Medical Group, Department of Otolaryngology-Head and Neck Surgery, Illinois, USA

Maria CS
Department of Ear Sciences, The University of Western Australia, Nedlands, Western Australia, Australia

Maria PLS
Ear Science Institute Australia, Subiaco, Western Australia, Australia

Ajay Manickam, Shaswati Sengupta and SK Basu
Department of ENT, RG Kar Medical College, Kolkata, India

Sudipta Pal
Department of ENT, Calcutta National Medical College, Kolkata, India

PK Gure
Department of ENT, North Bengal Medical College, Siliguri, India

Somnath Saha
Department of ENT, NRS Medical College, Sushrutanagar, west of Siliguri, India

Omakobia E and Micallef A
Department of ENT and Head & Neck Surgery, University College Hospital, London

Henrique Furlan Pauna
Resident at Otolaryngology, Head and Neck Department, UNICAMP, Brazil

Guilherme Machado de Carvalho, Eder Barbosa Muranaka, Alexandre Caixeta Guimarães and Luiz Henrique Schuch
ENT Doctor at Otolaryngology, Head and Neck Department, UNNICAMP, Brazil

Walter Adriano Bianchini and Arthur Menino Castilho
ENT Doctor, Otologist, Head Otology, Audiology and Implantable Ear Prostheses, UNICAMP, Brazil

Agrício Nubiato Crespo
ENT Doctor, Head of Otolaryngology, Head and Neck Department, UNICAMP, Brazil

Edi Lucia Sartorato
Head of CBMEG, UNICAMP, Brazil

Mohammad Shamim Ansari
Department of Speech and Hearing, Ali Yavar Jung National Institute for the Hearing Handicapped, K.C. Marg, Bandra (W), Mumbai-40050 Maharashtra, India

Rangasayee Raghunathrao
Technical Department, Dr. S.R. Chandrasekhar Institute of Speech and Hearing, Hennur Main Road, Lingarajapuram, Bnagalore-560084 Karnataka, India

Mohammad A Hafiz Ansari
Department of Physiology, Grant Medical College and Sir J. J. Groups of Hospital, Mumbai-400008, India

Index

A

Allergic Rhinitis, 23-28, 62, 70-74, 102, 104, 145-150, 152

Amniotic Membrane, 162-164

Amoxicillin, 109

Aryepiglottic Folds, 134, 136-137

Aspergillus Terreus, 123-124, 127-130

B

Basal Cell Adenocarcinoma, 1-2, 4-5

Basophil Activation Test, 102-103, 105

Behavioural Disorders, 59

Benign Tumour, 12, 14

C

Carotid Artery Injury, 51, 53

Cholesteatoma, 163-164

Chronic Rhinosinusitis, 91, 127, 129, 153

Cochlear Implant, 116, 122, 165-168, 172-175

Concomitant Chemoradiotherapy, 91, 112

Cranial Nerve, 12, 51, 177

Cystic Fibrosis, 153

D

Dendritic Cell, 78, 83-84

Dermatophagoides Pteronyssinus, 23, 28

Desmoid Fibromatosis, 6-8

Distant Metastasis, 4, 10, 35-37, 114

Dymista, 148, 152

Dysphagia, 1, 12, 14, 45, 48-51, 66, 91, 114, 135-136

Dyspnea, 75-77, 134-137

E

Ectopic Parathyroid, 66-68

Elective Neck Irradiation, 112-115

Endoscopic Gastrostomy, 88, 91

Endotracheal Tube, 38, 41, 43, 171

Epiglottic Vallecula, 45, 48-49

Epistaxis, 9, 11, 14, 39

Epithelial Tumor Cells, 54

Esthesioneuroblastoma, 9-11, 125

F

Fluticasone Propionate, 145-146, 152

Fungal Rhinosinusitis, 123, 127, 129-130

G

Gestational Diabetes, 106

H

Haemophilus Influenza, 78

Hearing Implant Sound Quality Index, 116-119, 122

Human Papillomavirus, 75

I

Intracochlear Membrane Rapture, 138

L

Laryngeal Injuries, 38, 41, 43, 169-171

Laryngeal Papillomatosis, 75-77

Laryngeal Trauma, 134, 169-171

M

Magnetic Resonance Image, 12, 85

Maxillary Sinus, 11, 14, 112-115, 126, 142-144

Melanotic Neuroectodermal, 6-8

Mucociliary Clearance, 153-155

N

N-acetyl Cysteine, 153, 155

Nasal Inspiratory Peak Flow, 145-146, 148

Nasopharyngeal Notochondroma, 85, 87

O

Obstructive Sleep Apnea, 59-60, 63-65, 136-137

Olfactory Neuroblastoma, 9-11, 125

Ostiomeatal Complex, 142

Otosclerosis, 92-97

P

Para Pharyngeal Space, 12-14

Paranasal Sinus, 53, 112, 114-115, 125

Parathyroid Adenoma, 66, 68-69

Percutaneous Endoscopic Gastrostomy, 88, 91

Perilymphatic Fistula, 92, 95, 132-133, 138

Pharyngeal Cancer, 35

Pyogenic Granuloma, 106

Pyriform Sinus, 45, 48-49

R

Retropharyngeal Abscess, 66, 68

S

Salivary Gland Neoplasms, 1

Salivary Immunoglobulins, 23-24, 28

Schwannomas, 12, 14

Seminal Fluid, 70, 74

Sensorineural Hearing Loss, 34, 93, 97, 131-133, 138, 140-141, 165, 175, 177, 180

Silent Sinus Syndrome, 142-144

Sphenoid Aspergilloma, 123, 126-127

Sphenoid Sinus, 51-53, 123, 126-129

Squamous Cell Carcinoma, 15, 21-22, 35-37, 54, 56-58, 112-113, 115

Supraglottic Collapse, 134, 136-137

T

Tinnitus Mechanisms, 29, 156

Total Thyroidectomy, 131, 133

V

Vasomotor Rhinitis, 70, 72, 74

Vertical Diplopia, 142-144

Vertigo, 92-93, 95-96

Vimentin Immunohistochemistry, 54, 56-57

W

White Birch Pollinosis, 102, 104

CPSIA information can be obtained
at www.ICGtesting.com
Printed in the USA
BVHW091756060322
630763BV00003B/45

9 781639 274123